Introduction to

Tui Na

World Century Compendium to TCM

Volume 1 Fundamentals of Traditional Chinese Medicine
by Hong-zhou Wu, Zhao-qin Fang and Pan-ji Cheng
(translated by Ye-bo He)
(Shanghai University of Traditional Chinese Medicine, China)
ISBN: 978-1-938134-28-9 (pbk)

Volume 2 Introduction to Diagnosis in Traditional Chinese Medicine
by Hong-zhou Wu, Zhao-qin Fang and Pan-ji Cheng
(translated by Chou-ping Han)
(Shanghai University of Traditional Chinese Medicine, China)
ISBN: 978-1938134-13-5 (pbk)

Volume 3 Introduction to Chinese Materia Medica
by Jin Yang, Huang Huang and Li-jiang Zhu
(translated by Yunhui Chen)
(Nanjing University of Chinese Medicine, China)
ISBN: 978-1-938134-16-6 (pbk)

Volume 4 Introduction to Chinese Internal Medicine
by Xiang Xia, Xiao-heng Chen, Min Chen and Yan-qian Xiao
(translated by Ye-bo He)
(Shanghai Jiaotong University, China)
ISBN: 978-1-938134-19-7 (pbk)

Volume 5 Introduction to Formulae of Traditional Chinese Medicine
by Jin Yang, Huang Huang and Li-jiang Zhu
(translated by Xiao Ye and Hong Li)
(Nanjing University of Chinese Medicine, China)
ISBN: 978-1-938134-10-4 (pbk)

Volume 6 Introduction to Acupuncture and Moxibustion
by Ren Zhang (translated by Xue-min Wang)
(Shanghai Literature Institute of Traditional Chinese Medicine, China)
ISBN: 978-1-938134-25-8 (pbk)

Volume 7 Introduction to Tui Na
by Lan-qing Liu, Jiang Xiao and Gui-bao Ke (translated by Azure Duan)
(Yueyang Hospital of Integrated Traditional Chinese and Western Medicine, Shanghai University of Traditional Chinese Medicine, China)
ISBN: 978-1-938134-22-7 (pbk)

World Century Compendium to TCM - Vol. 7

Introduction to Tui Na

Lan-qing Liu
Xiao Jiang
Gui-bao Ke
Yueyang Hospital of Integrated Traditional Chinese and Western Medicine, Shanghai University of Traditional Chinese Medicine, China

translated by
Azure Duan

World Century

Published by

World Century Publishing Corporation
27 Warren Street
Suite 401-402
Hackensack, NJ 07601

Distributed by

World Scientific Publishing Co. Pte. Ltd.

5 Toh Tuck Link, Singapore 596224

USA office: 27 Warren Street, Suite 401-402, Hackensack, NJ 07601

UK office: 57 Shelton Street, Covent Garden, London WC2H 9HE

Library of Congress Control Number: 2013001662

British Library Cataloguing-in-Publication Data
A catalogue record for this book is available from the British Library.

World Century Compendium to TCM
A 7-Volume Set

INTRODUCTION TO TUI NA
Volume 7

Published by arrangement with Shanghai Scientific & Technical Publishers.

Originally published in Chinese

ISBN 978-1-938134-34-0 (Set)
ISBN 978-1-938134-22-7 (pbk)

Typeset by Stallion Press
Email: enquiries@stallionpress.com

Printed in Singapore

CONTENTS

PREFACE TO THE SECOND EDITION

It has been more than a decade since the first title in the series *Mastering Traditional Chinese Medicine in 100 Days* appeared in 1996. Ten more titles have been published since then. The series has been well received by readers for several reasons: its unique style, its profound content written in simple language so that students find the subject easy to learn, and its practical use as a clinical reference book. All 11 titles have been reprinted repeatedly, with the most popular title selling over 100,000 copies.

From the end of the last millennium to the beginning of the 21st century, the spectrum of diseases has changed dramatically, resulting in a corresponding change in the clinical applications of traditional Chinese medicine (TCM) in terms of scope and methods. Therefore, we have carefully revised the series to help readers explore and grasp relevant information and techniques of TCM by inviting experts from various fields of TCM. We have kept the original style and format, removed obsolete or uncommon content and techniques, and added clinical treatment methods for more relevant diseases. As the publisher, our most sincere hope for the second edition of the series is that it makes its contribution in promoting traditional Chinese culture, advocating TCM, and popularizing related knowledge.

Shanghai Scientific and Technical Publishers
May 2006

A WORD FROM THE EDITORS

Tui na, one of the earliest Chinese medical treatment methods with a long history tracing back to ancient times, is an important component of TCM. With several thousand years of continual development, the maneuvers of tui na constantly enrich, the fundamentals of its efficacy are continuously discovered, and the clinical applications keep expanding.

With the complex state of health care today, more and more people are beginning to feel that relying on modern western medicine, with its emphasis on chemical medicines and surgery, is unsatisfactory. On the other hand, the advantages of traditional Chinese medicine in preventing and treating diseases are increasingly understood and gaining attention worldwide. Tui na is facing rapid development as a natural therapy, drawing international attention, and enjoying a surge in popularity because of its simplicity, convenience, safety, effectiveness and cost efficiency. It has become an important method of self-care at home.

We compiled this book in order to popularize tui na modality and make readers understand and master the fundamental theory, basic techniques, commonly used acupoints and parts, and diagnostic and treatment methods of diseases in a relatively short period of time. The book is a summary of clinical experience of tui na with practical content and detailed illustrations. Written in an easy-to-understand manner, it serves both to popularize tuina and to highlight advances in this field. The book is targeted at the following audience:

- Enthusiasts of tui na;
- Tuina therapists who have fundamental knowledge and clinical experience in tui na;
- Physicians practicing modern Western medicine who have an interest in tui na.

OVERVIEW

The book is arranged in such a way that each chapter (denoted as "Day") contains material that can be learned in a day. Six chapters make up one unit (denoted as "Week"). In the first two weeks of study, the reader will be introduced to fundamental tui na theory, commonly used acupoints and body areas, and basic maneuvers. For the following 12 weeks, the reader will learn the techniques in diagnosing and treating common diseases.

The book details 25 common maneuvers including manipulations in children, and more than 70 common diseases with diagnostic treatment and preventive methods. It contains 248 figures illustrating acupoints, maneuvers, and examination and treatment methods in order to help readers learn. The book covers 14 weeks, plus two days of extra content, adding up to one hundred days. Lastly, there are four indexes covering the following: Common Tui Na Aupoints and Areas, Common Tui Na Maneuvers, Common Examinations and Common Applicable Diseases and Symptoms.

After reading this book, readers will be able to understand the essence and basics of tui na and break away from the stereotyped view that tui na can only treat pain and movement disorders, when in fact it can be applied to a variety of diseases in the fields of internal medicine, gynecology, and pediatrics. Readers would also have built a solid foundation for further and in-depth grasp of the discipline.

Requirements of Study

It is unrealistic to expect to master the essence of the book in one sitting. For best results, readers should follow the suggestions below:

1. *Follow the proper sequence to make steady improvement and continually review previous sections.* The content in later chapters is often related to, and supplement, the previous ones. Therefore, it would be a good idea to follow the order of the book and make gradual improvement. By reviewing the knowledge obtained in a previous chapter while studying a new one, readers can gain new insights in both.
2. *Closely relate what you learned and apply it in clinical practice.* Tui na is an extremely practical subject requiring a lot of hands-on experience in clinical practice. Therefore, even during the course of study, learners need to try their best to practice it in clinical settings whenever possible. In some situations, such as acupoints and areas used in tui na, repetitive exercises using the human body are necessary. In other situations, learners need to continuously practice the operation of tui na maneuvers since correct manipulation directly determines the efficacy of tui na therapy. Furthermore, treatment applications are based on individual circumstances such as the scope of practice of the practitioner.
3. *Be perseverant and focus on several key points.* Learners should ideally spend an hour studying each chapter, excluding the time to memorize commonly used acupoints, their locations, and indications. Next, they need to practice tui na maneuvers often to get themselves

familiarized with the operational methods, efficacy, applicable diseases, and symptoms. Thirdly, learners should diligently complete the questions in the Everyday Exercises section to better absorb the material learned for that day. Engaging in self-tests is a good way to know how well one has mastered the content.

Sincerely,
The editors

WEEK 1

Day 1

A BRIEF HISTORY OF TUI NA

Tui na, also known as *an mo* in ancient times, refers to Chinese medical massage. It has a long history going back several thousand years.

A great deal of records in *an mo*, *dao yin* (mind-guided movements), *tu na* (breathing exercises) were found in silk books and inscribed bamboo and wooden slips unearthed from Ma Wang Dui Tombs in Changsha. These ancient medical records indicated that *an mo* had been widely practiced clinically in the Spring and Autumn periods (771 BCE–476 BCE) and the Warring States period (475 BCE–221 BCE) or even earlier in Chinese history.

The use of *an mo* to treat diseases originated in central China. According to *The Yellow Emperor's Inner Classic* (*Huáng Dì Nèi Jīng*, 黄帝内经), also known as *Inner Classic* (*Nèi Jīng*, 内经), the earliest classic masterpiece written more than 2,000 years ago, "the central land [of China] was flat and moist. The massive people living here ate diverse food and did not work very much. Therefore, flaccid paralysis (*wei*, 痿) and fainting (*jue*, 厥) were often prevalent. The appropriate treatment is *daoyin* (mind-guided movements) and *an qiao* (massage using hands and feet). Therefore, that was where *an qiao* originated." "Central land" is where the Luo Yang area of Henan Province is located today.

Bian Que, a famous physician in the Spring, Autumn, and Warring States periods, had successfully rescued a patient suffering from cadaverous syncope. As recorded in *Rites of Zhou — Miscellaneous Cases* (*Zhōu Lǐ Shū Àn*, 周礼疏案), one of the three ancient ritual books in classic Confucianism, "Bian Que was transiting in the State of Guo while the prince of Guo was having an episode of cadaverous syncope. [He] asked his student Zi Ming to prepare decoction, Zi Yi to feel the *shen* of pulse, and Zi You to perform *an mo*". With the combination of several methods, he successfully cured the disease of the prince of Guo.

In both the Qin and Han dynasties, *dao yin*, *tu na* and *gao mo* (massage with medicinal paste) were classified as preventive methods for health. Zhang Zhong-jing of Eastern Han Dynasty (25 CE–220 CE) wrote *Essentials from the Golden Cabinet* (*Jīn Guì Yào Lüè*, 金匮要略) based on many years of experience in medical practices. He thought "if a person carefully preserved his health, he would not allow pathogenic wind to attack the channels and collaterals. [Or he] would start the treatment when it just started to affect meridians and collaterals but not wait until it passed to the viscera and bowels. [He] would receive *dao yin*, *tu na*, acupuncture and moxibustion, and *gao mo* to avoid blockage of the nine orifices as soon as he sensed heaviness on his four limbs".

During the Sui and Tang eras (581 CE–907 CE), the classification of different subjects in Chinese medicine gradually improved as the result of advancement in productivity and civilization. *An mo* became a formal subject as part of the national education in medicine. The department specializing in *an mo* was established with *an mo* physicians and high-ranking doctors. As recorded in *Revised History of Tang Dynasty — Annals of Different Types of Officials* (*Xīn Táng Shū– Băi Guān Zhì*, 新唐书・百官志), "[it included] one *an mo* doctor and four massage therapists to teach the methods of *dao yin* as a way to treat diseases with the highest title equivalent to the ninth rank official." In other words, the ancient modality of *dao yin* had become part of the curriculum in formal medical training.

Between the Song and Jin periods (960–1234), the application of tui na expanded further. An infamous physician in the Song Dynasty named Pang An-shi employed tui na to expedite labor, and the record stated that "a pregnant woman in an ordinary family was about to deliver a baby. However, the baby was not delivered seven days after the expected date, with all modalities failing to speed up the labor ... [Dr. Pang] asked her family to warm up her waist and abdomen with warm herbal decoction, and he did *an mo* around the area. The woman felt slight abdominal pain, and delivered a baby boy while moaning." This was perhaps the world's earliest recorded medical case of using the tui na maneuver to aid labor during childbirth.

During the historic periods of the Ming and Qing dynasties (1368–1912), Chinese medicine made considerable strides, with tui na maturing at the same time. One major breakthrough was in pediatric tui na, while both orthopedic and wellness tui na developed into rich knowledge systems of their own. Many books on massage were published. One such book was *Acrane Techniques of Pediatric An Mo* (*Xiǎo Ér Àn Mó Jīng*, 小儿按摩经), the earliest specialty book in tui na. There were some 30 books published including *Encyclopedia of Pediatric Tui Na, Formulas, Pulse-taking and Rescuing Infants* (*Xiǎo Ér Tuī Ná Fāng Mài Huó Yīng Mì Zhǐ Quán Shū*, 小儿推拿方脉活婴秘旨全书) and *Secret Tips in Pediatric Tui Na* (*Xiǎo Ér Tuī Ná Mì Jué*, 小儿推拿秘诀), as the term "tui na" replaced *an mo*. The name change reflected the development of massage therapy and its recognition among the general public, which was a landmark in the history of Chinese medical massage.

The government of Emperor Qian Long in the Qing Dynasty composed a pandect named *Golden Mirror of the Medical Tradition — Key Points to the Hearty Methods of Bone Alignment* (*Yī Zōng Jīn Jiàn — Zhèng Gǔ Xīn Fǎ Yào Zhǐ*, 医宗金鉴 • 正骨心法要旨). A volume in this body of work was the systemic summarization in orthopedic massage and imperial experience in tui na around the country. It summarized the eight orthopedic methods: touching, connecting, supporting, lifting, pressing, rubbing, pushing, and grasping. As we can see, the publication of specialty books in tui na peaked in the Ming and Qing periods. Most of the classic tui na works existing now were produced during that period of time.

After the People's Republic of China was founded, tui na entered into another period of rapid development. In 1956, tui na formally became a major subject in the national educational system. A well-planned and formal academic education started as training programs, clinical departments, and specialty schools were established in Shanghai, and famous experts were invited to teach there. In the 1950's, outpatient Chinese medical massage facilities were divided into pediatric, internal, gynecologic, and locomotor departments. There were also departments in external medicine, otorhinolaryngology, ophthalmology, and stomatology.

Tui na schools carried out great efforts in investigating, studying, and organizing historical material and records to promote the modality. The therapeutic mechanisms and effects of tui na were investigated from a theoretical standpoint. The technical requirements of tui na manipulation maneuvers were also specified: maneuvers that are durable, strong, even, gentle, deep, and thorough.

In 1974, tui na came into its own when Shanghai College of Chinese Medicine first established the major disciplines of acupuncture, tui na, and orthopedic science. Between the end of the 1970's and the beginning of the 1980's, acupuncture and tui na were taught in combination in all TCM colleges. In 1987 the State Education Committee of China issued the *National List of Undergraduate Majors in Medicine for Higher Education,* which officially listed tui na as a major subject. From then on, most TCM colleges had separate departments in acupuncture and tui na. Shanghai University of Traditional Chinese Medicine was the first institution that offered a master's degree in tui na, marking the fact that tui na had formally entered the track of higher education.

Based on these achievements, research in tui na went even deeper and broader. Some performed tui na maneuvers to observe its effect prior to the surgery of removing the nucleus gelatinosus when the surgical area was completely exposed. Some applied computer technology to analyze tui na manipulation from a three-dimensional aspect. Some studied the biological mechanism of oblique pulling maneuvers in order to improve the correct use of strength while applying this maneuver. ECG studies were able to show that tui na could alter the S-T waves and left heart function of patients with coronary heart disease, while other studies were trying to prove tui na's efficacy in improving immunity by increasing the count of leukocytes. Lastly, studies on algogenic substances such as serum endorphin and 5-HT were carried out to try and discover the reason behind the antalgic effect of tui na.

In short, the ancient medical modality of tui na has proven that it is uniquely efficacious. With its integration into modern medical science, it will definitely make a greater contribution to the healthcare industry.

Day 2

FUNDAMENTAL KNOWLEDGE OF TUI NA

Subject 1 — The Mechanism behind the Effects of Tui Na Therapy

Basic Questions — Discussion of Pain (*Sù Wèn — Jǔ Tòng Lùn*, 素问 • 举痛论) states that "[when the pathogenic] cold qi invades the meridian [where] back *shu* points locate, it results in sluggish pulse and causes blood deficit. Blood deficit would result in pain transferring to the heart through its *shu* point and triggering the [chest] pain. By pressing the [affected] area, the warm qi arrives, so it would cease the pain." This paragraph in the classic book explained that when external cold qi invades certain acupoints on the back of the human body, it will block the meridians and collaterals, causing retardation of the qi (vital energy) and blood flow. The stagnation further causes the pain and even induces pain in the chest. Tui na will unblock the meridians and collaterals, free the qi and blood flows, and warm up the area. Thus, pain can be relieved by eliminating the obstruction, and cold pain can be reduced with warmth. In other words, tui na regulates the balance among *zang-fu* organs and tissues through points on meridians and collaterals to prevent and treat ailments by accelerating the metabolism and healing tissue damage. In the following paragraphs, we will discuss the different mechanisms of tui na as a medical modality.

The Effect on Skin Tissues

The skin, whose function is to regulate body temperature and protect the various structures beneath it from trauma, is the area of the body that directly accepts tui na treatment.

Tuina manipulations can promote secretion of sebaceous and sweat glands, remove necrotic epithelial cells, improve skin metabolism, soften scars, and increase the defensive ability of the skin. At the same time, they enhance the shininess and elasticity of the skin and delay its aging process.

Rubbing, kneading, scrubbing and patting-striking are able to dilate capillaries and increase skin temperature. A tui na physician applying excellent manipulation skill would not only increase temperature on the skin surface, but also that of the deeper structure, so that the maneuver could soften tense skin and relax adherence of subcutaneous tissue.

The Effect on Muscles

After intense exercise, a lot of lactic acid, an intermediate metabolic product, is produced and deposited in muscles, leading to cramps, pain and fatigue. Tui na can be used to treat muscle fatigue, improve the metabolism of lactic acid, and alleviate the pain. Therefore, athletes often accept preventive tui na to eliminate fatigue so as to quickly be in sportsman mode prior to competitions.

Tui na is capable of increasing the tensility and elasticity of the muscles and tendons to improve their constriction and strength, so that it is often used to treat muscle atrophy owing to disuse or sequelae of infantile poliomyelitis. It can also relieve the adherence of muscles and tendons to their surrounding tissues.

Enhancing the Recovery of Joint Injuries

When the joints of the bone are injured, the local circulation of blood and lymphatic fluid slows down due to inactivity of the affected muscles and joints. It results in edema of the tissue and adhesive liquids are formed due to serous fibrin exudates, leading to tissue adherence that causes dysfunction of joints and muscularatrophy. Appropriate tui na treatment speeds up the blood and lymphatic circulation to reduce swelling, relax adherence, and improve the range of motion of dysfunctional joints gradually to or close to its normal level. Thus, tui na is beneficial for the recovery of injured joints.

Adjusting Anatomic Displacement

Tui na maneuvers can adjust anatomic abnormalities such as joint malposition and tendon dislocation. For example, pediatric dislocation of capitulum radii causes a forced position due to the impaired arm; with proper maneuvers, the bone can be adjusted and snapped back in place. With regard to unbearable pain from synovial membrane incarceration of the lumbar intervertebral joints, tui na maneuvers can have instant effect as well. In addition, it can change the relationship between the protruded nucleus pulposus and affected nerve root in patients with a herniated disc, so that waist and leg pain can be alleviated.

Improving Blood Circulation

Some workers in a dye chemical factory had fatigue and decreased total blood indices because of exposure to poisonous chemical substances. After tui na treatment, such as pressing and kneading the Four-Gate Points and *zú sān lǐ* (ST 36), and pinching along the spine, the total blood picture among the workers improved considerably. Studies showed that tui na can significantly increase the number of capillary vessels and blood circulation, promote the rebuilding of the vascular network of tissue lesions, recover elasticity of vessel walls, improve the transporting function of vessels, and decrease peripheral resistance of blood circulation. Since tui na manipulations are capable of improving the blood and circulatory systems, it is a great supplementary therapy in clinical practice for treating hypertension, coronary heart disease, and cerebrovascular insufficiency.

Promoting Digestion

Some experiments have shown that stomach peristalsis could be increased by performing tui na on *pí shū* (BL 20) and *wèi shū* (BL 21) for one to two minutes, and decreased with *zú sān lǐ* (ST 36). It is worth mentioning that *zú sān lǐ* regulates the digestive system in both ways: stimulating and inhibiting. When stomach peristalsis is overly excited, applying tui na on *zú sān lǐ* can reduce it; otherwise, it can increase it. Other experiments proved that tui na reduces the secretion of gastrin and increases the absorptive function of the small intestine. Consequently, it has great treatment effect on digestive dysfunctions.

Regulating the Nervous System

Tui na decreases the excitability of peripheral sensory nerve endings, so that it is often used to relieve pain caused by disorders such as neuritis and neuralgia. Gentle maneuvers are able to stimulate motor nerves to improve the excitability of the muscles while stronger manipulations are applied in treating muscle spasms and enhancing the recovery process of impeded functions. Abdominal tui na stimulates the secretion of digestive glands, improves digestion and absorption, and regulates peristalsis of the bowels through autonomic nerves.

Tui na on back *shū* points affects the regulatory function of the spinal cord and the brain via neural reflexes, resulting in alteration in the functions of corresponding organs. Examples are the impact of *fèi shū* (BL 13) on the respiratory system, *pí shū* (BL 20) and *wèi shū* (BL 21) on the digestive system, and *bā liào* (BL 31 to 34, eight *liào*) on the genitourinary system.

Improving Mood

Gentle and soft manipulations can help patients to relax, calm down, or reduce negative psychological reactions to diseases, as well as alleviate depression and anxiety. Along with the accumulative effect of the treatment, the confidence of the patients can gradually increase to actively cooperating with the treatment. Therefore, tui na is an effective therapy for not only organic disorders, but also psychological imbalances.

To sum up, tui na is certainly a handy and practical therapeutic method with dependable efficacy. It is extremely important, however, to master the correct manipulation techniques, acupoints, anatomic location, and appropriate clinical application of each technique. If one wants to reach a high proficiency, one must study hard, rehearse diligently, think about it repeatedly, and practice it over a certain period of time until he or she gets the grasp of the techniques.

Everyday Exercise

Express your understanding of how tui na treats diseases.

Day 3

Subject 2 — Meridians, Collaterals, and Acupuncture Points

The meridian and collateral theory is one of the fundamental theories in Chinese medicine, and is a system formed through continual clinical practices, summarization, accumulation, distillation, and drawing conclusions. It has significant meaning in guiding clinical efforts.

Meridians and collaterals connect the upper and lower body, the exterior and the interior, and different *zang-fu* organs. They also smoothen the transportation of qi and blood. *Inner Classic* declaims that the 12 regular meridians "pertain to interior *zang-fu* [organs] and relate exterior limbs and artus", with physiological functions of "moving qi and blood, nourishing yin and yang, moistening sinews and bones and benefiting joints." It also deems that when pathogenic qi attacks the human body, it "must offend the skin first. [If it] lingers but is not removed, [it will] invade the minute collaterals. [If it] lags but is not dispelled, [it will] penetrate to the meridians and vessels, transmit to the interior organs, and disseminate to the intestines and the stomach." This is the pathologic process of how pathogenic qi spreads to the five *zang* and six *fu* organs via the meridians and collaterals, with the skin as the starting point. Certainly, pathologic changes of internal organs in turn can be reflected at the superficial level through the connected meridians and collaterals. For example, the ascendant hyperactivity of liver *yang* has symptoms of red eyes and headache while a distended chest and palpitations reflect heart diseases. When the spleen systems is diseased, the patient is bothered by "dampness" — he or she suffers from fatigue and a sense of heaviness, while a problematic kidney system causes soreness and weakness of the waist and lower extremities.

The meridian and collateral theory is the guiding principle for tui na modality in treating diseases in TCM, especially for internal and gynecological illnesses. In tui na, acupuncture points (also known as "acupoints") are determined near its circulating pathway of pathological changes, or on the affected meridians, collaterals, and *zang-fu* organs; and the stimulation of maneuvers, qi, and blood along a meridian or its collateral is adjusted to achieve the treatment outcome. Examples are treating *taiyang* headache with *fēng chí* (GB 20), *yangming* headache with *hé gǔ* (LI 4), epigastric pain with *zú sān lǐ* (ST 36), and chest pain with *nèi guān* (PC 6). As we can see, meridians, collaterals and their associated acupoints together serve as important guides in the clinical application of tui na treatment.

The system of meridians and collaterals consists of two parts: the meridian vessels and collateral vessels. Meridian vessels (or meridians) are relatively thicker vessels with a wider longitudinal distribution. Collateral vessels (or collaterals) are the relatively smaller branches that are either superficially or deeply distributed, serving as the network between the meridians. Meridians include the 12 regular meridians, eight extraordinary vessels, 12 divergent vessels, 12 meridian sinews, and 12 cutaneous segments. Collaterals include divergent collaterals, superficial collaterals, and minute collaterals. The 12 regular meridians, collectively the main meridians, and the eight extraordinary vessels, collectively the extraordinary vessels combined, make the major part of the meridian and collateral system. The 12 meridians plus *du mai* and *ren mai* are collectively known as the 14 meridians.

Acupoints are where the qi of *zang-fu* organs, meridians, and collaterals infuses and gathers toward the surface of the body. The majority of acupoints are along the pathway of meridians and collaterals, and are fairly sensitive when pricked, pressed or poked, with therapeutic results. Therefore, we cannot discuss meridians and collaterals on their own without mentioning acupoints. Meridians and collaterals are based on acupoints and serve as their conduits. Take railroads as the analogy — if the meridians and collaterals are like the rails, acupoints can be seen as the stations. There are three categories of acupoints: 14 meridian points, extraordinary points, and *ā shì xué*.

The 14 meridian points (or simply, "meridian points") are located along the 14 meridians, and make up the major proportion of all acupoints. Acupoints on a certain meridian have mutual indications for diseases of their corresponding meridian. Extraordinary acupoints (or simply, "extra points") have fixed names and locations, but are not part of the meridian system. They each have a unique treatment effect on certain diseases. *Ā shì xué*, also known as the "heavenly response points," do not have fixed names or locations, but are rather determined as tender or sensitive spots when touched, and are used to treat illnesses accordingly.

Twelve Regular Meridians

1. *Naming and classification* The 12 regular meridians are named and classified in accordance with the yin or yang nature of the *zang* or *fu* organ, and the circulating path on the body that each of them pertains to, so that there are three hand yin, three hand yang, three foot yin and three foot yang meridians. All yin meridians pertain to the *zang* organs that circulate on the medial aspect of the limbs while all yang meridians pertain to the *fu* bowels that travel along the lateral side of the limbs. See details in Tables 1 and 2.
2. *Circulating directions and connections* The three hand yin meridians start from the chest and run to the hands while the three hand yang meridians run toward the head from the hands. The three foot yang meridians take off from the head and travel to the feet while the three foot yin meridians start from the feet and return to the abdomen or the chest. Thus, they form a circulation pathway with "yin connecting to yang, as a circle without an end."

Table 1 Classification of the Yin meridians connecting the five *Zang* organs

Three hand yin meridians (medial aspect of the upper limbs)	Three foot yin meridians (medial aspect of the lower limbs)
Hand *Taiyin* Lung meridian	Foot *Taiyin* Spleen meridian
Hand *Jueyin* Pericardium meridian	Foot *Jueyin* Liver meridian
Hand *Shaoyin* Heart meridian	Foot *Shaoyin* Kidney meridian

Table 2 Classification of the yang meridians connecting the six *fu* bowels

Three hand yang meridians (lateral side of the upper limbs)	Three foot yang meridians (lateral side of the lower limbs)
Hand *yangming* large intestine meridian	Foot *yangming* stomach meridian
Hand *shaoyang sanjiao* meridian	Foot *shaoyang* gallbladder meridian
Hand *taiyang* small intestine meridian	Foot *taiyang* bladder meridian

Yang controls the exterior, and yin governs the interior. Related yin and yang meridians link to each other via the collaterals to form the following interior-exterior pairs:

- The interior hand *taiyin* Lung pairs with the exterior hand *yangming* large intestine meridian
- The interior hand *jueyin* pericardium pairs with the exterior hand *shaoyangsanjiao* meridian
- The interior hand *shaoyin* heart pairs with the exterior hand *taiyang* small intestine meridian
- The interior foot *taiyins* pleen pairs with the exterior foot *yangming* stomach meridian
- The interior foot *jueyin* liver pairs with the exterior foot *shaoyang* gallbladder meridian
- The interior foot *shaoyin* kidney pairs with the exterior foot *taiyan* gall bladder meridian

Figure 1 shows the circulation direction and connections of the 12 regular meridians.

Qi and blood in the 12 regular meridians circulate with no end. The path starts from hand *taiyin* Lung meridian all the way to the foot *jueyin* liver meridian, circulates back to the lung meridian as one complete cycle of infusion, and starts over again. Figure 2 shows the flow sequence of the 12 regular meridians.

Eight Extraordinary Vessels

The eight extraordinary vessels are the collective name for *du mai* (governing vessel), *ren mai* (conception vessel), *chong mai* (penetrating vessel), *dai mai* (girdling vessel), *yinwei mai* (yin linking vessel), *yangwei mai* (yang linking vessel), *yinqiao mai* (yin motility vessel), and *yangqiao mai* (yang motility vessel). *Ren mai* pertains to yin while *du mai* pertains to yang meridians. They both originate from *huì yīn* (RN 1, the perineum, 会阴) and run through the front and back midlines of the torso respectively. All *zang* meridians of yin nature connect and converge with *ren mai*, and all *fu* meridians of yang nature cross and merge with *du mai*.

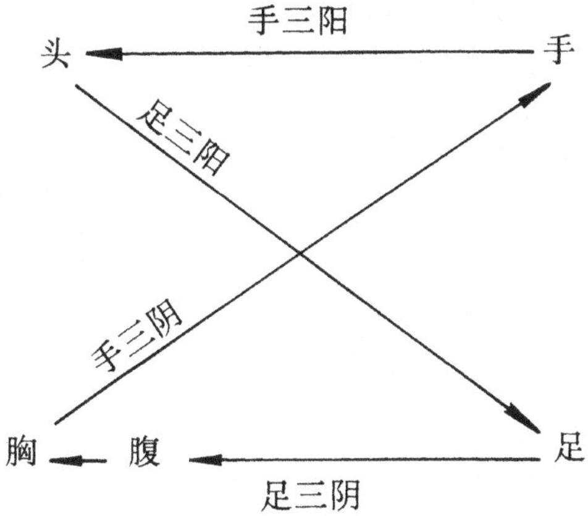

头	-	head
手三阳	-	three hand yang
手	-	hand
足三阳	-	three foot yang
手三阴	-	three hand yin
胸	-	chest
腹	-	abdomen
足三阴	-	three foot yin
足	-	foot

Figure 1 Circulation direction and connections of the 12 regular meridians

Because of the fact that *ren mai* and *du mai* are closely related to the 12 regular meridians, they are commonly called the 14 meridians and vessels.

Everyday Exercises

1. What are the so-called meridian and collateral system and fourteen meridians and vessels?
2. What is an acupoint? How many categories of acupoints are there?
3. Memorize the full name, direction, sequence, and connection pattern of the 12 regular meridians.

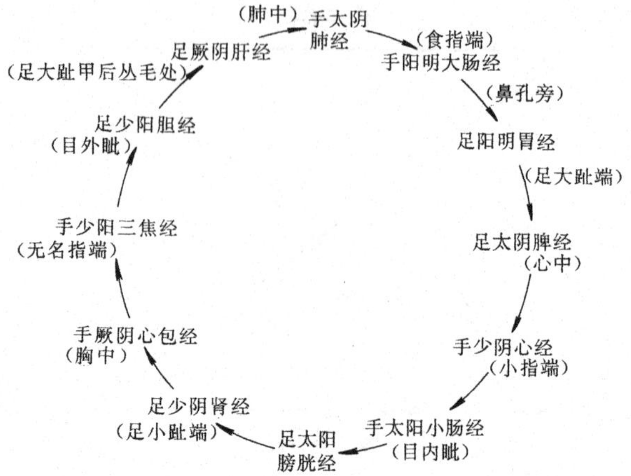

手太阴肺经	-	Hand *Taiyin* Lung Meridian
(食指端)	-	tip of the index fingers
手阳明大肠经	-	Hand *Yangming* Large Intestine Meridian
(鼻孔旁)	-	beside the nostrils
足阳明胃经	-	Foot *Yangming* Stomach Meridian
(足大趾端)	-	tip of the big toes
足太阴脾经	-	Foot *Taiyin* Spleen Meridian
(心中)	-	inside of the heart
手少阴心经	-	Hand *Shaoyin* Heart Meridian
(小指端)	-	tip of the little fingers
手太阳小肠经	-	Hand *Taiyang* Small Intestine Meridian
(目内眦)	-	inner canthus
足太阳膀胱经	-	Foot *Taiyang* Bladder Meridian
足少阴肾经	-	Foot *Shaoyin* Kidney Meridian
(足小趾端)	-	tip of the little toes
手厥阴心包经	-	Hand *Jueyin* Pericardium Meridian
(胸中)	-	center of the chest
手少阳三焦经	-	Hand *Shaoyang Sanjiao* Meridian
(无名指端)	-	tip of the ring fingers
足少阳胆经	-	Foot *Shaoyang* Gallbladder Meridian
(目外眦)	-	outer canthus
足厥阴肝经	-	Foot *Jueyin* Liver Meridian
(足大趾甲后丛毛处)	-	the hairy area behind the nails of the big toes
(肺中)	-	inside the lungs

Figure 2 Flow sequence of the 12 regular meridians

Day 4

CIRCULATION PATHWAYS OF THE 14 MERIDIANS AND VESSELS

Hand *Taiyin* Lung Meridian

"The lung hand *taiyin* vessel originates from the middle *jiao*, goes down to link up with the large intestine, returns to the entrance of the stomach, travels upwards through the diaphragm to pertain to the lung; [then,] it passes by its connecting components (i.e., trachea and throat), traverses from the axillary, follows the inner side of the upper arm in front of the *shaoyin* heart, goes down to the elbow, runs through the inner side of the bone of the lower arm, and reaches [where] the *cun* pulse palpates. [From this point,] it directs its way to the thenar eminence and exits at the tip of the thumb. Its branch comes out of the wrist to reach the tip of the index finger via its inner side."(See Figure 3.)

Hand *Yangming* Large Intestine Meridian

"The large intestine hand *yangming* vessel originates from the tip of the index finger, runs along its dorsal side, comes out between the two bones [where] *hé gǔ* (LI 4) is located, enters in between the two tendons and follows the dorsum of the lower arm to the lateral elbow; [then,] it reaches the lateral side of the upper forelimb, continues its way to the shoulder, exits from the front of the acromion. It travels to the seventh cervical vertebra to the crossing point [of *dà zhuī* (DU 14)], goes down to *quē pén* (ST 12) and connects the lung, passes through the diaphragm and pertains to the large intestine; its branch starts from *quē pén*, goes along the neck, penetrates from the cheek, reaches the lower teeth, returns to circle around the mouth, crosses at *rén zhōng* (also known as *shuǐ gōu*, DU 26); the left meridian directs to the right while the right one goes to the left, and ends next to the naris."(See Figure 4.)

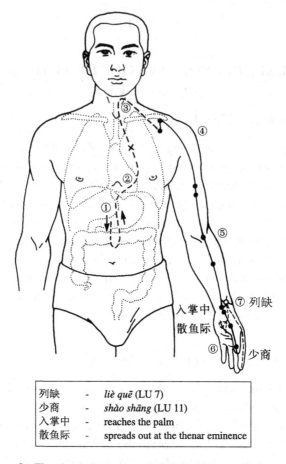

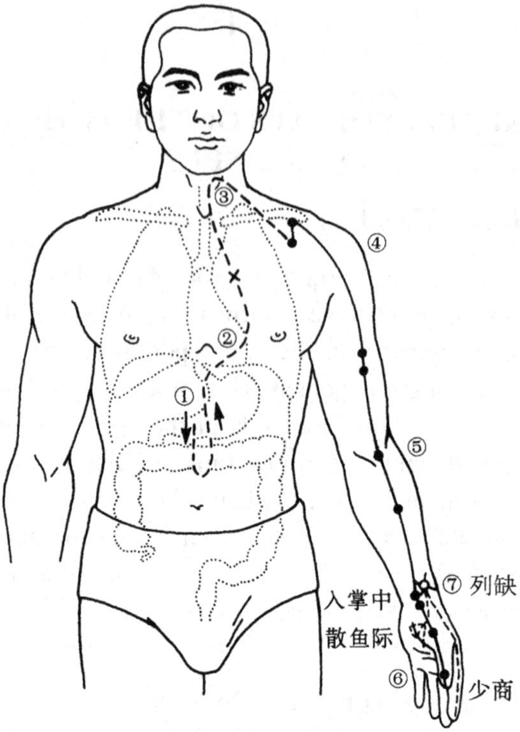

列缺	-	*liè quē* (LU 7)
少商	-	*shào shāng* (LU 11)
入掌中	-	reaches the palm
散鱼际	-	spreads out at the thenar eminence

Figure 3 The circulation pathway of the hand *Taiyin* lung meridian

Foot *Yangming* Stomach Meridian

"The stomach foot *yangming* vessel originates from both sides of the nose, crosses with the [foot] *taiyang* vessel, turns downwards along the outer side of the nose, enters the upper teeth, goes around the mouth, circles around the lips, and meets at *chéng jiāng* (RN 24); [then,] it returns and follows the edge of the lower mandible, comes out from *dà yíng* (ST 5) to *jiá chē* (ST 6), goes up in front of the ears, passes *kè zhǔ rén* (i.e., *shàng guān*, GB 3), follows the hairline and reaches the forehead; [one of] its branch begins from *dà yíng* (STS), goes down to *rén yíng* (ST 9),

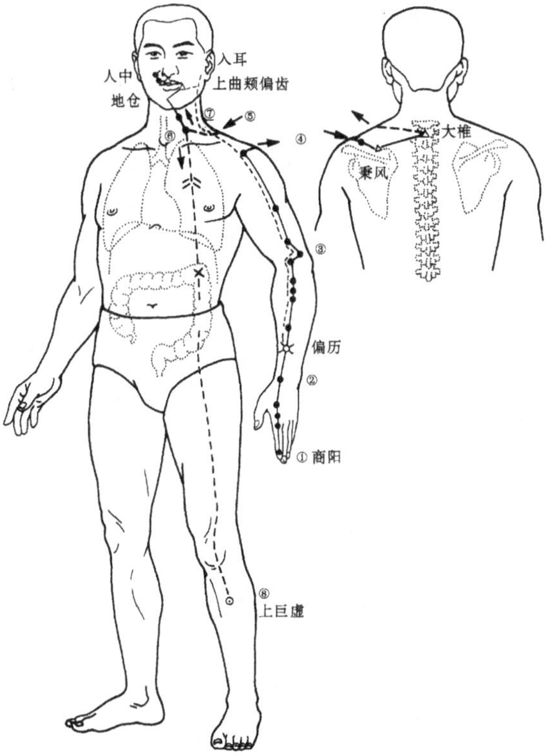

人中	-	*shuǐ gōu* (DU 26)
地仓	-	*dì cāng* (ST 4)
入耳	-	enters the ear
上曲颊偏齿	-	curves around the cheek to reach the teeth
偏历	-	*piān lì* (LI 6)
商阳	-	*shāng yáng* (LI 1)
上巨虚	-	*shàng jù xū* (ST 37)
秉风	-	*bǐng fēng* (SI 12)
大椎	-	*dàzhuī* (DU 14)

Figure 4 The circulation pathway of the hand *Yangming* large intestine meridian

follows the throat, enters *quē pén* (ST 12), runs down via the diaphragm, pertains to the stomach and links up with the spleen; the straight one starts from *quē pén*, goes down to the breasts, continues along the side of the navel and enters the *qì jiē* (i.e., *qì chōng*, ST 30); another one starts from the upper entrance of the stomach, makes its way down to the abdomen to meet with the previous one, goes down to *bì guān* (ST 31), passes *fú tù* (ST 32), continues downwards to the patella, follows the lateral side of the shin to the back of the foot, enters the inner aperture of the middle toe and exits to the tip of the second toe; another branch separates from three *cun* below the lower edge of the patella and goes down to the outer side of the middle toe; the last branch diverges from the back of the feet, and enters the gap of the big toe to its tip."(See Figure 5.)

Foot *Taiyin* Spleen Meridian

"The spleen foot *taiyin* vessel originates from the tip of the big toe, travels along the junction of the red and white skin on the medial aspect of the foot, passes the posterior side of the metatarsus prominence and goes upwards along the front edge of the medial mallelus; [then,] it continues on the medial aspect of the shank, travels along the posterior border of the tibia, crosses the [foot] *jueyin* and goes in front of it. Then, it passes the medial side of the knee and thigh, enters the abdomen, pertains to the spleen, networks with the stomach, crosses the diaphragm, passes along the pharynx, connects with the root of the tongue and spreads out underneath it. Afterwards, its branch comes out of the stomach, goes up to cross the diaphragm and infuses into the heart."(See Figure 6.)

Hand *Shaoyin* Heart Meridian

"The heart hand *shaoyin* vessel originates from the center of the heart, comes out and pertains to the heart vinculum; [then,] it goes down to network with the small intestine; its branch starts from the vinculum of the heart, goes up along the pharynx and connects to the pathway of the eyes; the straight branch [also] starts from the heart vinculum, travels to the lung, transverses to the oxter, goes down along the posterior medial aspect of the upper arm on the back side of the hand *taiyin* and *jueyin*; it continues along the posterior medial side of the elbow, reaches the end of the postular bone, enters the medial aspect of the palm, follows the medial side of the little finger and exits from its tip." (See Figure 7.)

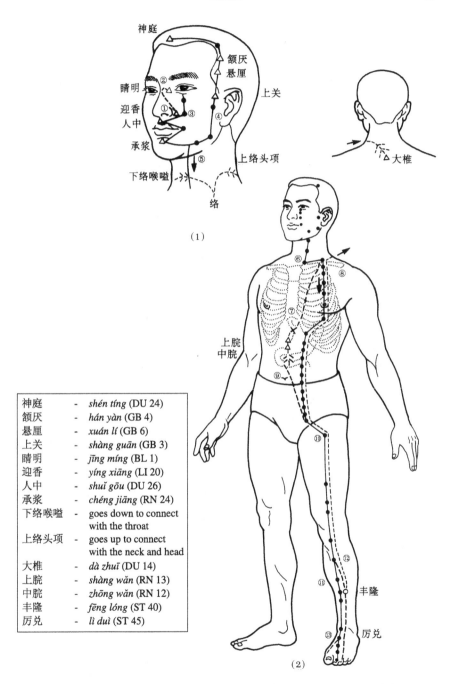

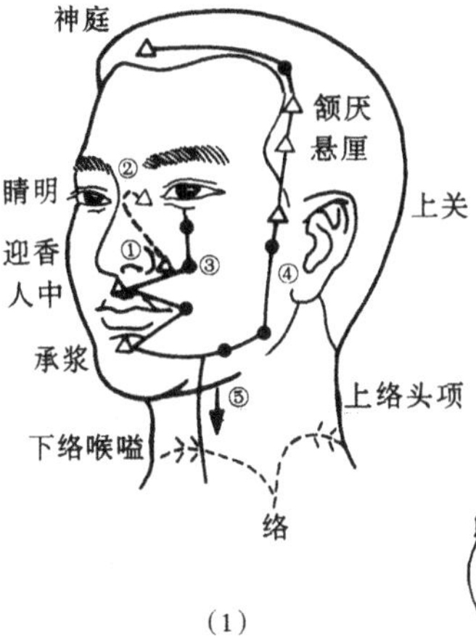

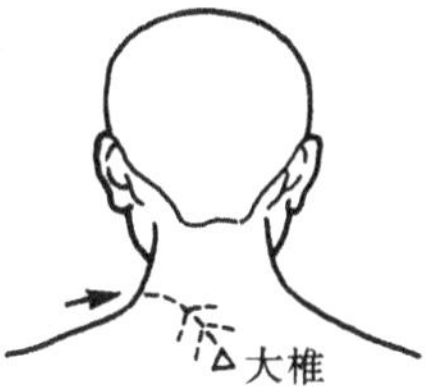

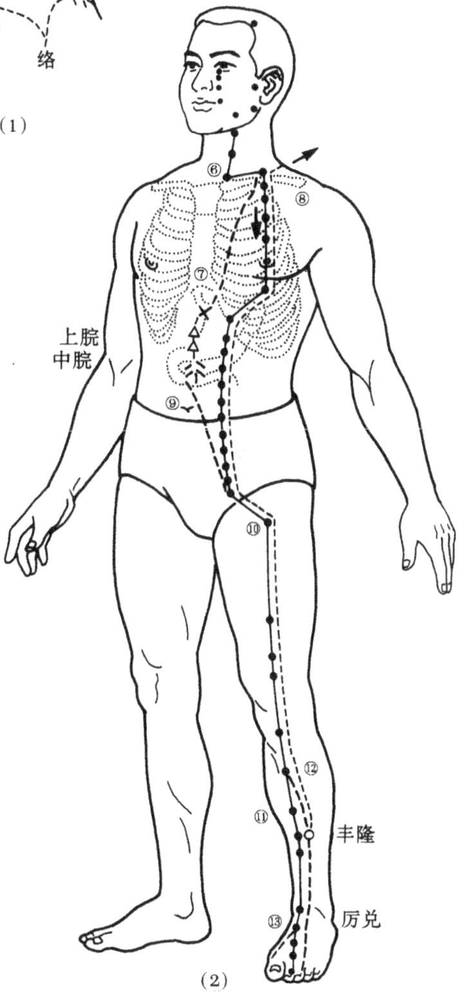

神庭	-	*shén tíng* (DU 24)
颔厌	-	*hán yàn* (GB 4)
悬厘	-	*xuán lí* (GB 6)
上关	-	*shàng guān* (GB 3)
睛明	-	*jīng míng* (BL 1)
迎香	-	*yíng xiāng* (LI 20)
人中	-	*shuǐ gōu* (DU 26)
承浆	-	*chéng jiāng* (RN 24)
下络喉嗌	-	goes down to connect with the throat
上络头项	-	goes up to connect with the neck and head
大椎	-	*dà zhuī* (DU 14)
上脘	-	*shàng wǎn* (RN 13)
中脘	-	*zhōng wǎn* (RN 12)
丰隆	-	*fēng lóng* (ST 40)
厉兑	-	*lì duì* (ST 45)

Figure 5 The circulation pathway of the foot *Yangming* stomach meridian

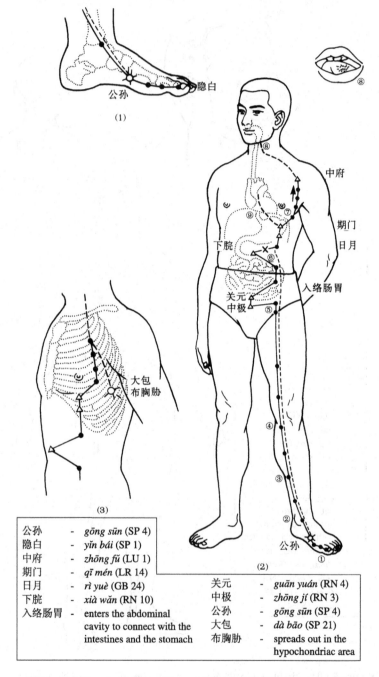

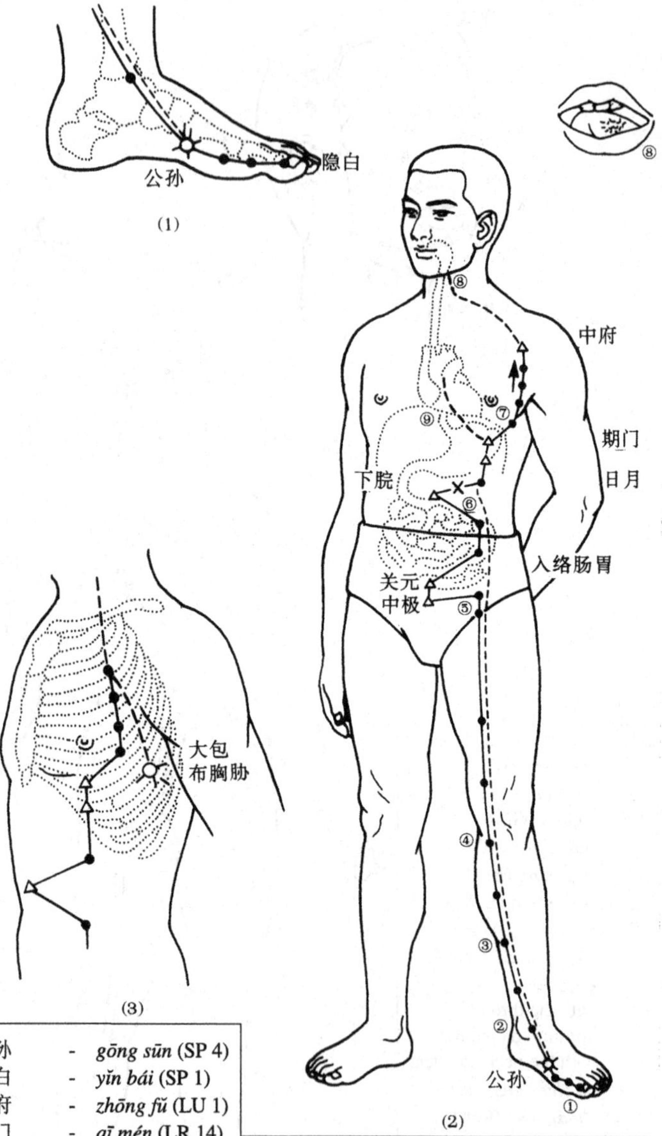

公孙	- *gōng sūn* (SP 4)
隐白	- *yǐn bái* (SP 1)
中府	- *zhōng fǔ* (LU 1)
期门	- *qī mén* (LR 14)
日月	- *rì yuè* (GB 24)
下脘	- *xià wǎn* (RN 10)
入络肠胃	- enters the abdominal cavity to connect with the intestines and the stomach
关元	- *guān yuán* (RN 4)
中极	- *zhōng jí* (RN 3)
公孙	- *gōng sūn* (SP 4)
大包	- *dà bāo* (SP 21)
布胸胁	- spreads out in the hypochondriac area

Figure 6 The circulation pathway of the foot *Taiyin* spleen meridian

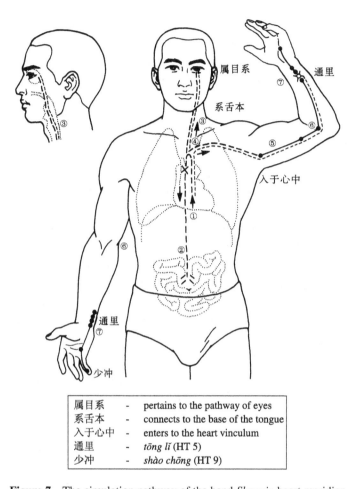

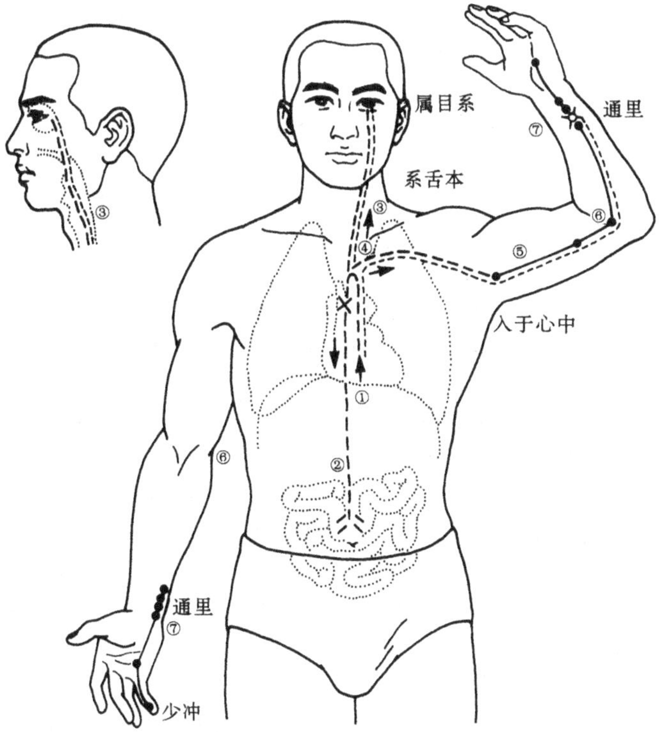

属目系	-	pertains to the pathway of eyes
系舌本	-	connects to the base of the tongue
入于心中	-	enters to the heart vinculum
通里	-	*tōng lǐ* (HT 5)
少冲	-	*shào chōng* (HT 9)

Figure 7 The circulation pathway of the hand *Shaoyin* heart meridian

Hand *Taiyang* Small Intestine Meridian

"The small intestine hand *taiyang* vessel originates from the tip of the little finger. It follows the lateral ulnar aspect of the hand to the wrist, and exits from the styloid process of the ulna. It [then] goes up along the posterior aspect of the ulna, passes the middle of the two bones, follows the posterior side of the upper arm to the back of the shoulder, zigzags around the scapula and reaches the upper shoulder; it enters from *quē pén* (ST 12) to network with the heart, follows the esophagus to the diaphragm and stomach, and pertains to the small intestine. Its branch starts from *quē pén*, follows the neck, travels up to the cheek, arrives at the outer canthus and enters the ear; another branch separates from the upper cheek, reaches the nose and inner canthus, and obliquely connects the cheekbone."(See Figure 8.)

Foot *Taiyang* Bladder Meridian

"The bladder foot *taiyang* vessel originates from the inner canthus, goes up to the forehead, and reaches the apex of the scalp. Its branch starts from the apex and arrives at the upper corner of the ear. A branch enters from the apex to connect with the brain, comes out, goes down along the neck and inside the shoulder, then follows the sides of the spinal cord, enters from the waist, goes inside along its muscle, networks with the kidney, and pertains to the urinary bladder. Another branch starts from the internal lumbar muscle, passes through the buttock and enters the popliteal fossa. A [last] branch penetrates through the inner side of shoulder blade, follows the sides of the spinal cord, travels to the greater trochanter, passes the lateral side of the thigh to reach its back, arrives at the popliteal fossa to meet the previous branch, goes down the calf, exits from the lateral malleolus, goes alongside of the fifth metatarsus bone, and arrives at the lateral side of the fifth toe."(See Figure 9.)

Foot *Shaoyin* Kidney Meridian

"The kidney foot *shaoyin* vessel originates under the little toe, obliquely goes towards the bottom of the foot, comes out from *rán gŭ* (KI 2). It goes along the medial malleolus with its branch entering the heel to reach the medial side of the calf and the popliteal space. [It then] passes through the spinal cord, pertains to the kidney and networks with the bladder. The straight branch passes through the liver and the diaphragm to reach inside of the lung; [then,] it follows the throat and travels on the side of the tongue. Its branch networks with the heart while it comes out from the lung, and [finally] infuses to the center of the chest."(See Figure 10.)

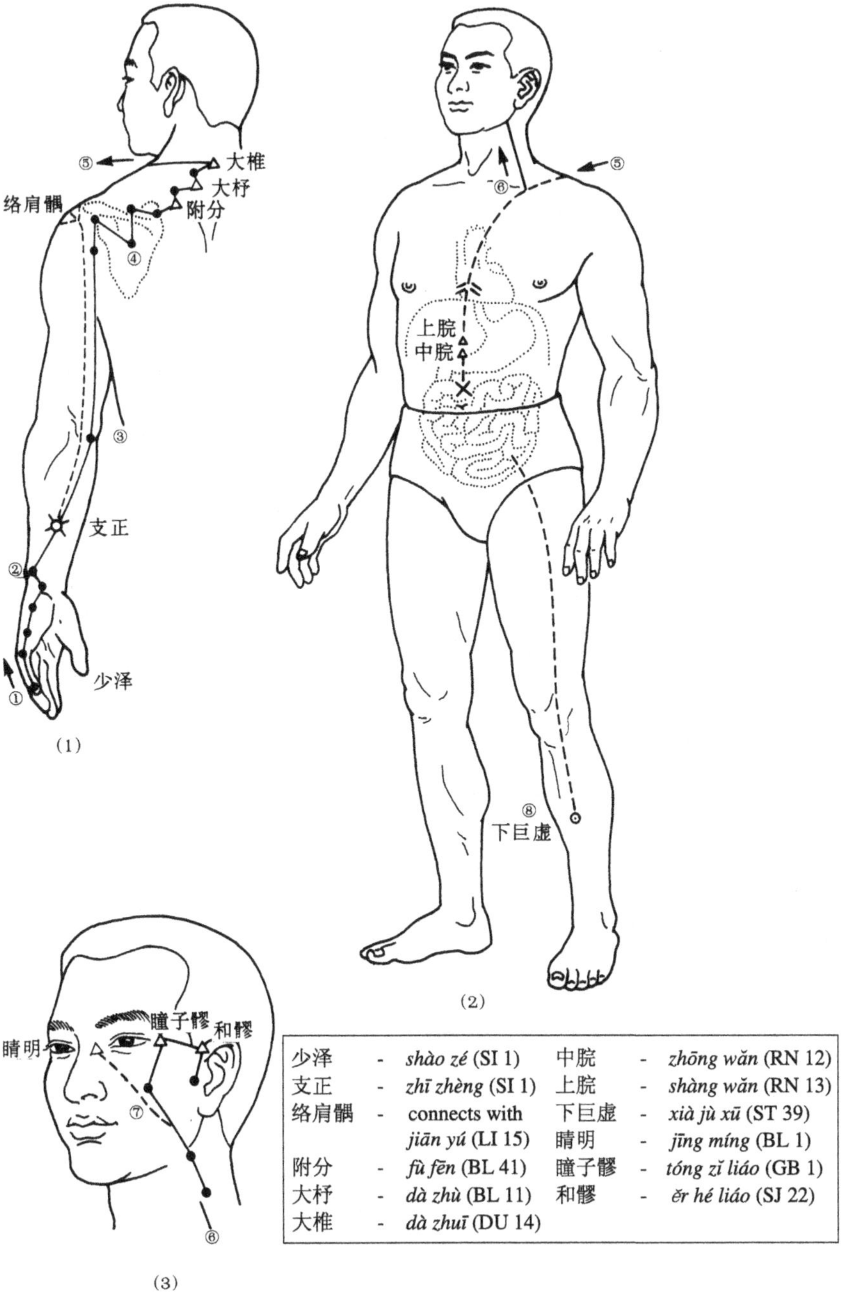

少泽	-	*shào zé* (SI 1)	中脘	-	*zhōng wǎn* (RN 12)
支正	-	*zhī zhèng* (SI 1)	上脘	-	*shàng wǎn* (RN 13)
络肩髃	-	connects with *jiān yú* (LI 15)	下巨虚	-	*xià jù xū* (ST 39)
			睛明	-	*jīng míng* (BL 1)
附分	-	*fù fēn* (BL 41)	瞳子髎	-	*tóng zǐ liáo* (GB 1)
大杼	-	*dà zhù* (BL 11)	和髎	-	*ěr hé liáo* (SJ 22)
大椎	-	*dà zhuī* (DU 14)			

Figure 8 The circulation pathway of the hand *Taiyang* small intestine meridian

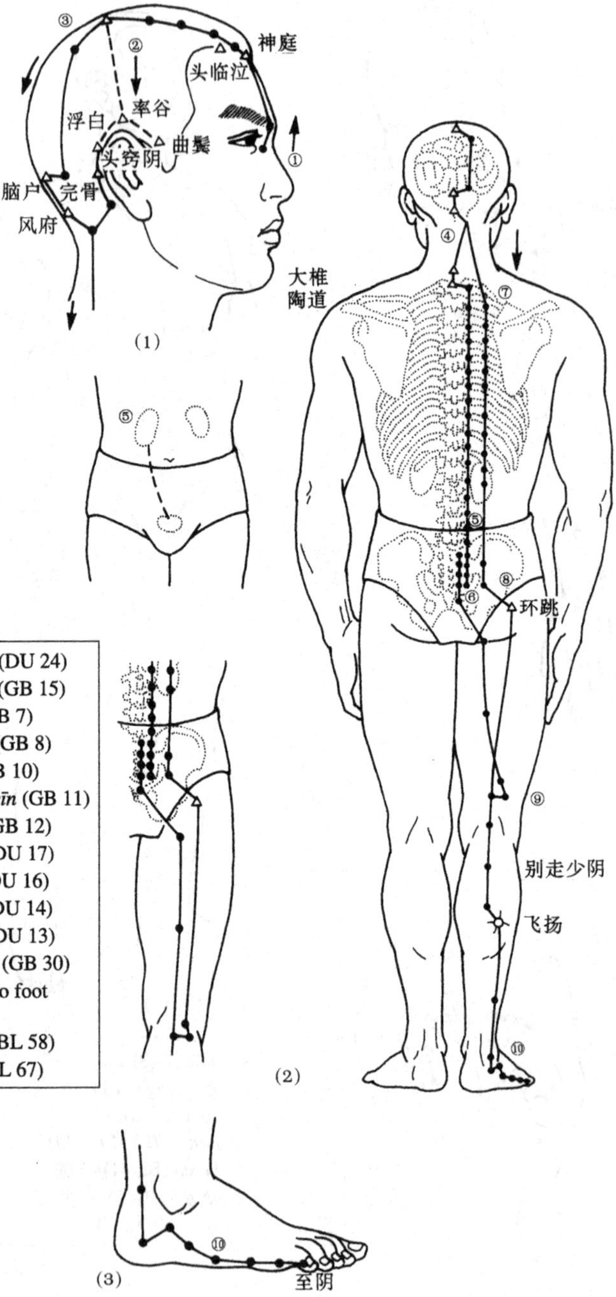

神庭	-	*shén tíng* (DU 24)
头临泣	-	*táo lín qì* (GB 15)
曲鬓	-	*qŭ bìn* (GB 7)
率谷	-	*shuài gŭ* (GB 8)
浮白	-	*fú bái* (GB 10)
头窍阴	-	*tóu qiào yīn* (GB 11)
完骨	-	*wán gŭ* (GB 12)
脑户	-	*năo hù* (DU 17)
风府	-	*fēng fŭ* (DU 16)
大椎	-	*dà zhuī* (DU 14)
陶道	-	*táo dào* (DU 13)
环跳	-	*huán tiào* (GB 30)
别走少阴	-	diverges to foot *shaoyin*
飞扬	-	*fēi yáng* (BL 58)
至阴	-	*zhì yīn* (BL 67)

Figure 9 The circulation pathway of the foot *Taiyang* bladder meridian

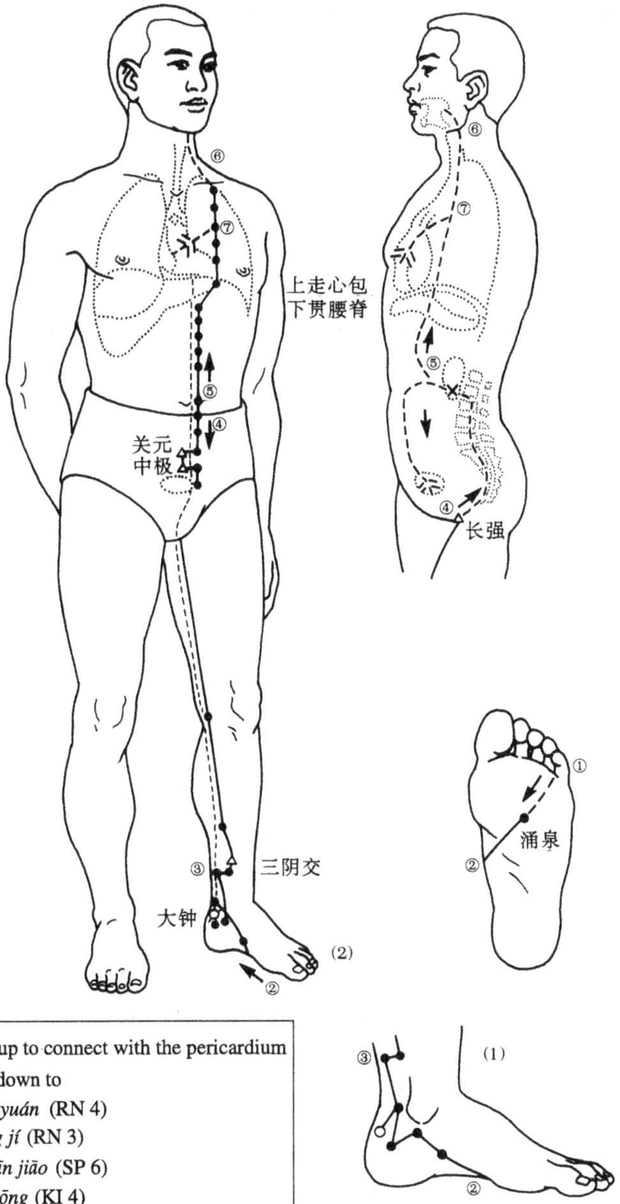

上走心包	-	goes up to connect with the pericardium
下贯腰脊	-	runs down to
关元	-	*guān yuán* (RN 4)
中极	-	*zhōng jí* (RN 3)
三阴交	-	*sān yīn jiāo* (SP 6)
大钟	-	*dà zhōng* (KI 4)
涌泉	-	*yǒng quán* (KI 1)

Figure 10 The circulation pathway of the foot *Shaoyin* kidney meridian

Hand *Jueyin* Pericardium Meridian

"The hand *jueyin* pericardium vessel, the master of the heart, originates from the center of the chest, comes out to pertain to the pericardium, goes down through the diaphragm to network with the three *jiao*. Its branch follows the ribs in the chest, goes down three cun from the axillary line, and goes up to the axillary. [Then,] it goes down along the medial side of the upper arm between hand *taiyin* and hand *shaoyin*, enters the middle of the cubital crease, continues in between the two tendons of the forearm to reach the middle of the palm, and exits out from the middle finger to arrive at its tip. Its branch exits out from the center of the palm and follows the fourth finger to its end."(See Figure 11.)

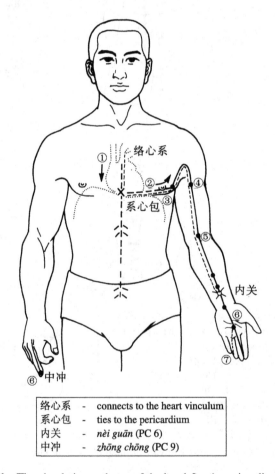

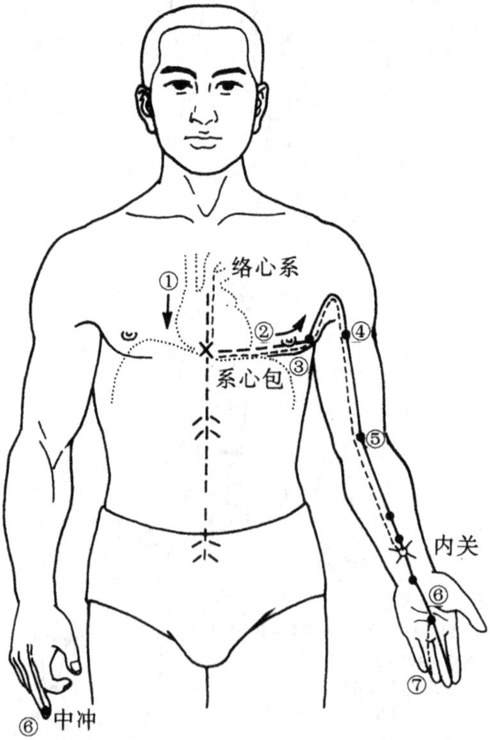

络心系	-	connects to the heart vinculum
系心包	-	ties to the pericardium
内关	-	*nèi guān* (PC 6)
中冲	-	*zhōng chōng* (PC 9)

Figure 11 The circulation pathway of the hand *Jueyin* pericardium meridian

Hand *Shaoyang Sanjiao* Meridian

"The *sanjiao* hand *shaoyang* vessel originates from the end of the fourth finger, goes up and comes out between the two fingers, follows the surface of the dorsum of the wrist, comes out from the lateral side of the two bones, passes through the elbow, follows the lateral upper arm to reach the shoulder, and crosses on the back of the foot *shaoyang*. [It then] enters *quē pén* (ST 12), distributes [its small branches] to *dàn zhōng* (RN 17), networks with the pericardium, and travels down and pertains to the three *jiao*. Its branch comes out from *dàn zhōng* and exits from *quē pén*, goes up along the neck to the back of the ear and its upper corner, and wanders down toward the cheek. Another branch enters the ear from its back, comes out to its front, passes in front of *shàng guān* (GB 3), crosses the cheek, and reaches the outer canthus."(See Figure 12.)

Foot *Shaoyang* Gallbladder Meridian

"The gallbladderfoot *shaoyang* vessel originates from the outer canthus, goes up to the frontal eminence of the head, turns down to the back of the ear, follows the neck, runs in front of the hand *shaoyang* vessel, reaches the shoulder, crosses to the back of the hand *shangyang* at this point, and enters *quē pén* (ST 12). Its branch enters inside of the ear from the back of the ear, exits to the front of the ear, and reaches the outer canthus. The second branch separates from the outer canthus, goes down to *dà yíng* (ST 5), joins hand *shaoyang*, arrives at [the spot] below the orbita, continues down to *jiá chē* (ST 6) and then to the neck and joins *quē pén*. From there, it travels down the center of the chest, passes the diaphragm, networks with the liver and pertains to the gallbladder, follows the inside of the rib, exits from [the abdominal] *qi-jie* (i.e., qi street), circles the hairy pubic area, and transverses to enter the pivot of the hip. The straight branch comes down from *quē pén* to the axillary, passes along the chest and hypochondriac region, goes down to the pivot of the hip, continues down to follow the lateral thigh, exits at the lateral side of the knee, goes down to the front of the fibula caput, then goes straight down to the tip of *juegu*, i.e., *xuán zhōng* (GB 39), passes the dorsum of the foot, and enters [the space] between the little and the fourth toe. Another branch separates

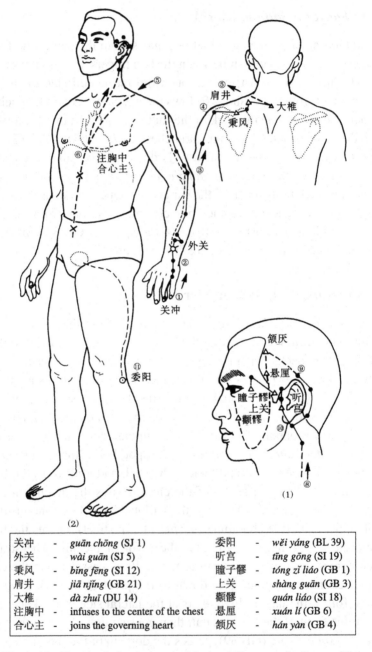

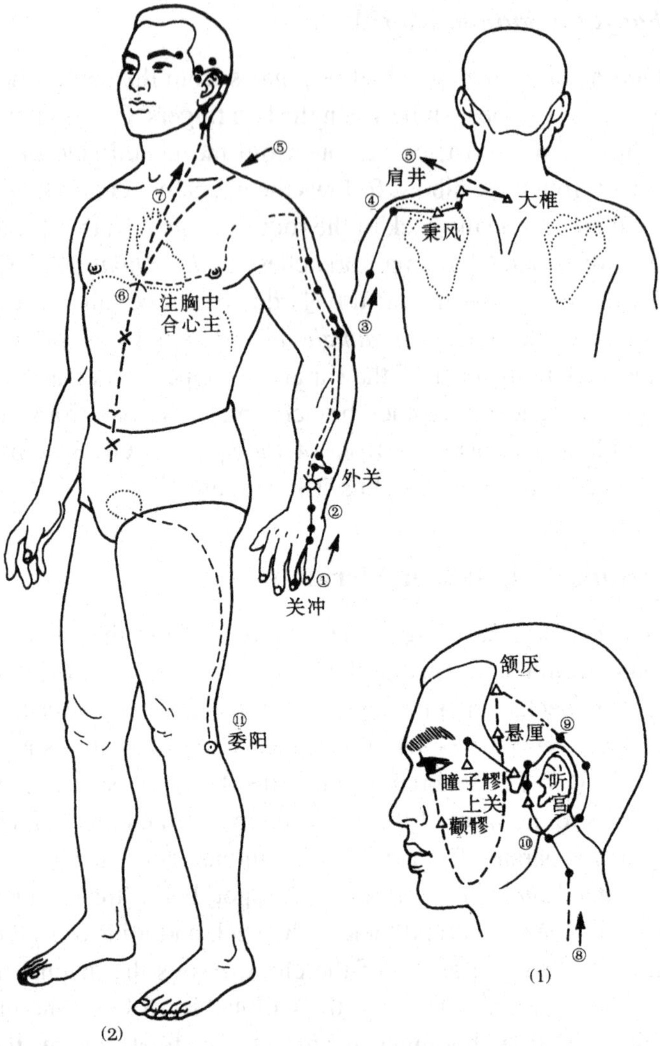

关冲	-	*guān chōng* (SJ 1)	委阳	-	*wěi yáng* (BL 39)
外关	-	*wài guān* (SJ 5)	听宫	-	*tīng gōng* (SI 19)
秉风	-	*bǐng fēng* (SI 12)	瞳子髎	-	*tóng zǐ liáo* (GB 1)
肩井	-	*jiā njǐng* (GB 21)	上关	-	*shàng guān* (GB 3)
大椎	-	*dà zhuī* (DU 14)	颧髎	-	*quán liáo* (SI 18)
注胸中	-	infuses to the center of the chest	悬厘	-	*xuán lí* (GB 6)
合心主	-	joins the governing heart	颔厌	-	*hán yàn* (GB 4)

Figure 12 The circulation pathway of the hand *Shaoyang Sanjiao* meridian

from the dorsum of the foot, enters [the space between] the big toe, goes between the big and second toe to the tip of the toe, returns to the nail base, and exits from *san-mao* (i.e., between the first and the second phalanx of the big toe)."(See Figure 13.)

Foot *Jueyin* Liver Meridian

"The vessel originates from the hairy area of the toe, runs up along the upper edge of the dorsum of the foot, arrives at [the spot] one cun from the medial malleolus, continues up and crosses to the back of the [foot] *taiyin* [at the spot] eight cun from the [medial] malleolus. [Then,] it travels to the medial side of the popliteal crease, follows the medial thigh to enter the hairy pubic area, circles around the external genital organs, arrives at the lower abdomen, passes along the side of the stomach, pertains to the liver and networks with the gallbladder. It [then] penetrates the diaphragm [with its small branches], disseminates in the hypochondria, passes the back of the throat, goes up to the head of the throat, connects the eye, exits on the forehead, and joins with the *du mai* on the apex [of the head]. Its branch starts from the eye area, goes down to the cheek, and circles the lips internally. Another branch diverges from the liver, transverses the diaphragm, and goes up to infuse the lung."(See Figure 14.)

Du Mai

It originates inside of the abdomen, goes down to the perineum, wanders toward the back, goes along the internal path of the spinal cord, travels up to reach *fēng fŭ* (DU 16), enters into the brain, goes up to the apex, and makes its way down the bridge of the nose.(See Figure 15.)

Ren Mai

It originates inside of the abdomen, goes down to the perineum, turns up to follow the hairy pubic area, travels along the internal abdomen, goes up while passing points including *guān yuán* (RN 4), and arrives at the throat. Then, it travels up further circling the mouth, passes the facial area, and enters the orbita at *chéng qì* (ST 1). (See Figure 16.)

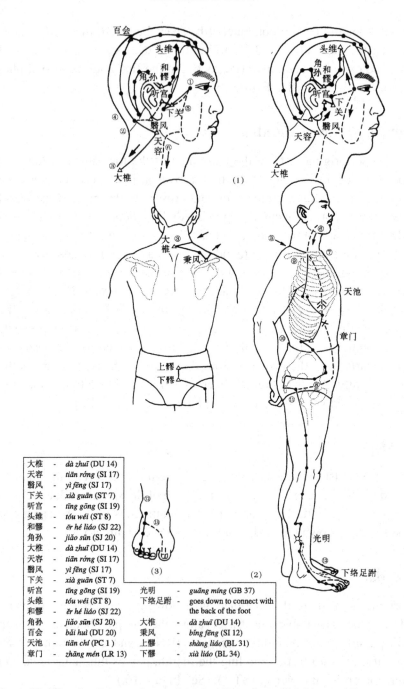

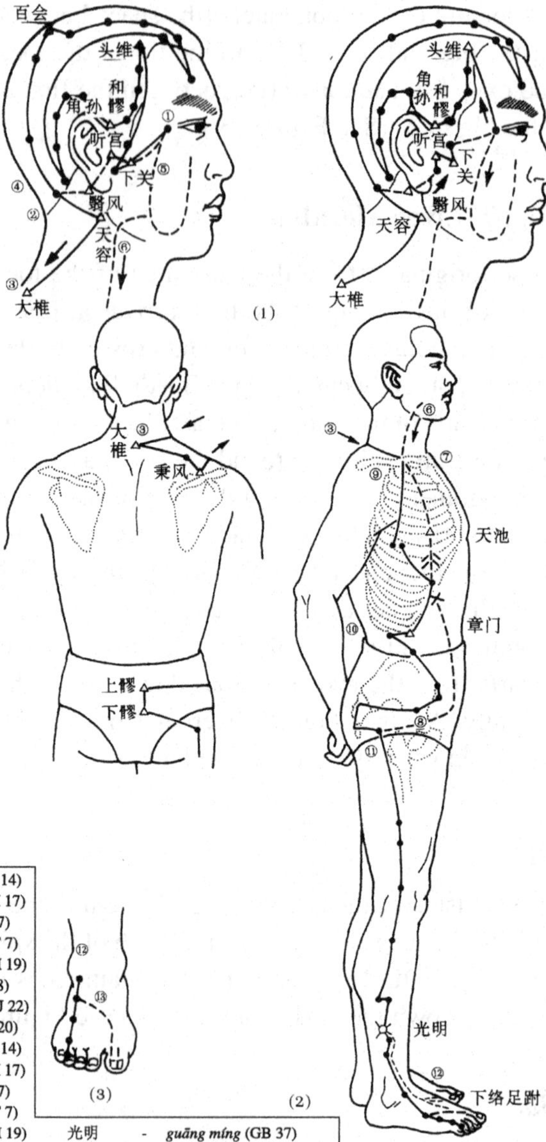

大椎	*dà zhuī* (DU 14)		
天容	*tiān róng* (SI 17)		
翳风	*yì fēng* (SJ 17)		
下关	*xià guān* (ST 7)		
听宫	*tīng gōng* (SI 19)		
头维	*tóu wéi* (ST 8)		
和髎	*ěr hé liáo* (SJ 22)		
角孙	*jiǎo sūn* (SJ 20)		
大椎	*dà zhuī* (DU 14)		
天容	*tiān róng* (SI 17)		
翳风	*yì fēng* (SJ 17)		
下关	*xià guān* (ST 7)		
听宫	*tīng gōng* (SI 19)	光明	*guāng míng* (GB 37)
头维	*tóu wéi* (ST 8)	下络足跗	goes down to connect with the back of the foot
和髎	*ěr hé liáo* (SJ 22)		
角孙	*jiǎo sūn* (SJ 20)	大椎	*dà zhuī* (DU 14)
百会	*bǎi huì* (DU 20)	秉风	*bǐng fēng* (SI 12)
天池	*tiān chí* (PC 1)	上髎	*shàng liáo* (BL 31)
章门	*zhāng mén* (LR 13)	下髎	*xià liáo* (BL 34)

Figure 13 The circulation pathway of the foot *Shaoyang* gallbladder meridian

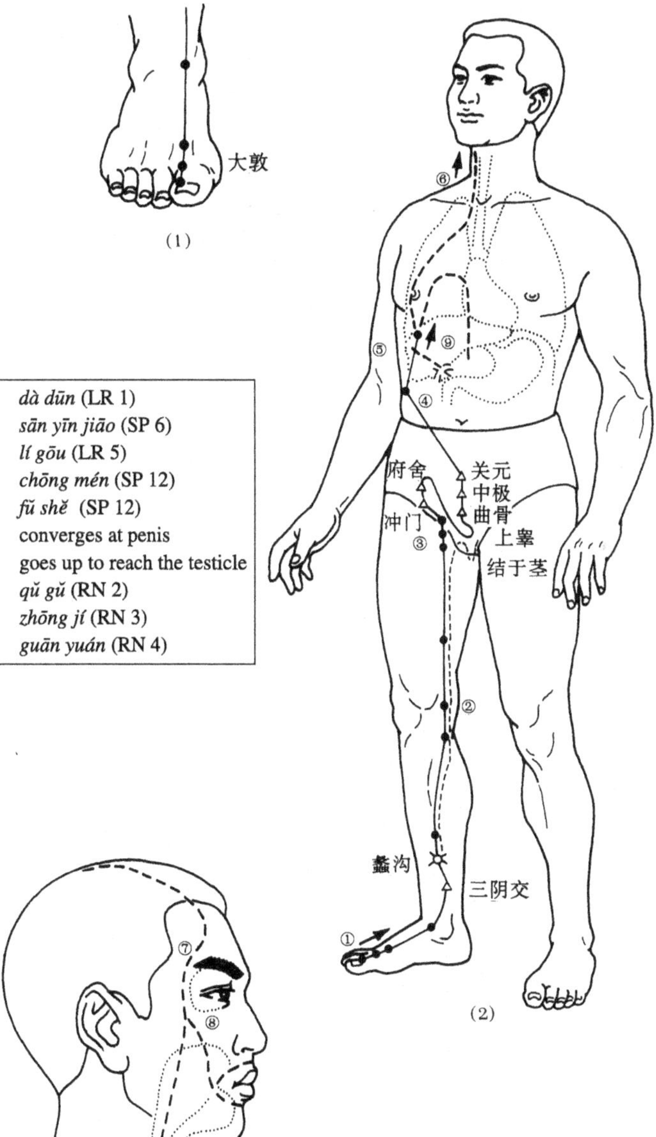

大敦	-	*dà dūn* (LR 1)
三阴交	-	*sān yīn jiāo* (SP 6)
蠡沟	-	*lí gōu* (LR 5)
冲门	-	*chōng mén* (SP 12)
府舍	-	*fŭ shě* (SP 12)
结于茎	-	converges at penis
上睾	-	goes up to reach the testicle
曲骨	-	*qŭ gŭ* (RN 2)
中极	-	*zhōng jí* (RN 3)
关元	-	*guān yuán* (RN 4)

Figure 14 The circulation pathway of the foot *Jueyin* liver meridian

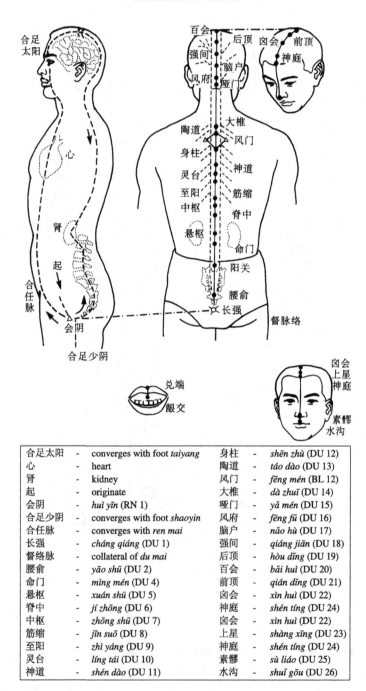

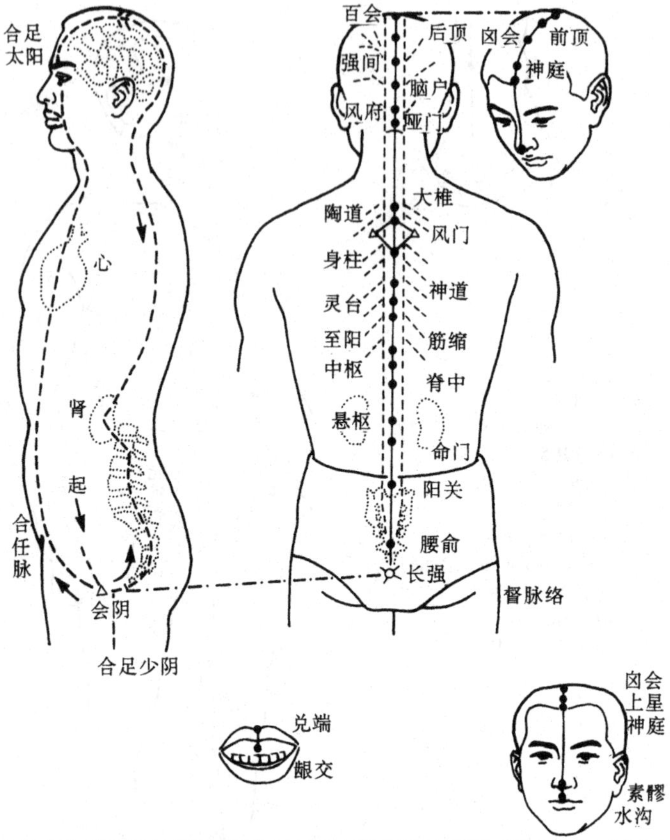

合足太阳	-	converges with foot *taiyang*	身柱	-	*shēn zhù* (DU 12)
心	-	heart	陶道	-	*táo dào* (DU 13)
肾	-	kidney	风门	-	*fēng mén* (BL 12)
起	-	originate	大椎	-	*dà zhuī* (DU 14)
会阴	-	*huì yīn* (RN 1)	哑门	-	*yǎ mén* (DU 15)
合足少阴	-	converges with foot *shaoyin*	风府	-	*fēng fǔ* (DU 16)
合任脉	-	converges with *ren mai*	脑户	-	*nǎo hù* (DU 17)
长强	-	*cháng qiáng* (DU 1)	强间	-	*qiáng jiān* (DU 18)
督络脉	-	collateral of *du mai*	后顶	-	*hòu dǐng* (DU 19)
腰俞	-	*yāo shū* (DU 2)	百会	-	*bǎi huì* (DU 20)
命门	-	*mìng mén* (DU 4)	前顶	-	*qián dǐng* (DU 21)
悬枢	-	*xuán shū* (DU 5)	囟会	-	*xìn huì* (DU 22)
脊中	-	*jí zhōng* (DU 6)	神庭	-	*shén tíng* (DU 24)
中枢	-	*zhōng shū* (DU 7)	囟会	-	*xìn huì* (DU 22)
筋缩	-	*jīn suō* (DU 8)	上星	-	*shàng xīng* (DU 23)
至阳	-	*zhì yáng* (DU 9)	神庭	-	*shén tíng* (DU 24)
灵台	-	*líng tái* (DU 10)	素髎	-	*sù liáo* (DU 25)
神道	-	*shén dào* (DU 11)	水沟	-	*shuǐ gōu* (DU 26)

Figure 15 The circulation pathway of *Du Mai*

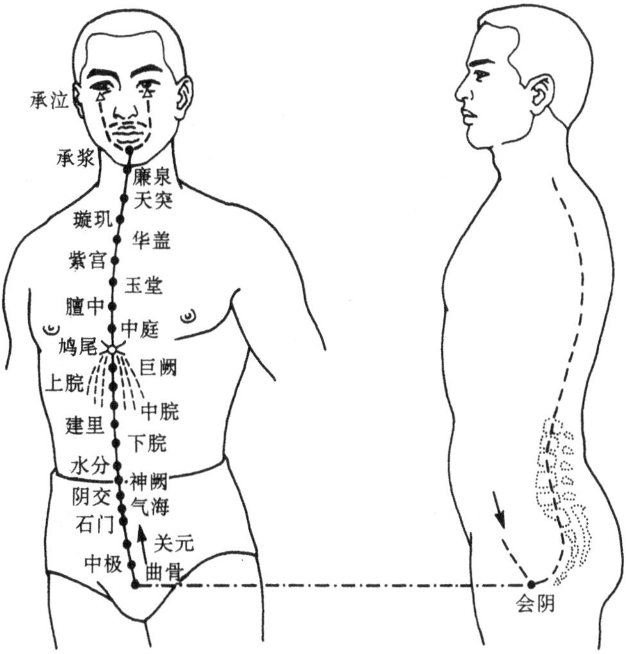

会阴	-	*huì yīn* (RN 1)	巨阙	-	*jù què* (RN 14)
曲骨	-	*qǔ gǔ* (RN 2)	鸠尾	-	*jiū wěi* (RN 15)
中极	-	*zhōng jí* (RN 3)	中庭	-	*zhōng tíng* (RN 16)
关元	-	*guān yuán* (RN 4)	膻中	-	*dàn zhōng* (RN 17)
石门	-	*shí mén* (RN 5)	玉堂	-	*yù táng* (RN 18)
气海	-	*qì hǎi* (RN 6)	紫宫	-	*zǐ gōng* (RN 19)
阴交	-	*yīn jiāo* (RN 7)	华盖	-	*huá gài* (RN 20)
神阙	-	*shén què* (RN 8)	璇玑	-	*xuán jī* (RN 21)
水分	-	*shuǐ fēn* (RN 9)	天突	-	*tiān tū* (RN 22)
下脘	-	*xià wǎn* (RN 10)	廉泉	-	*lián quán* (RN 23)
建里	-	*jiàn lǐ* (RN 11)	承浆	-	*chéng jiāng* (RN 24)
中脘	-	*zhōng wǎn* (RN 12)	承泣	-	(ST 1)
上脘	-	*shàng wǎn* (RN 13)			

Figure 16 The circulation pathway of *Ren Mai*

Everyday Exercises

Study the text and use the figures as reference to master the pathways of the 14 meridians and vessels.

Day 5

Commonly Used *Shu Xue* (Acupoints), Part I

Shu-xue, also known as *xué wèi* or *xué dào*, is the Chinese name for an acupoint. *Shu* means to transport and infuse while *xue* means interstice and gathering.

There are different methods used to locate acupoints, including using anatomic landmarks on the surface of the body, bone-length cun determination, and body cun (also known as finger cun) determination. Cun is the standard unit of measurement for the body used in acupuncture. Figure 17 shows the determination methods of common bone-length cun and body cun.

The accuracy of acupoint identification has a direct impact on the treatment effect. Clinically, we can use specific striations, tendons, groove, creases, prominence or depression to locate certain points in addition to common anatomic landmarks. It requires careful observation, practice, and experience to reach a certain level of competence.

With regard to acupoint selection and combination, one can rely on criteria such as indications of the acupoints, the meridian they belong to, and whether they are distal or local, front-*mu* or back-*shu*, upper or lower, and left or right. Tables 3 to 7 show the commonly used acupoints associated with five of the 12 meridians.

Everyday Exercises

Try to memorize the commonly used acupoints of the Lung, Large Intestine, Stomach, Spleen, and Heart meridians.

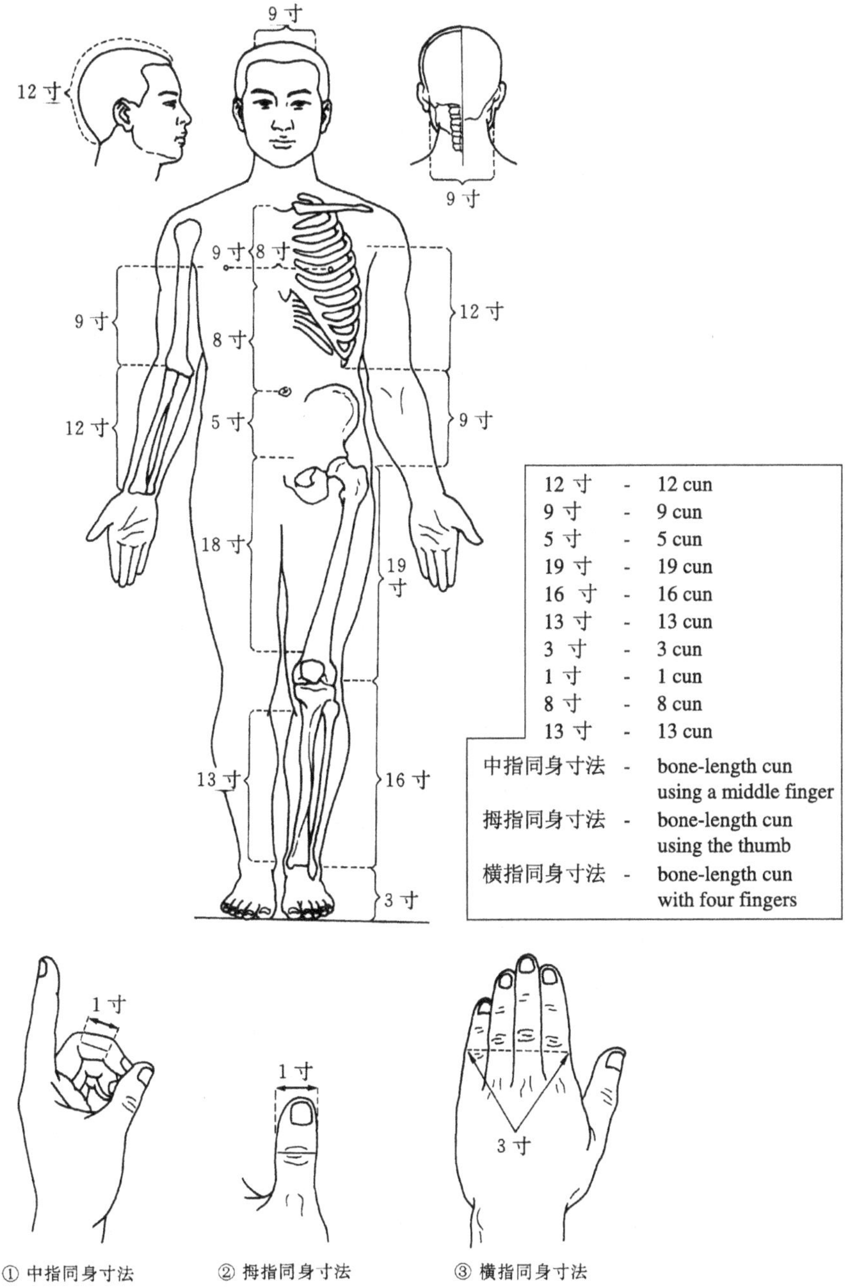

Figure 17 Common bone-length cun and body cun determination methods

Table 3 Common acupoints of the hand *Taiyin* lung meridian

Name	Location	Indications	Common Manipulations
zhōng fǔ (LU 1, 中府)	6 cun from the midline of the chest, level with the first intercostal space	Cough, asthma, suppressed chest, bronchitis	Pushing, kneading, rubbing
yún mén (LU 2, 云门)	1 cun directly above *zhōng fǔ*	Cough, asthma, chest pain	Kneading, rubbing
chǐ zé (LU 5, 尺泽)	At the cubital crease, on the radial side of the tendon of biceps brachii	Cough, asthma, spasm or pain of the elbow and arm, infantile convulsion	Pressing, kneading, grasping
liè quē (LU 7, 列缺)	Right above the styloid process of the radius, 1.5 cun from the transverse crease of the wrist	Stiffness of the neck, pain of the head and neck, cough	Pressing, kneading
tài yuān (LU 9, 太渊)	On the radial end of the transverse crease of the wrist and radial artery	Cough, asthma, sore throat, wrist pain	Pressing, nailing
yú jì (LU 10, 鱼际)	At the midpoint of the palmar side of the thumb, on the junction of the red and white skin	Wheezing, asthma, cough, pain on the chest and upper back	Kneading, nailing
shào shāng (LU 11, 少商)	On the radial side of the thumb, 0.1 cun from the corner of the nail base	Infantile convulsion, cough	Nailing

Table 4 Common acupoints of the hand *Yangming* large intestine meridian

Name	Location	Indications	Common Manipulations
hé gŭ (LI 4, 合谷)	Between the first and second metacarpal bones, approximately in the middle of the second metacarpal bone	Headache, toothache, fever, facial nervous paralysis, pain of the arm, pain and spasm of the finger	Grasping, kneading
yáng xī (LI 5, 阳溪)	On the radial side of the dorsal crease of the wrist, between the tendons of extensor pollicis longus and brevismuscles	Headache, redness of the eyes, toothache, wrist pain	Pressing, kneading
piān lì (LI 6, 偏历)	On the line connecting *yáng xī* and *qŭ chí* (LI 11), 3 cun above *yáng xī*	Nosebleed, red eyes, deafness, tinnitus, arthritic pain of the arms	Pressing, kneading, grasping
shŏu sān lĭ (LI 10, 手三里)	2 cun below the transverse cubital crease and *qŭ chí* (LI 11)	Spasm and restricted range of motion of the elbow, numbness, soreness and pain of the arm	Grasping, pressing, kneading
qŭ chí (LI 11, 曲池)	With the elbow flexed, the point is on the lateral end of the transverse cubital crease	Fever, hypertension, pain of the elbow, paralysis of the upper extremities	Grasping, kneading
jiān yú (LI 15, 肩髃)	Anterior and inferior to the acromion, in the depression of the shoulder with the arm lifted	Pain of the shoulder and arm, restricted motion of the shoulder joint, hemiplegia	Kneading, pressing
yíng xiāng (LI 20, 迎香)	0.5 cun from the border of the ala nasi, in the nasolabial groove	Rhinitis, nasal congestion, wry mouth and eyes	Kneading, nailing

Table 5 Common acupoints of the foot *Yangming* stomach meridian

Name	Location	Indications	Common Manipulations
sì bái (ST 2, 四白)	Directly below the pupil in the depression of the infraorbital foramen	Facial nervous paralysis; red, itchy, and painful eyes	Pushing, kneading
dì cāng (ST 4, 地仓)	0.4 cun lateral to the corner of the mouth	Salivation, wry mouth and eyes	Pushing, kneading
jiá chē (ST 6, 颊车)	In the depression 1 middle-finger-width anterior and superior to the lower angle of the mandible, at the prominence of the masseter muscle when the teeth are clenched	Wry mouth and eyes, toothache, swelling cheek	Pushing, kneading
xià guān (ST 7, 下关)	In the depression between the zygomatic arch and the condyloid process of the mandible while the mouth is closed, and it disappears when the mouth opens	Facial paralysis, toothache	Pushing, kneading, pressing
tóu wéi (ST 8, 头维)	0.5 cun directly above the hairline at the corner of the forehead	Headache	Pushing, kneading, wiping
rén yíng (ST 9, 人迎)	1.5 cun lateral to the Adam's apple	Swelling and sore throat, labored breathing, scrofula, goiter, swelling neck	Kneading, grasping
quē pén (ST 12, 缺盆)	In the middle of the supraclavicular fossa, 4 cun lateral to the anterior midline	Fullness of the chest, cough, asthma, stiffness of the neck	Pressing, plucking

(*Continued*)

Table 5 (*Continued*)

Name	Location	Indications	Common Manipulations
tiān shū (ST 25, 天枢)	2 cun lateral to the umbilicus	Diarrhea, constipation, abdominal pain, irregular menstruation	Pushing, kneading, rubbing
bì guān (ST 31, 髀关)	On the line connecting the anterior superior iliac spine and the lateral border of the patella, level with the lower border of the symphysis pubis	*Bì* and *wěi* patterns of the lower extremities, spasm of the tendons, restricted range of motion of the leg	Pressing, plucking
fú tù (ST 32, 伏兔)	6 cun above the upper lateral border of the patella	Paralysis of the lower extremities, pain, coldness, and numbness of the knee	Pressing, plucking
liáng qiū (ST 34, 梁丘)	Two cun above the upper lateral border of the patella	Coldness and numbness of the knee	Pressing, grasping
dú bí (ST 35, 犊鼻)	On the lower lateral border of the patella, in the depression lateral to the patella ligament	Coldness, numbness, restricted motion of the knee	Pressing, kneading, point pressing
zú sān lǐ (ST 36, 足三里)	3 cun below *dú bí*, one middle-finger width lateral to the anterior crest of the tibia	Abdominal pain, diarrhea, constipation, *bi* and pain of the lower extremities, hypertension	Pressing, point pressing, pushing
shàng jù xū (ST 37, 上巨虚)	3 cun below *zú sān lǐ*	Abdominal pain, diarrhea, and distention of the abdomen	Pressing, point pressing
xià jù xū (ST 39, 下巨虚)	3 cun below *shàng jù xū*	Pain of the intercostal nerves, enteritis	Pressing, point pressing

(*Continued*)

Table 5 (*Continued*)

Name	Location	Indications	Common Manipulations
fēng lóng (ST 40, 丰隆)	At the midpoint between the lower lateral border of the patella and the external malleolus	Headache, excessive phlegm and saliva, constipation, numbness, pain, *bi* and *wei* patterns of lower extremities	Pressing, grasping, point pressing
jiě xī (ST 41, 解溪)	At the midpoint of the transverse crease of the ankle, between the tendons of muscle extensor hallucis longus and digitorum longus	Injury of the ankle joint, numbness of the toes	Kneading, pressing, point pressing
chōng yáng (ST 42, 冲阳)	1.5 cun below *jiě xī*, at the highest point of the dorsum of the foot where the dorsal artery of the foot pulsates	Stomachache, pain of upper teeth, restricted motion of the foot	Pressing, point pressing, kneading

Table 6 Common acupoints of the foot *Taiyin* spleen meridian

Name	Location	Indications	Common Manipulations
tài bái (SP 3, 太白)	Proximal to the first metatarsal bone, at the junction of the red and white skin	Gastric pain, abdominal distention, diarrhea, constipation, hemorrhoids	Nailing, kneading
gōng sūn (SP 4, 公孙)	Distal to the base of the first metatarsal bone, at the junction of the red and white skin	Gastric pain, indigestion, epigastric pain, diarrhea	Nailing, kneading

(*Continued*)

Table 6 (*Continued*)

Name	Location	Indications	Common Manipulations
sān yīn jiāo (SP 6, 三阴交)	3 cun above the medial malleolus, on the posterior border of the medial aspect of tibi	Insomnia, distention and pain of the lower abdomen, enuresis, dysuria, gynecopathy	Kneading, point pressing, grasping
yīn líng quán (SP 9, 阴陵泉)	In the depression on the inferior border of the medial tibial condyle	Soreness and pain of the knee, dysuria	Pressing, point pressing, grasping
xuè hăi (SP 10, 血海)	2 cun above the upper border of the medial patella	Pain of the knee, irregular menstruation	Pressing, point pressing, grasping
dà héng (SP 15, 大横)	4 cun lateral to the umbilicus	Constipation, diarrhea due to deficient coldness, pain of the lower abdomen	Pushing, rubbing, kneading

Table 7 Common acupoints of the hand *Shaoyin* heart meridian

Name	Location	Indications	Common Manipulations
jí quán (HT 1, 极泉)	At the midpoint of the axillary fossa, medial to where the axillary artery palpates	*Bi* pattern and pain of the arm and elbow, pain on the ribs	Plucking
shào hăi (HT 3, 少海)	In the depression on the ulnar aspect of the cubital crease end when the elbow is flexed	Pain of the elbow joint, tremor of the hand, spasm of the elbow	Plucking, kneading
shén mén (HT 7, 神门)	At the ulnar end of the transverse crease of the wrist, on the depression of the radial side of the tendon of the flexor carpi ulnaris	Palpitation, insomnia, poor memory	Kneading, pressing
shào chōng (HT 9, 少冲)	On the radial aspect of the little finger, 0.1 finger cun from the base of the nail	Palpitation, heart pain, hypochondriac pain, manic psychosis	Nailing

Day 6

Commonly Used *Shu Xue*, Part II

Tables 8–12 show the acupoints of five more meridians.

Table 8 Common acupoints of the hand *Taiyang* small intestine meridian

Name	Location	Indications	Common Manipulations
shào zé (SI 1, 少泽)	On the ulnar side of the little finger, 0.1 finger cun from the nail base	Apoplectic coma, swelling and pain of the throat, fever	Nailing
hòu xī (SI 3, 后溪)	Make a loose fist, on the ulnar side, proximal to the metacarpophalangeal joint, at the junction of the red and white skin	Stiffness and pain of the neck; pain of the arm, shoulder, and waist; tinnitus; deafness	Nailing
xiǎo hǎi (SI 8, 小海)	In the depression between the ulnar olecranon and the medial epicondyle of the humerus	*Bì* pattern pain of the upper extremity, pain of the neck, toothache	Grasping
jiān zhēn (SI 9, 肩贞)	1 finger cun above the posterior end of the axillary fossa	Periarthritis of the shoulder; numbness, soreness, and pain of the upper extremity	Pressing, point pressing
tiān zōng (SI 11, 天宗)	In the depression in the center of the subscapular fossa	Pain in the shoulder joint, pain and heavy sensation in the back	Pressing, point pressing, kneading
jiān wài shū (SI 14, 肩外俞)	3 cun lateral to the lower border of the spinous process of T1	Soreness and pain of the shoulder and back, stiff neck, coldness and pain of the upper limb	Point pressing, pressing
jiān zhōng shū (SI 15, 肩中俞)	2 cun lateral to the lower border of the spinous process of C7	Pain in the shoulder and back, cough, asthma	Point pressing, pressing
quán liào (SI 18, 颧髎)	Directly below the outer canthus of the eyes, in the depression of the lower border of the malar bone	Wry mouth and eyes	Pushing, pressing, kneading

Table 9 Common acupoints of the foot *Taiyang* bladder meridian

Name	Location	Indications	Common Manipulations
jīng míng (BL 1, 睛明)	0.1 cun lateral and superior to the inner canthus	Disease of the eyes	Pressing
cuán zhú (BL 2, 攒竹)	In the depression of the medial end of the eyebrow	Pain on the superciliary ridge, red and painful eyes, headache, insomnia	Pressing, kneading
tiān zhù (BL 10, 天柱)	In the depression 1.3 cun lateral to *yǎ mĕn* and 0.5 cun above the posterior hair margin	Occipital pain, stiff and painful neck, sore throat, stuffy nose	Grasping, pressing
dà zhù (BL 11, 大杼)	1.5 cun lateral from the depression of the spinous process of T1	Fever, cough, stiff neck, scapular pain	Pressing, point pressing, kneading
fēng mén (BL 12, 风门)	1.5 cun lateral from the depression of the spinous process of T2	Cough caused by externally contracted wind, stiff neck, pain in the chest and back	Pressing, point pressing, kneading
fèi shū (BL 13, 肺俞)	1.5 cun lateral from the depression of the spinous process of T3	Cough, asthma, distention of the chest, degenerative damage of the back muscle	Pushing, kneading, kneading
xīn shū (BL 15, 心俞)	1.5 cun lateral from the depression of the spinous process of T5	Insomnia, palpitations	Pushing, kneading
gé shū (BL 17, 膈俞)	1.5 cun lateral from the depression of the spinous process of T7	Vomiting, hiccups	Pressing, point pressing, kneading
gān shū (BL 18, 肝俞)	1.5 cun lateral from the depression of the spinous process of T9	Hypochondriac pain, liver diseases, blurred vision	Pushing, pressing, kneading

(*Continued*)

Table 9 (*Continued*)

Name	Location	Indications	Common Manipulations
dǎn shū (BL 19, 胆俞)	1.5 cun lateral from the depression of the spinous process of T10	Hypochondriac pain, gallbladder diseases	Pushing, pressing, point pressing
pí shū (BL 20, 脾俞)	1.5 cun lateral from the depression of the spinous process of T11	Distention and pain of the epigastric area, indigestion, fatigue, sleepiness, lassitude	Pushing, pressing, kneading
wèi shū (BL 21, 胃俞)	1.5 cun lateral from the depression of the spinous process of T12	Gastric pain, poor appetite, indigestion	Pushing, pressing, kneading, point pressing
sān jiāo shū (BL 22, 三焦俞)	1.5 cun lateral from the depression of the spinous process of L1	Stiffness and pain of the waist muscles, vomiting, distention of the abdomen	Pushing, pressing, kneading
shèn shū (BL 23, 肾俞)	1.5 cun lateral from the depression of the spinous process of L2	Pain in the waist, lassitude, spermatorrhea, enuresis, irregular menstruation	Pushing, kneading
dà cháng shū (BL 25, 大肠俞)	1.5 cun lateral from the depression of the spinous process of L4	Diarrhea, waist and leg pain	Pushing, pressing, kneading
páng guāng shū (BL 28, 膀胱俞)	1.5 cun lateral from the depression of the spinous process of S2	Dysuria, enuresis, stiff and painful waist muscle	Pushing, pressing, kneading

(*Continued*)

Table 9 (*Continued*)

Name	Location	Indications	Common Manipulations
bā liào (BL 31 to 34, eight *liào*, 八髎)	*shàng liào* (BL 31), *cì liào* (BL 32), *zhōng liào* (BL 33), and *xià liào* (BL 34) are located in the 1st, 2nd, 3rd, and 4th sacral foramens respectively. With one on each side, they total up to eight acupoints	Lower back pain, genitourinary disorders	Pressing, kneading, point pressing
yīn mén (BL 37, 殷门)	On the posterior aspect of the thigh, 6 cun below the gluteal fold	Sciatica, paralysis of the lower limb	Point pressing, heavy pressing
wěi zhōng (BL 40, 委中)	In the midpoint of the popliteal	Waist and back pain, restricted motion of the knee, hemiplegia	Grasping, kneading, plucking
zhì biān (BL 54, 秩边)	3 cun lateral from the lower border of the 4th sacral foramen	Pain in the waist and buttocks, *bì* and *wěi* patterns of the lower limb, dysuria	Pressing, point pressing, heavy pressing
chéng shān (BL 57, 承山)	Extending the foot straight, the point is at the apex of the depression where a reversed "V" presents in the middle of the posterior calf	Waist and back pain, spasm of the gastrocnemius, hemorrhoids	Grasping, pressing
kūn lún (BL 60, 昆仑)	At the midpoint between the tip of the lateral malleolus and the Achilles tendon	Sciatica, stiff neck	Grasping, pressing
shēn mài (BL 62,申脉)	In the depression at the posterior border of the lateral malleolus	Soreness and pain of the waist and leg	Point pressing, pressing,

Table 10 Common acupoints of the foot *Shaoyin* kidney meridian

Name	Location	Indications	Common Manipulations
yǒng quán (KI 1, 涌泉)	On the sole, in the depression when the foot is in plantar flexion, at the anterior 1/3 and the posterior 2/3 of the line from the web between the 2nd and 3rd toes	Hypertension, headache	Pressing, kneading
tài xī (KI 3, 太溪)	At the midpoint between the tip of the medial malleolus and the Achilles tendon	Cystitis, spermatorrhea, enuresis, irregular menstruation	Pushing, pressing, kneading
zhào hǎi (KI 6, 照海)	1 cun directly below the tip of the medial malleolus	Irregular menstruation	Pressing, kneading
zhù bīn (KI 9, 筑宾)	5 cun directly above *tài xī*, 2 cun lateral to the medial aspect of the tibia	Cramps of the calf, epilepsy, pain caused by hernia	Pressing, kneading, grasping

Table 11 Common acupoints of the hand *Jueyin* pericardium meridian

Name	Location	Indications	Common Manipulations
qǔ zé (PC 3, 曲泽)	On the transverse crease of the elbow, on the ulnar side of the tendon of the biceps brachii	Palpitation, elbow pain, hand tremor	Grasping, pressing, kneading
jiān shǐ (PC 5, 间使)	3 cun above the transverse crease of the wrist, between the tendons of palmaris longus and flexor carpi radialis	Heart pain, palpitation, vomiting	Grasping, pressing, kneading

(*Continued*)

Table 11 *(Continued)*

Name	Location	Indications	Common Manipulations
nèi guān (PC 6, 内关)	2 cun above the transverse crease of the wrist, between the tendons of palmaris longus and flexor carpi radialis	Palpitation, gastric pain, vomiting	Grasping, pressing, kneading
láo gōng (PC 8, 劳宫)	Make a fist — the point is where the tip of the middle finger lands	Palpitation, apoplectic coma	Nailing

Table 12 Common acupoints of the hand *Shaoyang* sanjiao meridian

Name	Location	Indications	Common Manipulations
zhōng zhǔ (SJ 3, 中渚)	In the depression between the 4th and 5th metacarpal bones, proximal to the 4th metacarpophalangeal joint	Migraine, tinnitus, deafness, pain of the palm and fingers	Pressing, kneading
yáng chí (SJ 4, 阳池)	On the dorsal transverse crease of the wrist, in the depression on the ulnar side of the tendon of extensor digitorum communis	Wrist, arm, and shoulder pain	Pressing, heavy pressing, kneading
wài guān (SJ 5, 外关)	2 cun above the dorsal transverse crease of the wrist, between the ulna and radius	Joint pain and restricted motion of the upper limb	Pressing, kneading
zhī gōu (SJ 6, 支沟)	1 cun above *wài guān*	Soreness and pain of the arm and shoulder, constipation	Pressing, kneading
sān yáng luò (SJ 8, 三阳络)	1 cun above *zhī gōu*	Deafness, toothache, *bi* pattern and pain of the upper limb	Pressing, kneading
sī zhú kōng (SJ 23, 丝竹空)	In the depression at the lateral end of the eyebrows	Eye problems, migraine, facial nerve paralysis	Pushing, pressing, kneading

Everyday Exercises

Try to memorize the commonly used acupoints of the Small Intestine, Bladder, Kidney, Pericardium and Sanjiao meridians.

WEEK 2

Day 1

Commonly Used *ShuXue*, Part III

Tables 13 and 14 show the acupoints of the remaining two meridians.

Table 13 Common acupoints of the foot *Shaoyang* Gallbladder Meridian

Name	Location	Indications	Common Manipulations
fēngchí (GB 20, 风池)	Below the occiput, in the depression between the upper portion of sternocleidomastoideus and trapezius muscles	External contractions, headache, stiff neck, hemiplegia	Pushing, grasping, pressing
jiānjǐng (GB 21, 肩井)	At the midpoint between *dàzhuī* and the acromion	Shoulder and back pain, stiff neck	Grasping, pressing, kneading
jūliào (GB 29, 居髎)	At the midpoint between the anterior iliac spine and the great trochanter of the femur	Waist and leg pain, hip soreness and pain	Rolling, point pressing, heavy pressing, pressing
huántiào (GB 30, 环跳)	At the junction of the lateral 1/3 and medial 2/3 on the line connecting the greater trochanter and the sacralhiatus	Waist and leg pain, hemiplegia	Rolling, point pressing, heavy pressing, pressing
fēngshì (GB 31, 风市)	At the point where the tip of the middle finger touches while standing erect with the hands hanging down close to the sides	*Bi* pattern and pain of the lower limb, paralysis	Rolling, pressing

(*Continued*)

Table 13 *(Continued)*

Name	Location	Indications	Common Manipulations
yánglíngquán (GB 34, 阳陵泉)	In the depression anterior and inferior to the head of the fibula	Soreness and pain of the knee, hypochondriac pain	Pressing, kneading, grasping
guāngmíng (GB 37, 光明)	5 cun directly above the lateral malleolus, on the anterior border of the fibula	Myopia, night blindness, pain on the lateral side of the lower leg	Pressing, kneading
xuánzhōng (a.k.a. *juégǔ*, GB 39, 悬钟)	3 cun directly above the lateral malleolus, on the posterior border of the fibula	Hypochondriac pain, stiff neck, soreness and pain of the lower limb	Pressing, kneading, grasping
qiūxū (GB 40, 丘墟)	Anterior and inferior to the lateral malleolus, in the depression on the lateral side of the tendon of extensor digitorumlongus muscle	Pain of the ankle joint, hypochondriac pain	Pushing, pressing, kneading

Table 14 Common acupoints of the Foot *Jueyin* liver meridian

Name	Location	Indications	Common Manipulations
tàichōng (LR 3, 太冲)	On the dorsum of the foot, in the depression proximal to the space between the 1st and 2nd metatarsus	Headache, dizziness, hypertension	*Pushing, pressing, kneading*
lígōu (LR 5, 蠡沟)	5 cun directly from the tip of the medial malleolus, at the midpoint on the medial aspect of the tibia	Pain owing to *bi* pattern of the shin, dysuria, irregular menstruation	*Pressing, kneading, grasping*
zhāngmén (LR 13, 章门)	At the anterior end of the 11th rib	Chest distention, hypochondriac pain	*Pushing, rubbing, kneading*
qīmén (LR 14, 期门)	Directly below the nipple, in the 6th intercostal space	Hypochondriac pain	*Pushing, rubbing, kneading*

Tables 15 and 16 show the acupoints of the *du* and *ren* vessels.

Table 15 Common acupoints of *Du Mai* (*Du* vessel)

Name	Location	Indications	Common Manipulations
chángqiáng (DU 1, 长强)	0.5 cun below the tip of the tail bone	Diarrhea, constipation, rectal prolapse	Pressing, kneading
yāoyángguān (DU 3, 腰阳关)	In the depression inferior to the spinous process of L4	Lumbosacral pain	Pressing, kneading, palm scrubbing
mìngmén (DU 4, 命门)	In the depression inferior to the spinous process of L2	Asthenia (deficiency)	Pressing, kneading, palm scrubbing
shēn zhù (DU 12, 身柱)	In the depression below the spinous process of T3	Stiffness and pain of the spine	Pressing, point pressing, palm scrubbing
dà zhuī (DU 14, 大椎)	In the depression below the spinous process of C7	Common cold, fever, acute stiff neck while awake (laozhen)	Pushing, point pressing, kneading
fēngfŭ (DU 16, 风府)	1 cun directly above the hair margin on the posterior midline	Headache, stiff neck	Pressing, grasping
bǎihuì (DU 20, 百会)	At the apex of the head, in the midpoint between the apex of the two ears	Headache, dizziness, hypertension, fainting	Pushing, pressing, kneading
shuǐgōu, also known as *rénzhōng* (DU 26, 水沟, 人中)	At the junction of the superior 1/3 and inferior 2/3 of the philtrum	Fainting, wry mouth and eyes	Nailing

Table 16 Common acupoints of *Ren Mai* (*Ren* vessel)

Name	Location	Indications	Common Manipulations
guānyuán (RN 4, 关元)	3 cun below the umbilicus	Abdominal pain, menstrual pain, enuresis	Pushing, rubbing, kneading
shímén (RN 5, 石门)	2 cun below the umbilicus	Abdominal pain, diarrhea	Pushing, rubbing, kneading
qìhăi (RN 6, 气海)	1.5 cun below the umbilicus	Abdominal pain, irregular menstruation, spermatorrhea	Pushing, rubbing, kneading
shénquè (RN 8, 神阙)	At the center of the umbilicus	Abdominal pain, diarrhea	Rubbing, kneading
zhōngwăn (RN 12, 中脘)	4 cun above the umbilicus	Gastric pain, vomiting, indigestion	Pushing, rubbing, kneading
dànzhōng (RN 17, 膻中)	On the anterior midline, level with the 4th intercostal space	Cough, asthma, distention and pain of the chest	Pushing, rubbing, kneading
tiāntū (RN 22, 天突)	In the center of the suprasternal fossa	Cough, asthma, difficulty of coughing up phlegm	Pressing, kneading
chéngjiāng (RN 24, 承浆)	In the depression at the midpoint of the mentolabial groove	Wry mouth and eyes, toothache	Nailing, pressing, kneading

Commonly Used Extraordinary Non-Meridian and Non-Vessel Points

Table 17 shows some common extraordinary non-meridian and non-vessel points.

Table 17 Common extraordinary points

Name	Location	Indications	Common Manipulations
sìshéncōng (EX-HN 1, 四神聪)	1 cun anterior, posterior, left and right respectively to *bǎihuì* (DU 20)	Headache, dizziness, amnesia, epilepsy	Pushing, pressing, kneading
yìntáng (EX-HN 3, 印堂)	At the midpoint between the two medial ends of the eyebrow	Headache, rhinitis, insomnia	Pushing, wiping, pressing, kneading
yúyāo (EX-HN 4, 鱼腰)	In the depression at the midpoint of the eyebrow	Pain on the superciliary ridge, red, swelling and painful eyes	Pushing, pressing, wiping
tàiyáng (EX-HN 5, 太阳)	1 cun lateral from the midpoint between the lateral end of the eyebrow and the outer canthus	Headache, common cold, eye diseases	Pushing, wiping, pressing, kneading
qiáogōng (bridge arch, 桥弓)	Unique to tui na, between the back of the ear to *quēpén*, equivalent to the sternocleido-mastoid muscle emerging on the body surface	Headache, dizziness, hypertension	Wiping, grasping
dìngchuǎn (EX-B 1, 定喘)	0.5 cun lateral to *dàzhuī*	Cough, asthma, pain of the shoulder and back	Pushing, kneading
huàtuójiájǐ, also known as *jiájǐ* (EX-B 2, 华陀夹脊, 夹脊)	0.5 cun lateral to the lower border of each spinous process from the T1 to L5	Stiffness and pain of the spine, diseases of corresponding zang and *fu* organs	Pushing, pressing, kneading, point pressing

(*Continued*)

Table 17 (*Continued*)

Name	Location	Indications	Common Manipulations
jiānnèiling, also known as *jiānqián* (肩内陵,肩前)	Midway between the anterior axillary fold and *jiānyú* (LI 15) when the arm is naturally hanging down	Periarthritis of the shoulder	Pushing, pressing, kneading, grasping
làozhěn, also known as *wàiláogōng* (EX-UE 8, 落枕, 外劳宫)	On the dorsum of the hand, between the 2nd and 3rd metacarpal bones, 0.5 cun proximal to the 2nd metacarpophalangeal joint	Neck rigidity after sleeping, pain of the hand and the arm	Point pressing, nailing
shíxuān (EX-UE 11,十宣)	At the tip of the ten fingers, 0.1 cun from the upper nail border	Coma, epilepsy	Nailing
hèdǐng (EX-LE 2,鹤顶)	At the midpoint of the upper border of the patella	Paralysis, weakness of the lower limb, knee pain	Pressing, kneading, point pressing
xīyǎn (EX-LE 5, 膝眼)	In the depressions on both the inferior borders of the patella	Knee pain	Pressing, kneading, point pressing
lánwěi (EX-LE 7, 阑尾)	2 cun below *zúsānlǐ* where a tender spot can be felt by the patient	Appendicitis	Point pressing, pressing
dǎnnáng (EX-LE 6, 胆囊)	2 cun below *yánglíngquán* where a tender spot can be felt by the patient	Cholecystitis, gallstones, ascariasis of biliary tract	Point pressing, pressing
āshìxué (i.e., tenderness or reactive spot, 阿是穴)	Any tender or sensitive spot felt by a patient	Relieving local pain or other ailments	Point pressing, pressing, kneading

Everyday Exercises

Try to memorize the commonly used acupoints of the Gallbladder and Liver meridians, *dumai* and *renmai*, and the extraordinary non-meridian and non-vessel points.

Day 2

Subject 3 — Common Diagnostic Methods for Tui Na

Tui na therapy is mostly used to treat pain in the neck, shoulder, waist and legs, as well as problems of the joints, muscles, and nerves of the four limbs. In order to prevent unnecessary medical accidents from happening, it is completely acceptable to learn from and integrate modern diagnostic methods. In this way we can obtain a clearer diagnosis of the disease and we can rule out problems like tumors, which cannot be treated with tui na.

In this book, we will only focus on introducing the most basic yet practical physical examination methods of the joints on the four limbs and the spinal column, because there are so many modern diagnostic methods available, and new techniques are continually being developed.

Examination of the Upper Extremities

Shoulder

1. *Inspection* It is mandatory to examine and compare both shoulders owing to the fleshy muscles around the shoulders. Both shoulders need to be exposed so that the examiner can observe if they are symmetrical in shape and height, and if there is deformity, swelling, sinus, lumps, venous engorgement, or muscular atrophy. A normal shoulder should be evenly rounded in shape. If the bulge of the deltoid has disappeared and the shape of the shoulder appears square, it may indicate a dislocation of the shoulder or atrophy of the deltoid. If the shoulder blades appear to be hunched, the problem is most probably a congenital one.

   It is necessary to observe the patient not only when the patient is still, but also when he or she is in motion. The examiner should ask the patient to move the shoulder in all directions to see if there is any abnormal condition. For example, paralyzed cost oscapularis would cause a winged scapula when the patient lifts the arm to the level of the shoulder.
2. *Palpation* First of all, we need to identify the bony marks of the shoulder. The bony prominence on the lateral side of the shoulder is the acromion. The major tubercle of the humerus is inferior to it while

anterior to it is the lateral end of the clavicle. Lastly, the coracoid is located one middle-finger-crease width below the junction of the middle 1/3 and lateral 1/3 of the clavicle.

Secondly, we need to examine the temperature of the skin of the affected area and note if there is any swelling. If there is a lump, we need to feel its hardness and how it is related to the surrounding tissue. Tenderness is another important aspect we need to watch for. The following are some common tender points of the shoulder area and what they indicate:

(a) In the intertubercular groove of the humerus: tendinous synovitis of the long head of biceps brachii muscle.
(b) At the apex of the major tubercle: injury of tendon of supraspinatus muscle.
(c) On the acromion: subacromial bursitis.

Besides the tenderness, abnormal activities should be assessed. For instance, if there is a snap while pressing the lateral end of the clavicle, it indicates a dislocation of the acromioclavicular joint. Another example is that a bouncing tendon can be felt in the tubercle sulcus when the long head of the biceps tendon has slipped away.

3. *Range of motion examination of the shoulder* We need to pay attention to the movement pattern, range of motion, and any pain or restriction felt while checking the shoulder joint, especially that of the scapula, to avoid misinterpretation of a false range of motion owing to the confounding factor of the scapular activities. Figure 18 shows the normal range of motion of the shoulder.
4. *Special assessments*
   (a) *Dugus test* With the elbow of the affected arm flexed, place the hand to the opposite shoulder. If the elbow cannot touch the chest wall tightly, the test is positive, indicating dislocation or adhesion of the shoulder joint.
   (b) *Longhead of bicepstension test* Ask the patient to flex the elbow and use the forearm to perform a posterior (backward) rotation while you apply resistance to the patient's forearm. The test is positive when there is pain on the intertubercular groove, indicating tendinous synovitis of the long head of the biceps brachii muscle.

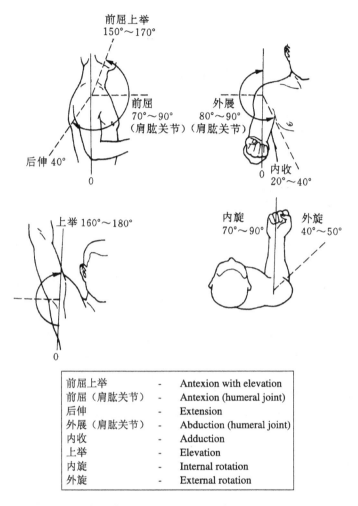

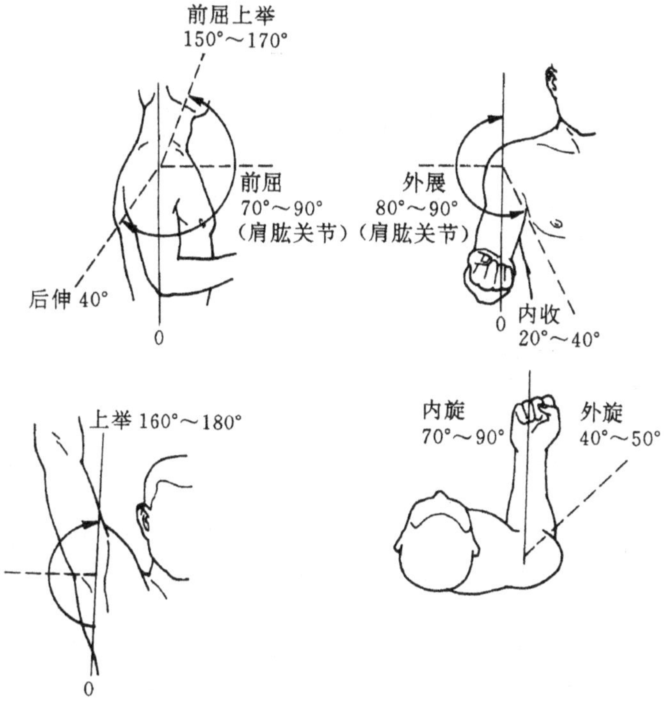

前屈上举	-	Antexion with elevation
前屈（肩肱关节）	-	Antexion (humeral joint)
后伸	-	Extension
外展（肩肱关节）	-	Abduction (humeral joint)
内收	-	Adduction
上举	-	Elevation
内旋	-	Internal rotation
外旋	-	External rotation

Figure 18 Range of motion of the shoulder

The neutral position of the shoulder: arms naturally hanging down, elbows flexed to 90°, and upper limbs pointing to the front.
Flexion: 70° to 90°
Extension: 40°
Abduction: 80° to 90°
Adduction: 80° to 90°
Internal rotation: 70° to 90°
External rotation: 40° to 50°
Elevation: 160° to 180° (the combination of flexion, abduction, and scapular rotation)

(c) *Ruler test* (*Hamilton's test*) The acromion of a normal person is located on the medial side of the line connecting the external condyle and the greater tuberosity of the humerus. The test is positive for a dislocated shoulder joint when the edge of a ruler placed along the humerus can touch the external condyle and the acromion at the same time.

Elbow

1. *Inspection* The first thing is to look for any deformity. When a normal elbow is extended straightly, there is a 5° to 15° carrying angle. In general, the angle is slightly greater in women than in men. If the angle exceeds this range, the condition is called cubitus valgus; if the angle is less than this range, the condition is called cubitusvarus. Contour changes can be observed if necessary repair has not been made for conditions such as intercondylar fracture of the humerus, or dislocation of the elbow or the capitulum radii. Secondly, we need to see if there is any swelling on the elbow. If the swelling is at the joint, tendons on both sides of the triceps brachii muscle posterior to the elbow are bulged. The swelling is more localized when the fracture is internal to the humerus or at the lateral epicondyle. If the fracture is at the capitulum radii, the skin depression on the radial aspect of the olecranon disappears.
2. *Palpation* The most important thing to pay attention to is the location of the tenderness on the elbow. If it is at the outer condyle of the humerus, it usually indicates external humeral epicondylitis, while tenderness at the inner condyle of the humerus indicates internal humeral epicondylitis. A tender point of the ulnar olecranon with membranous sac is often a sign of olecranon bursitis. Moreover, we need to assess such factors as the tensility of the skin around the elbow; pulsation of the brachial artery; rigidity and width of the ulnar nerve; the presence, size, hardness, and location of any lumps; relativity to different motions, and swelling of the supratrochlear lymph nodes.
3. *Range of motion examination of the elbow joint*
   Figure 19 shows the normal range of motion of the elbow.

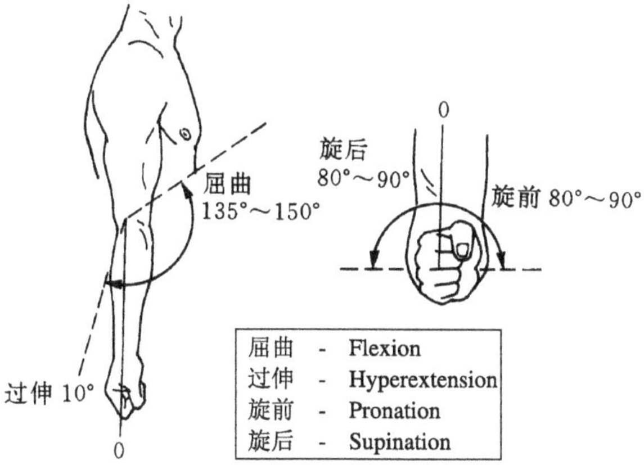

Figure 19 Range of motion of the elbow

Neutral position of the elbow joint: forearm extends straight down
Flexion: 135° to 150°
Hyperextension: 10°
Pronation: 80° to 90°
Supination: 80° to 90°

4. *Special assessments*
   (a) *Tennis elbow test, also known as the wrist extensor tension test* The patient extends the elbow straight and does pronation of the forearam to cause the passive flex of the wrist. If there is pain on the outer condyle of the humerus, the test is positive, indicating external humeral epicondylitis.
   (b) *Elbow eversion and compression test* Ask the patient to extend the elbow straight. The examiner uses one hand to fix the lateral elbow and everts the it. The test is positive when there is pain, indicating a fracture of the capitulum radii.
   (c) *Elbow triangle test* The three bony landmarks — the external and internal condyle of the humerus, plus the ulnar olecranon — should be on the same straight line when a normal elbow completely extends. On the other hand, when the elbow completely flexes, the three landmarks should form an isosceles triangle. If the triangular relationship of the three is different from what is stated, it is an indication of bone fracture or dislocation. Figure 20 shows the elbow triangle.

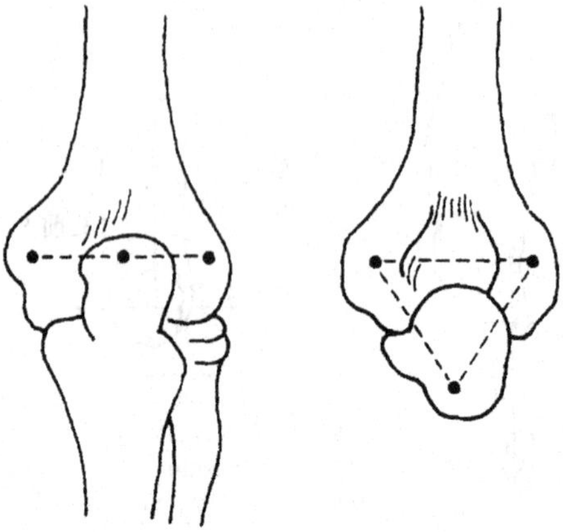

Figure 20 The elbow triangle

Wrist and Hand

1. *Inspection* Compare and examine both wrists and hands to see whether there is any deformity, swelling, or tremor. Common deformities included inner fork wrist caused by a distal radius fracture, the hand deformity known as monkey paw due to thenar atrophy as a result of median nerve injury, dropping wrist due to radial nerve damage, and claw-hand because of hypothenar and interosseous atrophy resulting from ulnar nerve injury. Other deformities include polydactyly, boutonniere deformity, and gooseneck deformity.

   Wrist swelling is usually more obvious on both sides of the dorsal aspect of the primary extensor tendon. The disappearance of the snuffbox is often an indication of scaphoid fracture. Rheumatoid arthritis is a common factor resulting in swelling on both sides of the wrist, with multiple and symmetrical prism swelling of the interphalangeal joints. Phalanx swelling is commonly seen in phalanx tuberculosis or enchondroma. Mallet fingers indicate pulmonary osteoarthropathy. A localized swelling on the dorsum of the wrist or metacarpophalangeal joints lateral to the palm that feels like sacs, which does not adhere to the skin but attaches to the deeper tissue, is often the sign of ganglion cyst.

Finger tremors are often seen in conditions such as hyperthyroidism, shaking palsy, or chronic alcoholic intoxication. Tremors with "pill-rolling" movements that are more severe while the patient is at rest than when he or she is engaged in physical activities commonly indicates Parkinson's disease (shaking palsy).

2. *Palpation* The examiner needs to check the location and degree of the tender spots of the wrists and hands along the line from the distal radial end to the phalanx, including swelling, radiating pain, and paresthesia. The thenar and hypothenar tendons of the flexor of the palm need to be examined for tenderness, local swelling, and whether the swelling moves along with the tendon. During finger flexion, if you hear a snap, the condition is known as trigger finger, or stenosing tenosynovitis of the flexor tendon. If a snap is heard on the lower radioulnar articulation while rotating the forearm, it is normally due to disc damage of the triangular fibrocartilage.
3. *Range of motion examination of the joints of the wrist and hand* Figure 21 shows the normal range of motion of the wrist and hand joints.
4. *Special assessments*
   (a) *Fist ulnar deviation test* Ask the patient to make a fist with the thumb underneath the other fingers. The examiner will hold the fistto represent a passive movement toward the ulna. The test is positive if there is pain on the styloid process of the radius, seen in stenosis of the radial styloid tenosynovitis. (See Figure 22.)
   (b) *Friction test of the radial wrist extensor tendon* The examiner holds the distal end of the forearm of the patient with the palm on the radial side of the forearm dorsum, and requests the patient to continuously flex the wrist or make a fist and relax. If there is an obvious sound of friction under the palm of the examiner, then it is a positive test result, seen in the peripheral inflammation of the radial wrist extensor tendon.
   (c) *The ulnar aspect of the wrist compression test* Have the patient's wrist in a neutral position. The examiner then applies pressure to have it leaning toward the ulnar side. The test is positive when the patient feels pain on the lower radioulnar articulation, which is

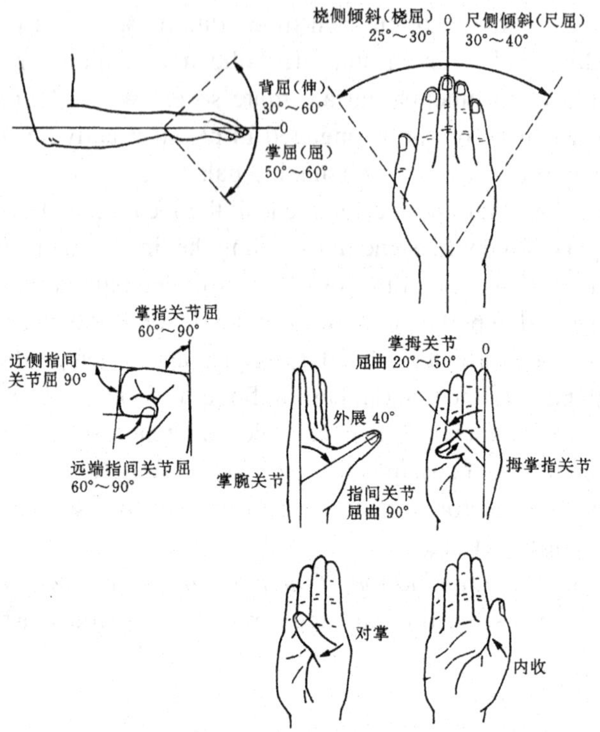

背屈(伸)	- Dorsiflexion (extension) 30° to 60°	掌拇关节屈曲	- Flexion of the thumb-metacarpal joint 20° to 50°
掌屈	- Palmar flexion 50° to 60°	拇掌指关节	- Metacarpophalangeal joint of the thumb
桡侧倾斜	- Radial tilt 25° to 30°	指间关节屈曲	- Flexion of the interphalangeal joint 90°
尺侧倾斜	- Ulnar tilt 30° to 40°	掌腕关节	- carpometacarpal joint
掌指关节屈	- Flexion of the Metacarpophalangeal joint 60° to 90°	外展	- Abduction 40°
近节指间关节屈	- Flexion of the proximal interphalangeal joint 90°	对掌	- Opposition
远节指间关节屈	- Flexion of the distal interphalangeal joint 60° to 90°	内收	- Adduction

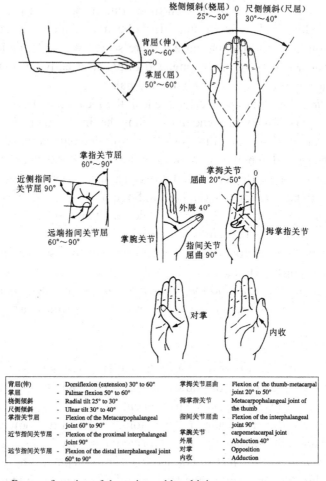

Figure 21 Range of motion of the wrist and hand joints

(a) Neutral position of the wrist: the hand and forearm in a straight line with palm facing down
Dorsiflexion (extension): 30° to 60°
Palmar flexion: 50° to 60°
Radial tilt: 25° to 30°
Ulnar tilt: 30° to 40°

(b) Neutral position of the phalangeal joints: straight extension
Metacarpophalangeal joints: 0° on extension, 60° to 90° on flexion
Proximal interphalangeal joint: 0° on extension, up to 90° on flexion
Distal interphalangeal joint 0° on extension, 60° to 90° on flexion

(c) Neutral position of the thumb: straight extension towards the index finger
Abduction: up to 40°
Flexion: 20° to 50° for thumb-metacarpal joint, up to 90° for interphalangeal joint
Opposition: not easy to measure, pay attention to how far it can cross the palm
Adduction: capable of attaching the radial side of the index finger

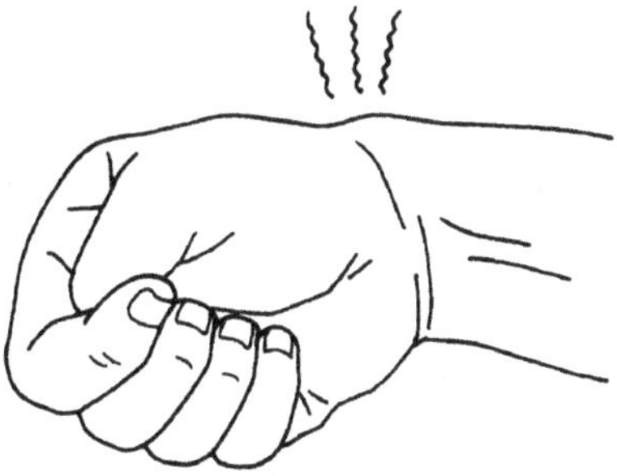

Figure 22 First ulnar deviation test

seen in disc damage of the triangular fibrocartilage or fracture of the styloid process of the ulna.

Everyday Exercises

Try to memorize the physical examination methods for the upper limb– the shoulder, elbow, hand, and wrist.

Day 3

EXAMINATION OF THE LOWER EXTREMITIES

Hip

1. *Inspection* Examine the patient as the patient stands, to see whether there is hip deformity, muscle atrophy, increased compensatory lumbar lordosis, and deepened skin folds of the thigh. Things to watch out for in the lower limbs include deformities in adduction, abduction, internal and external rotations, and shrunken or increased length of the limb. At the same time, observe whether the iliac crest and gluteal folds on both sides are level. Examine the patient as the patient walks, to see if he or she can carry weight normally, and whether the gait is even and stable. Describe the characteristics of the gait.
2. *Palpation* The tensility of the surrounding skin increases if there is swelling of the hip joint. For dislocation of the hip, the caput femoris or weaker pulsation of the femoral artery on the affected area can be felt. A tense girdle-like structure can be felt if gluteal muscle contracture and spasms present. Snapping hip syndrome can be detected when you hear a snapping sound when the patient moves his leg. You will also feel tics of the tendon at the trochanter when you touch it. Tenderness toward the surface at the greater trochanter, associated with a cystic mass, is probably an indication of trochanteric bursitis.
3. *Range of motion examination of the hips*
   Figure 23 shows the normal range of motion of the hips
4. *Special assessments*
   (a) *Trendelenberg test* The patient is in upright standing position with the back facing the doctor. Get the patient to stand on his healthy limb and lift up the affected limb by flexing the hip and knee. Normally, a negative test result is indicated when the pelvis tilts to the contralateral side with the folds of the other hip lifted up. If the pelvis of the non-affected side and the folds of the hip are at a lower level, the test is positive, seen in the pathologic changes of the hip, and muscle paralysis of the mesoglutaeus or the gluteus minimus. (See Figure 24.)

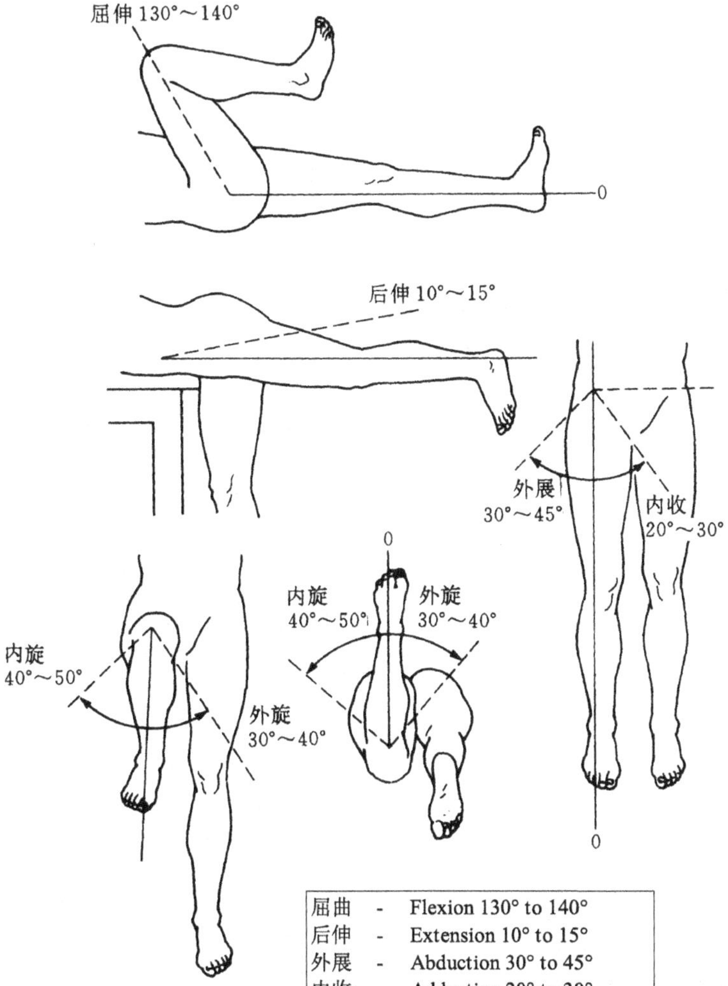

屈曲	-	Flexion 130° to 140°
后伸	-	Extension 10° to 15°
外展	-	Abduction 30° to 45°
内收	-	Adduction 20° to 30°
内旋	-	Internal rotation 40° to 50°
外旋	-	External rotation 30° to 40°

Figure 23 Range of motion of the hips

Neutral position: hip joints extend straight and patella facing upwards

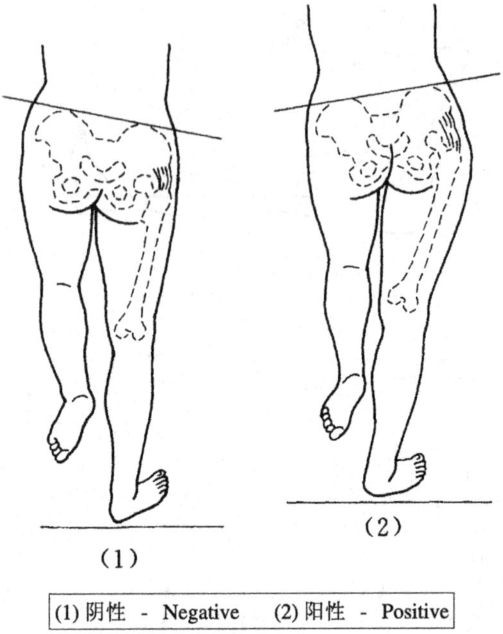

Figure 24 Trendelenberg test

(b) *Barlow test* The patient should be in a supine position with his legs straight. Use one hand to hold the lower leg of the patient, pushing up along the vertical axis of the body, while with your other hand, palpate the ipsilateral greater trochanter. If there is the sense of a piston-like activity, the test is positive for a congenital hip dislocation, with more obvious signs seen especially in young children.

(c) *FABER/Patrick test* With the patient in a supine position, ask him or her to flex the hip and knee, and rotate the hip externally, so that the lateral malleolus is on top of the knee of the contra lateral lower limb, shaped like the figure of "4". If the patient cannot complete a "4" figure and experience ship pain while attempting it, there is a problem with the hip. If the "4" shape can be completed, apply pressure to the contralateral anterior superior iliac spine with one hand, while with your other hand, press down on the medial knee. If there issacroiliac joint pain, the test is positive, often seen in sacroiliac lesions including sacroiliac arthritis. (See Figure 25.)

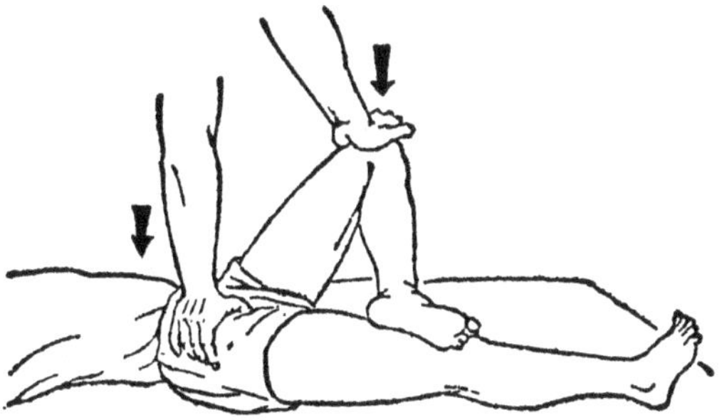

Figure 25 FABER/Patrick test

(d) *Bilateral flexion of knees and hips and separation test* Have the patient liein a supine position, with both lower legs flexed and externally rotated to have the pelmas facing each other. Place one hand on each of his knees, and separate his legs. If there is medial side thigh pain, the test is positive, suggesting adductor spasms.

(e) *Heel percussion test* Have the patient supine with both the lower limbs straight. Use one hand to slightly elevate the affected limb, and with your other hand, tap the heel along the longitudinal axis of the body. If the result is shaking hip pain, the test is the positive, indicating a hip fracture, inflammation, or lower limb fractures.

(f) *Neutral standing position test* With the patient in a supine position and legs straight, hold the heel of the affected leg. If the foot is externally rotated, the test is positive for a femoral neck fracture.

(g) *Iliotibial band contracture test* Ask the patient to lie down in a lateral position on his unaffected side, and flex the contralateral hip and knee to have the knee as close as possible to the chest. Stand behind the patient with one hand holding the pelvis in place, and with your other hand, hold the affected limb above the ankle and flex the knee to 90°. Make sure that the affected hip is flexed and abducted; then, extend it straight. Next, let it fall freely. If there is iliotibial band contracture, the limb can passively remain abducted, signifying a positive test result. In this situation, the contracted iliotibial band can be felt between the iliac crest and the great trochanter. (See Figure 26.)

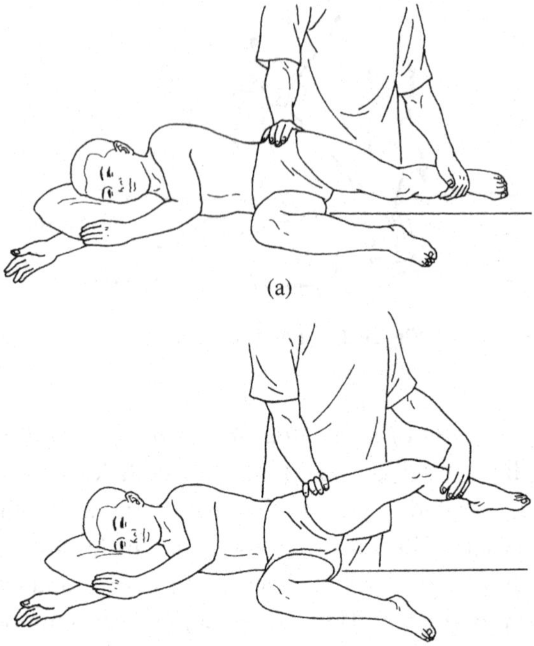

(a)

(b)

Figure 26 Iliotibial band contracture test

(h) *Thomas test* Have the patient lie supine with the contralateral hip and knee flexed to its extreme, so that the thigh closely aligns along the trunk. Ask the patient to use both hands to cling to the knee, and make the waist affixed to the bed. If the hip is not completely straight, or it is straight but with anterior waist protrusion, the test is positive. The angle of the hip flexion should be recorded. The condition manifests itself as hip stiffness, spinal tuberculosis, or iliopsoas spasms. (See Figure 27.)

Knee

1. *Inspection* Compare both sides of the quadriceps; in particular, note whether there is dramatic atrophy in the medial head of the quadriceps. When the knee is flexed, if the patellar ligament on both sides of the

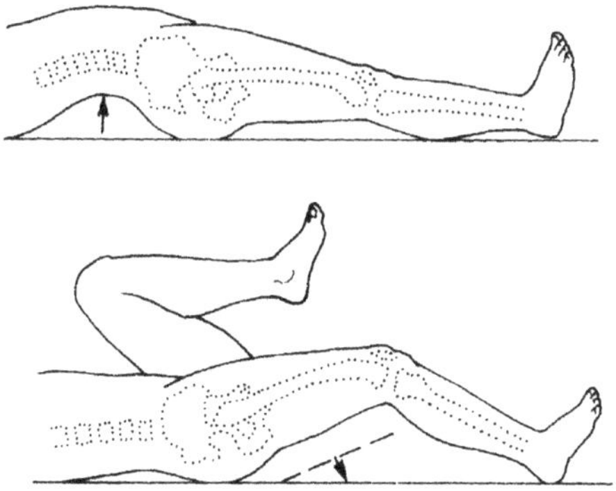

Figure 27 Thomas test

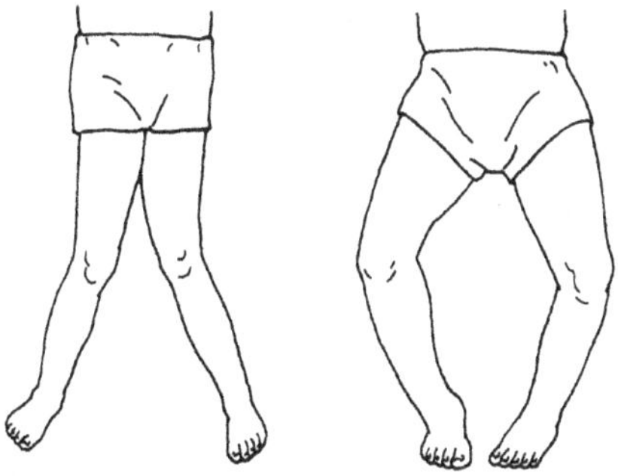

膝内翻	-	Knee Varus
膝外翻	-	Knee Valgus

Figure 28 Knee valgus deformities

"knee eye" disappears, it indicates joint swelling. The medial femoral condyles and malleolus on both sides should touch each other while the patient stands with legs together. If the two medial malleolus separate, the condition is called knee varus, also known as X-shaped legs; if the two condyles separate, it is called knee valgus, also known as O-shaped legs (see Figure 28). Knee varus and valgus deformities are common in rickets, lower femur or upper tibia fractures, osteomyelitis, cartilage dysplasia, and asymmetric growth of the epiphyseal plate. While the patient is standing, if the knee is obviously hyperextended, the condition is known as recurvation or saber leg (see Figure 29),

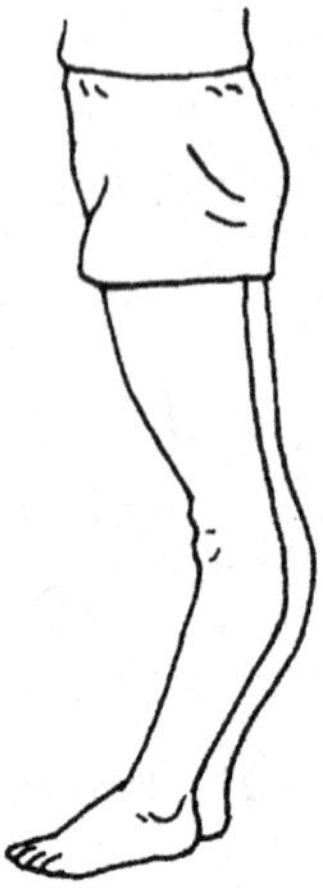

Figure 29 Saber leg

commonly seen in polio sequelae. Lastly, localized swelling of the femur or the condyle on either the medial or lateral side indicates the possibility of tumors.

2. *Palpation* It is very important to determine the location of the tenderness in diagnosing knee disorders. Common knee tenderness points are shown in Figure 30. If any masses are found, including those in the popliteal fossa, check its size, hardness, depth, whether there is tenderness, and its relationship with the surrounding tissue and the knee joint. Synovial thickening and a tougher feeling around the knee suggests chronic synovitis. The rustling friction sound and spasmic pain experienced by the patient when you push the patella up and down or left to right indicates patella chondromalacia. A crisp snapping sound accompanied by pain upon knee movement suggests meniscus injury.
3. *Range of motion examination of the knee*
The neutral position of the knee is to extend it straight. Figure 31 shows the normal range of motion of the knee.
4. *Special assessments*
    (a) *Floating patella test* Have the patient lie in a supine position with the affected leg straight and relaxed. Place the web between your

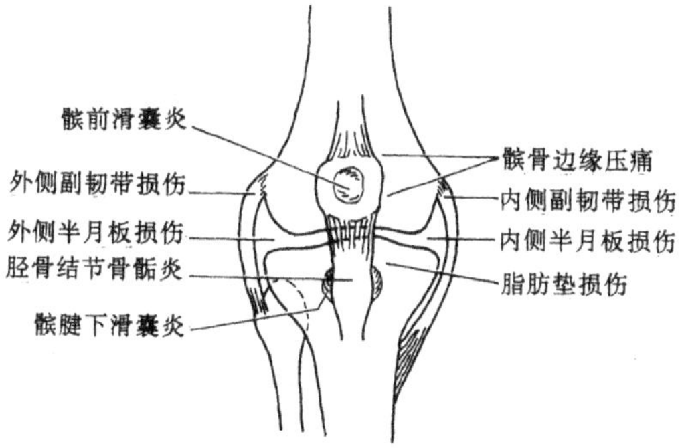

髌前滑囊炎	-	prepatellar bursitis
外侧副韧带损伤	-	injury of the lateral collateral ligament (LCL)
外侧半月板损伤	-	injury of the lateral meniscus
胫骨结节骨骺炎	-	epiphysitis of tibial tuberosity
髌腱下滑囊炎	-	patellar tendon bursitis
髌骨软化症	-	patella chondromalacia
髌骨边缘压痛	-	tenderness on the edge of the patellar
内侧副韧带损伤	-	injury of the medial collateral ligament (MCL)
内侧半月板损伤	-	injury of the medial meniscus
脂肪垫损伤	-	injury of fat pad

Figure 30 Common tenderness points of the knee

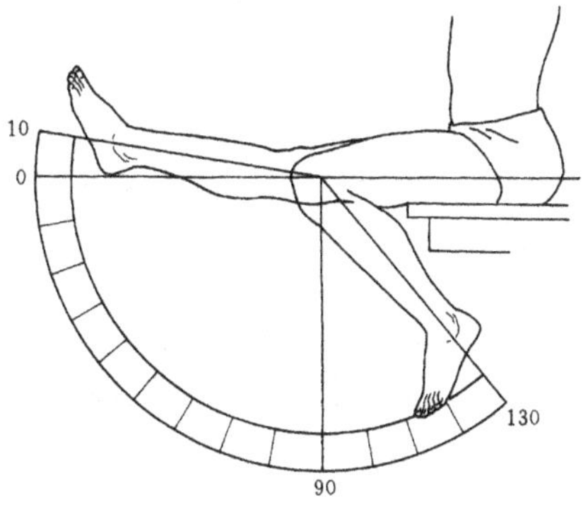

Figure 31 Range of motion of the knee

Flexion: 120° to 150°
Hyperextension: 5° to 10°
Internal rotation (approx.): 10°
External rotation (approx.): 10°

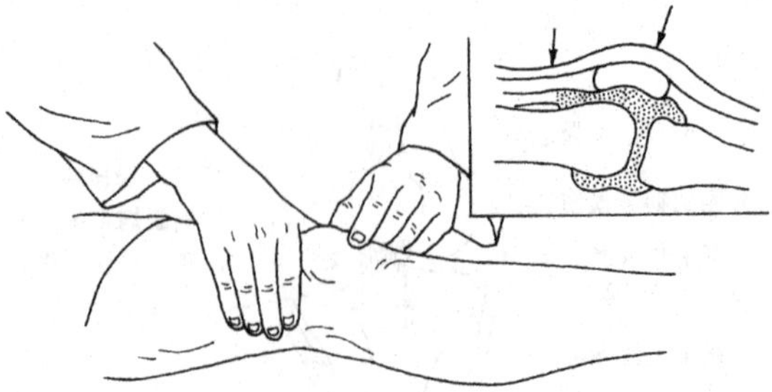

Figure 32 Floating patella test

thumb and index finger of one hand against the patella of the patient, with the palm down on the suprapatellar pouch, so that the joint fluid gathers under the patella. Then, use the index finger of your other hand (as shown) to vertically extrude the patella and quickly release it. If it feels like the patella is floating or striking the femoral condyle, the test result is positive, suggesting that there is fluid inside the knee joint. (See Figure 32.)

(b) *Patella friction test* Have the patient lie in a supine position with the affected leg straight and relaxed. Hold the patella and press down on it with one hand, moving it up, down, left, and right on the surface of the femoral condyle articular. If friction sound or pain presents, the test is positive, indicating patellar chondromalacia.

(c) *McMurray test/sign* Have the patient lie in a supine position. Hold the foot of the affected leg with one hand, and hold the medial knee joint and lateral joint space with the thumb and four fingers of the other hand, respectively. First, flex the knee to its extreme, and make the lower leg adduct, then rotate externally, and gradually straighten the knee. If there is pain or a snapping sound on the medial side, it signifies a medial meniscus injury. Next, make the lower leg abduct, rotate internally, and gradually straighten the knee. If there is pain or a snapping sound on the lateral side, it is an indication of lateral meniscus injury. (See Figure 33.)

(d) *Apley grind test* This test is designed to identify lateral collateral ligament injury and meniscal injury. The patient lies prone with legs straightened out, and knee flexed to 90°. Get an assistant to

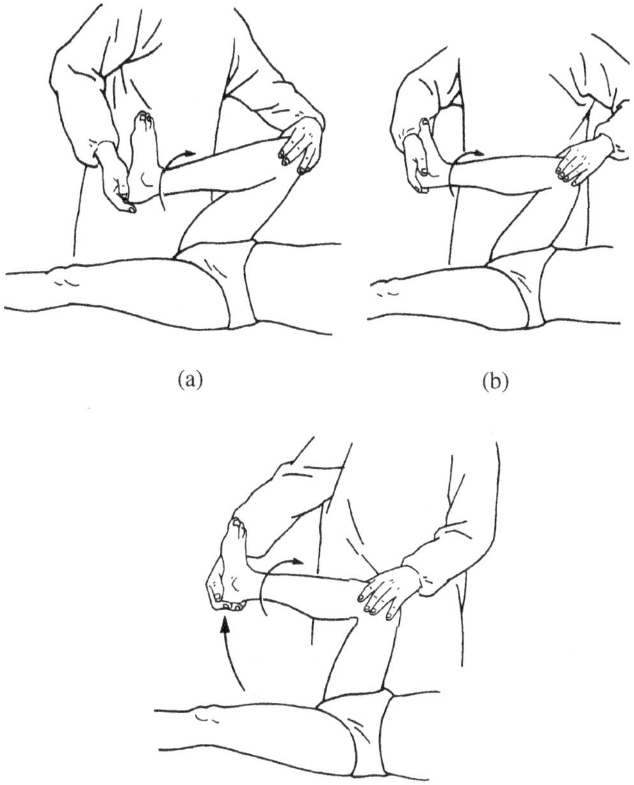

(a) (b) (c)

Figure 33 McMurray test

hold down the patient's thigh so that it does not rotate. Use both your hands to hold the ankle, lift the leg up along the longitudinal axis of the leg, and then rotate the leg internally and externally. At this point the lateral collateral ligament would be in a tense state. Pain upon rotation suggests injury of the lateral collateral ligament. Next, press the foot using both hands and rotate the lower leg internally and externally. Pain suggests meniscus injury. (See Figure 34.)

(e) *Valgus stress test* The patient lies supine with legs straightened. Use one hand to hold the ankle and apply pressure toward the

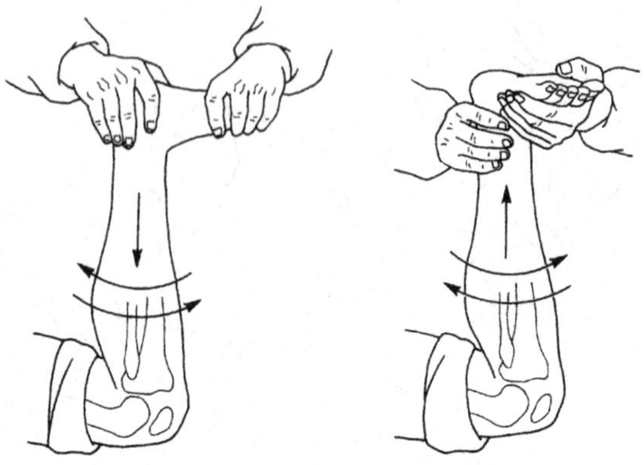

按压旋转	-	Press and rotate
提拉旋转	-	Lift, pull and rotate

Figure 34 Apley grind test

lateral side, while with the other hand, press the knee toward the medial side so that the patient's medial collateral ligament withstands valgus tension. If there is pain or side movement, the test is positive, suggesting medial collateral ligament injury. On the other hand, if there is pain or lateral movement when the pressure is applied in the opposite direction on the knee with the lateral collateral ligament withstanding varus tension, it indicates lateral collateral ligament injury. (See Figure 35.)

(f) *Hyperextension test* The patient lies supine with knees straightened. Use one hand to lift up the lower leg, while with the other hand, press the knee to have it passively hyperextended. If there is pain, the test is positive, seen in conditions such as anterior horn injury of the meniscus, femoral condyle cartilage injury, or fat pad hypertrophy and injury.

(g) *Drawer test* The patient lies supine with knees flexed to 90° and the feetlying flat on the examination table. Stabilize the patient's foot, and use both hands to pull it forward, then push it backwards. If the knee can be pulled, it indicates injury of the anterior cruciate ligament.

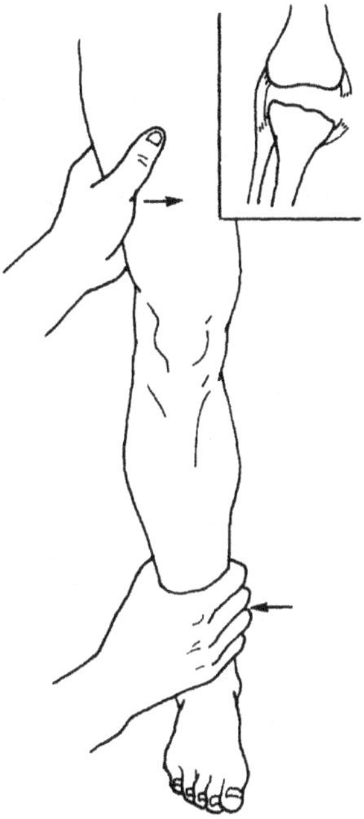

Figure 35 Valgus stress test

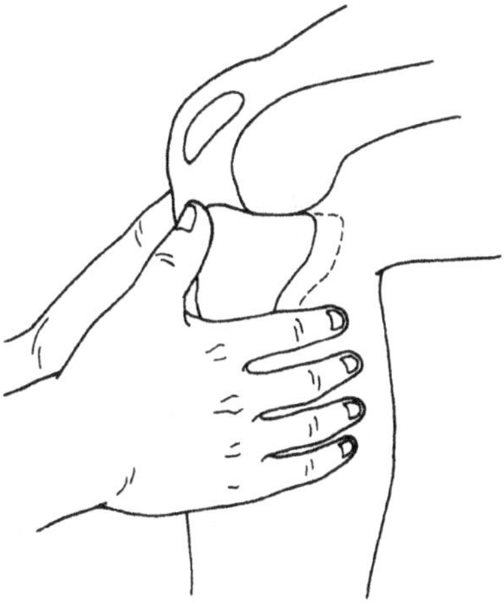

Figure 36 Drawer test

Ankle and Foot

1. *Inspection* The contours are very clear for a normal medial and lateral malleolus. There is also a depression on each side of the Achilles tendon, which might not be easy to see in obese women. The extensor tendon can be seen underneath the skin upon ankle dorsiflexion. When the ankle is swollen, all of the above contours would disappear. In addition, some common foot deformities are as the follows (see Figure 37):
   - (a) *Flat feet*: collapsed longitudinal arch, heel valgus, first half of the foot abducted.
   - (b) *Clubfoot*: plantar flexion of the ankle joint resulting in the tendency of toe-walking of the affected foot.

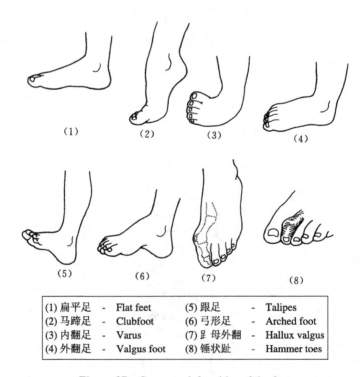

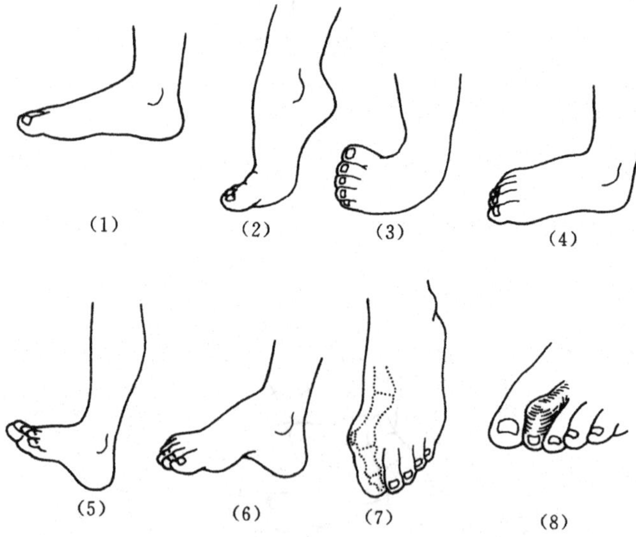

(1) 扁平足	-	Flat feet	(5) 跟足	-	Talipes
(2) 马蹄足	-	Clubfoot	(6) 弓形足	-	Arched foot
(3) 内翻足	-	Varus	(7) 𧾷 母外翻	-	Hallux valgus
(4) 外翻足	-	Valgus foot	(8) 锤状趾	-	Hammer toes

Figure 37 Common deformities of the foot

(c) *Varus foot*: an increased foot arch often accompanied by varus
(d) *Valgus foot*: often accompanied by arch flattening.
(e) *Talipes*: in contrast with clubfoot, the affected foot has a tendency of heel-standing.
(f) *Arched foot*: contrary to flat feet, the longitudinal arch of the affected foot is higher than normal.
(g) *Halluxvalgus*: lateral deflection the long axis of the toe, often accompanied by a widened first half feet, severe valgus with the second toe attached on top of the big toe, and bursitis on the lateral side of the first metatarsal head.
(h) *Hammer toes*: due to proximal interphalangeal joint contracture, the toe is shaped like a hammer.

2. *Palpation* The soft tissue of the ankle and foot is thin; therefore, localized tender points are often the location of the lesion. Tenderness at the end of the Achilles tendon is perhaps tendon bursitis. If it is slightly posterior to the middle of the plantar surface of the calcaneus, it suggests heel spur or fat pad lesions. Upon rupture of the Achilles tendon, a horizontal groove can be felt underneath of the skin. Slip of peroneal tendons can cause bouncing of the tendon. Moreover, the examiner needs to carefully compare the pulse on both sides of the dorsalispedis and posterior tibial arteries.
3. *Range of motion examination of the ankle and foot* The neutral position of the ankle is a 90° angle between the foot and the leg, without varus or valgus. The neutral position of the foot is not easy to determine. Figure 38 shows the normal range of motion of the ankle and foot.
4. *Special assessments*

(a) *Triceps surae pinching test* Ask the patient to lie prone with the feet hanging off the edge of the bed. Squeeze the belly of the triceps surae. Normally, it will result in plantar flexion. Otherwise, it is a positive result, suggesting rupture of the Achilles tendon.
(b) *Lateral compression test on the anterior aspect of the foot* Have the patient lie in a supine position. Use both hands to laterally squeeze both sides of the front part of the affected foot. The pain indicates a positive test result, suggesting metatarsal fractures or plantar interosseous muscle injury.

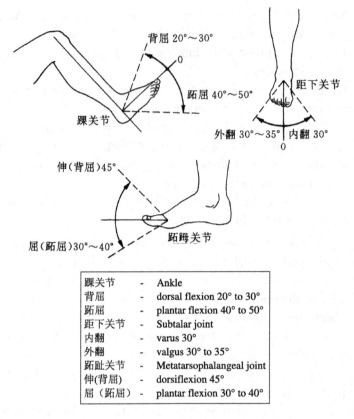

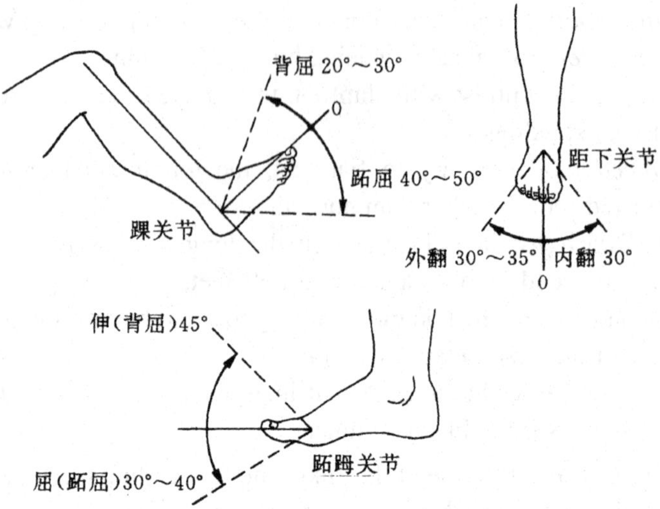

踝关节	-	Ankle
背屈	-	dorsal flexion 20° to 30°
跖屈	-	plantar flexion 40° to 50°
距下关节	-	Subtalar joint
内翻	-	varus 30°
外翻	-	valgus 30° to 35°
跖趾关节	-	Metatarsophalangeal joint
伸(背屈)	-	dorsiflexion 45°
屈（跖屈）	-	plantar flexion 30° to 40°

Figure 38 Range of motion of the ankle and the foot

Everyday Exercises

Try to memorize the physical examination methods for the lower body — the hips, knees, and ankles.

Day 4

EXAMINATION OF THE TORSO

Neck

1. *Inspection* Have the patient sit and loosen his collar; if necessary, have him take off his shirt for a thorough inspection. Check whether there are any scars or sinuses in an odd location. Check the posterior pharyngeal abscess if cervical tuberculosis is suspected. If acute stiff neck (*laozhen*) occurs, the patient may maintain a torticollis posture owing to the pain. Cervical fracture and dislocation can result in a forced neck position.
2. *Palpation*
   (a) *Tenderness* If one side of the neck has sudden trapezius spasms and obvious tenderness, most likely it is *laozhen*. Tenderness on the cervical supraspinal ligament with subcutaneous beam-like changes or paraspinal tenderness along C4 to C7 often indicate cervical vertebral disease. Tenderness on the posterior triangle is mostly anterior scalene muscle syndrome. Soft tissue strain on the nape of the neck, on the other hand, has a broader range of tenderness.
   (b) *Lumps* Unilateral spindle-shaped masses at the mastoid neonatal sternoclavicular in newborns are mostly congenital muscular oblique. If the side of the neck has any masses, the examiner should distinguish them from conditions such as swollen neck lymph nodes, cold abscesses, cystic hygroma, or branchial cleft cysts.
3. *Range of motion examination of the neck*
   The neutral position of the neck is as follows: facing the front, looking straight ahead, and chin adducted. Figure 39 shows the normal range of motion of the neck.
4. *Special assessments*
   (a) *Linder test* With the patient lying supine, place one hand on the chest, another hand on the occipital area to lift the head up, and flex the neck passively toward the chest. If the chin cannot touch the sternum or there is resistance and pain, the test is positive for cervical spondylosis, lumbar disc herniation, meningitis, meningeal irritation, and other nervous system disorders. (See Figure 40.)

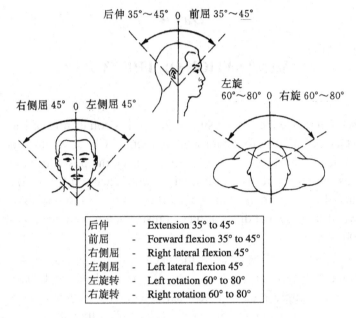

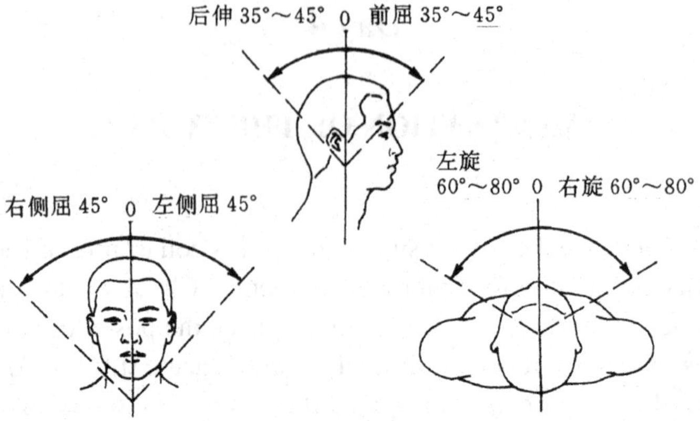

后伸	-	Extension 35° to 45°
前屈	-	Forward flexion 35° to 45°
右侧屈	-	Right lateral flexion 45°
左侧屈	-	Left lateral flexion 45°
左旋转	-	Left rotation 60° to 80°
右旋转	-	Right rotation 60° to 80°

Figure 39 Range of motion of cervical vertebrae

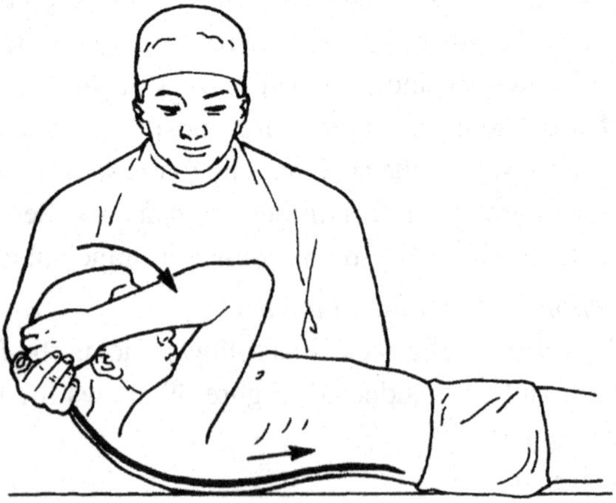

Figure 40 Linder test

(b) *Head tapping test* With the patient sitting, and the neck, chest, and waist straight, chin adducted, firmly place the palm of one hand on the top of the patient's head, while with your other hand make a loose fist and gently tap the back of the first hand. If it causes radiating upper neck pain to the patient, the test is positive, often suggesting cervical spondylosis. (See Figure 41.)

(c) *Cervical foraminal compression test* With the patient sitting and head tilting to the back of the ipsilateral side, use both your hands to hold the top of the head of the patient, and apply pressure downward along the longitudinal axis of the neck. If it causes neck pain or associated radiating pain to the upper extremities, the test is positive, often suggesting cervical spondylosis. (See Figure 42.)

(d) *Brachial plexus traction test* With the patient sitting up straight, use one hand to push the patient's head to the contralateral side, while with the other hand, hold the wrist of the patient and pull it to the posterior lateral aspect. If it causes limb numbness or pain, the test is positive, often suggesting cervical spondylosis. (See Figure 43.)

(e) *Deep-breath test,* also known as Adson's test Have the patient in a sitting position with head slightly tilted toward the back and chin rotated to the affected side. Ask the patient to take a deep breath and

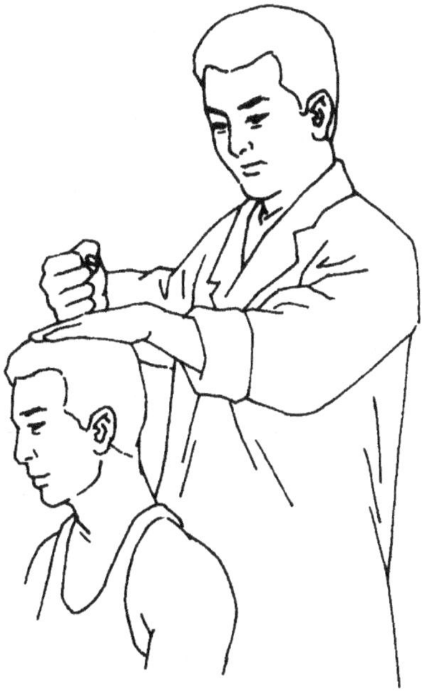

Figure 41 Head tapping test

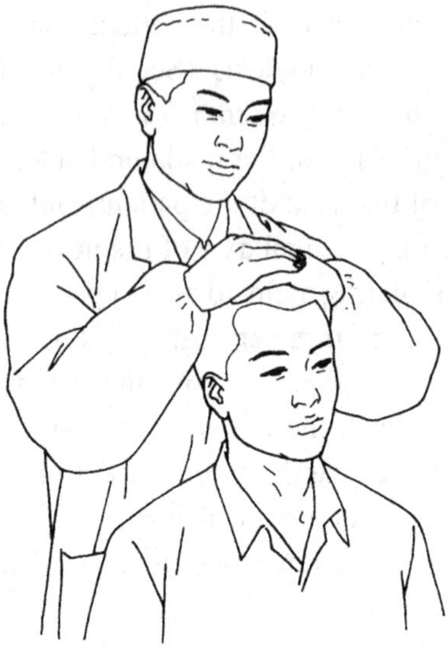

Figure 42 Cervical foraminal compression test

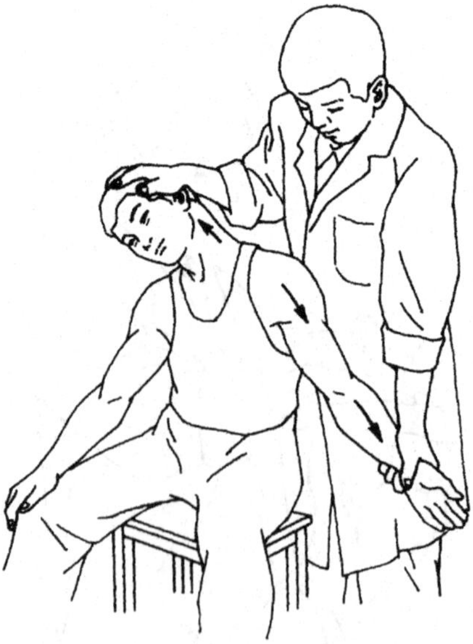

Figure 43 Brachial plexus traction test

hold it. Use one hand to apply resistance against the ipsilateral chin, and the other hand to palpate the ipsilateral radial artery. If the pulse is weakened or disappears, the test result is positive, usually indicating the anterior scalene muscle syndrome (thoracic outlet syndrome).

(f) *Chest expansion test* Ask the patient to sit up straight, with both shoulders abducted and arms extended toward the back. If the pulse of the radial artery weakens or disappears, the test result is positive, often signifying costoclavicular syndrome (thoracic outlet syndrome). (See Figure 44.)

(g) *Hyperabduction test* With the patient sitting and upper limbs naturally hanging down, hold the wrist of the ipsilateral side to sense the pulse of the radial artery. Making sure to have the patient's upper limbs straight, passively abduct and lift up the affected arm above the shoulder until it is level with the head. If the radial artery pulse weakens or disappears, the test is positive, often indicating hyper abduction syndrome (coracoid pectoralis minor muscle syndrome). (See Figure 45.)

(h) *Intermittent fluctuations test* Have the patient sit or stand upright with arms held flat and abducted to 90°, reaching the externally rotated position. Then ask the patient to quickly flex and extend his or her fingers. Within a few seconds, if the patient has discomfort, pain, or tiredness of the forearm with gradual drooping, the test is positive, suggesting thoracic outlet syndrome. If the patient can continuously perform the activity for more than a minute without changing the position of the upper limbs, then test is negative.

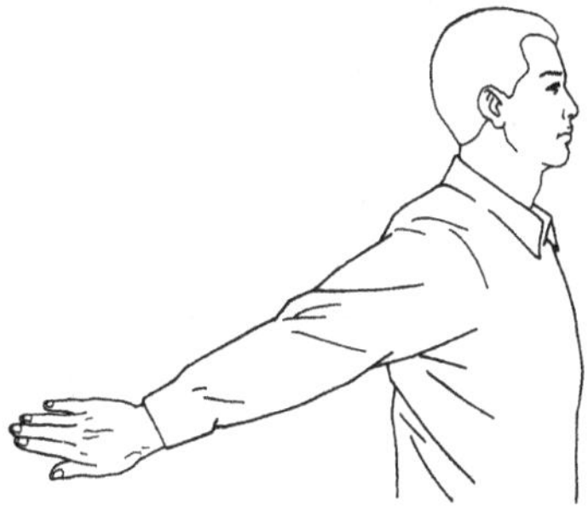

Figure 44 Chest expansion test

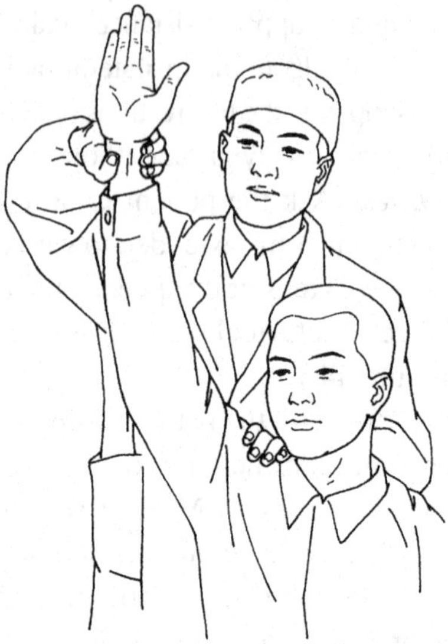

Figure 45 Hyper-abduction test

Back and Lumbar

1. *Inspection* Observe carefully to see if there are any abnormalities on the back and lumbar area along the spine. The spine should be in a straight line from top to bottom when observed from the back. If any scoliosis changes are found, use a colored pen to mark on the affected spinous processes, so that the degree of scoliosis and its direction are clear. From the lateral view, see whether there is any round-shaped kyphosis (in ankylosing spondylitis, etc.), or angular kyphosis (in spinal tuberculosis, etc.), whether the physiological lumbar protrusion is normal, and whether there is any increase, flatness or posterior protrusion. Moreover, you can observe the patient in a combination of different body positions such as sitting, standing, walking, and lying to see whether there are any posture changes at the lower back. Where there are muscle cramps or intense pain, the muscle can be seen raised in the affected area. Pigmentation or lumbosacral plexus hair is prevalent in insidious spina bifida. Last but not least, if there are any skin lesions, abscesses, or sinuses on the waist, they should be described. Figure 46 shows some common deformities of the back.

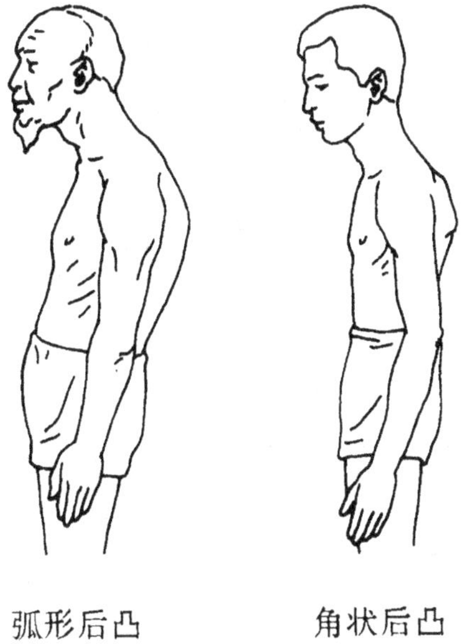

弧形后凸	-	archy kyphosis
角状后凸	-	angular kyphosis

Figure 46 Deformity of the back

2. *Palpation* It is important to examine tenderness points on the back and lumbar areas for diagnosing and locating the ailment. The following is a list of common tenderness points in clinical practice (see Figure 47):
   (a) *Tenderness above the spinous process* Found in supraspinal ligament injuries, spinous process bursitis, and fractures.
   (b) *Tenderness between the spinous process* Seen in interspinous ligament injury.
   (c) *Tenderness on the vertebrocostal angle* At the intersection of the 12th rib and the lateral edge of the sacrospinalis muscle, seen in renal diseases or fractures at the transverse process of L1.
   (d) *Tenderness on the lumbar muscle* There are localized tender spots on both sides of the sacral spine, often accompanied by increased muscle tensility and found in muscle strain.

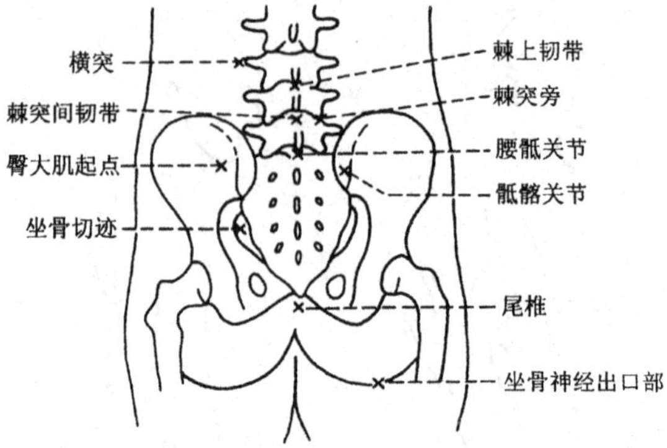

横突	-	transverse process
棘上韧带	-	supraspinal ligament
棘突间韧带	-	interspinous ligament
棘突旁	-	lateral to a spinous process
臀大肌起点	-	the head of gluteus maximus
腰骶关节	-	lumbosacral joint
坐骨切迹	-	ischiatic notch
骶髂关节	-	sacroiliac joint
尾椎	-	coccygeal vertebra
坐骨神经	-	the exit point of sciatic nerve

Figure 47 Common lumbosacral tenderness

(e) *Tenderness at the transverse process of L3* At the outer end of L3 transverse process, with beam-like texture while palpating, seen in the transverse process syndrome of L3.

(f) *Tenderness on the side of a spinous process* Bilateral tenderness along the spinous process that is 1.0 to 1.5 cm from the spine, with pain radiating to the affected limb. It is found in illnesses such as intraspinal canal diseases, herniated disc, and cancer.

(g) *Interspinal tenderness between L5 and S1* Seen in lumbosacral joint strain.

(h) *Sacroiliac joint tenderness* Seen in sacroiliitis. When it occurs in postpartum women, it is often seen in osteitis condensans ilii.

(i) *Piriformis tenderness* Equivalent to where *huántiào* (GB 30) is located on the hip, a horizontal strip of tenderness with pain radiating to the limbs, often seen in piriformis syndrome.

In addition to checking for tenderness on the lower back, we often need to combine the palpation with percussion using a medical hammer or fist to determine deeper tissue lesions, such as vertebral tuberculosis and cancer.

3. *Range of motion examination of the waist* It is not easy to determine the neutral position of the waist. Its normal range of motion is as follows (see Figure 48):
   (a) *Flexion* Have the patient in an upright standing position, with waist naturally flexed and arms and hands naturally hanging, fingertips pointing to the dorsum of the feet. Under normal circumstances, the waist is curved with a natural arc, without being rigid; usually it is 90°.
   (b) *Extension* Same position as the above. Ask the patient to naturally extend the back, usually at 30°.
   (c) *Lateral flexion* (bending) About 30° each side.
   (d) *Rotation* With the pelvis fixed, ask the patient to perform left and right rotation, and measure the angle between the shoulder line and the pelvis diameter; it is usually at 30°.

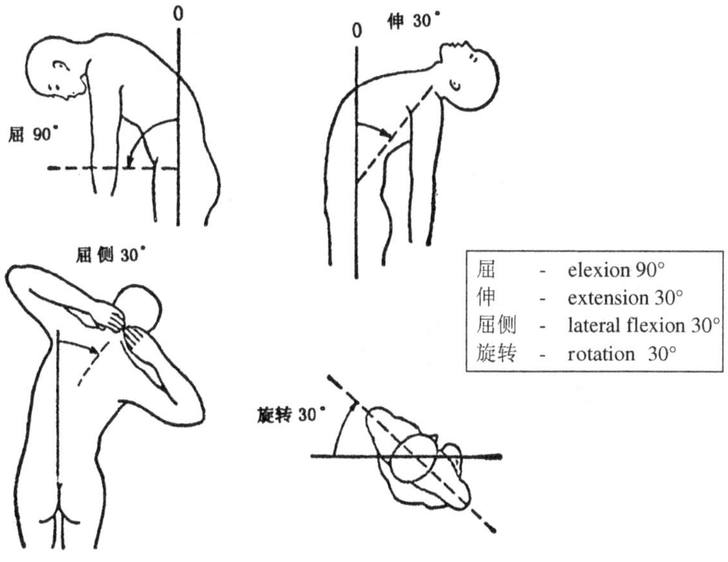

Figure 48 Range of motion of the lumbar vertebrae

4. *Special assessments*

(a) *Pick-up test* It may be a problem to get small children to cooperate. A good idea is to put toys on the ground and persuade the child to pick them up while observing if the child shows signs of any stiffness of the waist. If the child does not have any spine disease, he or she can quickly bend down to pick up the toy. On the other hand, a child with a rigid spine would use one hand to press the knee, since the only way for him or her to pick up things from the floor is to have the hips and knees flexed. Therefore, if the waist cannot flex, the test is positive for spinal tuberculosis. (See Figure 49.)

(b) *Children's waist stretch test* With the child in a prone position, lift both lower legs of the child. A normal child's waist is soft, and easy to be extended freely without pain. If the child suffers spinal tuberculosis, the lower back will be rigid and will leave the examination table as you lift the legs; the hips will be elevated, accompanied by pain. (See Figure 49.)

(c) *Straight leg raise test, also known as Lasègue test* The patient lies supine with both legs straight. With one hand, hold and press the knee of the patient to keep an extension position, while the other hand holds the ankle to gradually elevate the affected leg. If waist pain or sciatica occurs prior to it reaching 70°, the test is positive, suggesting spinal nerve root and sciatic nerve irritation. You need to record the angle when the pain appears. Based on the raised angle causing the pain, you can lower the angle by 5° to 10°, and passively perform dorsiflexion of the ankle. If it also causes pain, it further indicates that there is pressure on the intraspinal nerve. (See Figure 51.)

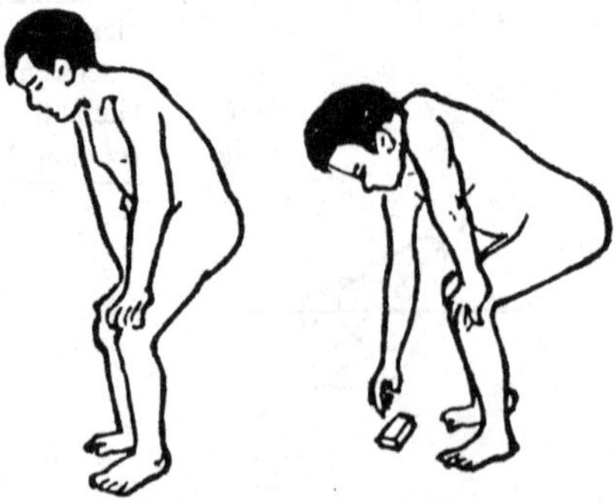

正常	- normal
僵直	- stiff

Figure 49 Pick-up test

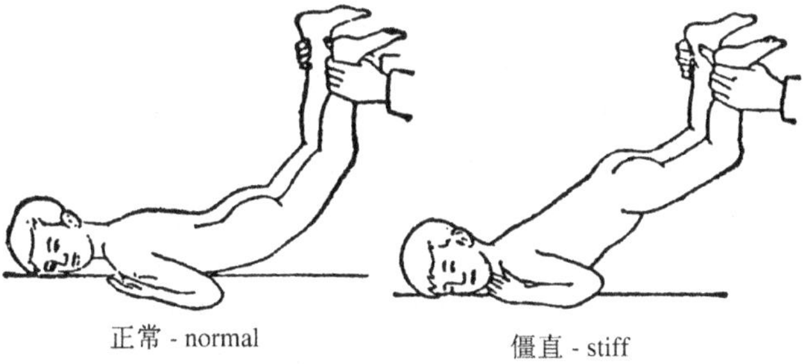

Figure 50 Waist stretch test

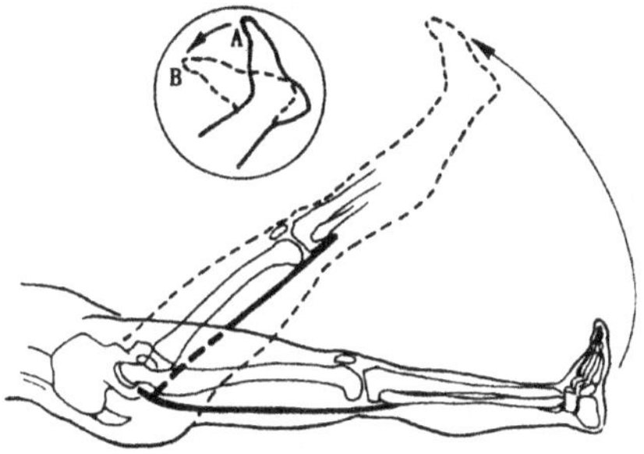

Figure 51 Straight leg raise test and enhanced test

(d) *Contralateral straight leg raise test* The test is performed after the straight leg raise test to check the unaffected leg using the same method. If it induces radiating pain at the sciatic nerve, the test result is positive, commonly seen in lumbar disc herniation.

(e) *Bowstring test/Cramm maneuver* With the patient sitting in a chair, upper body straight and legs hanging naturally, gradually raise the ipsilateral leg and straighten it out until the patient feels radiating pain on the lower extremity. Then, with the fingers of the other hand, press the middle of the popliteal fossa, where the tibial nerve is located. If the radiating pain is exacerbated, the test result is positive for lumbar disc herniation.

(f) *Femoral nerve traction test* The patient is in a prone position with knee flexed to 90°. Lift the lower leg or make the knee passively flexed. Radiating pain along the femoral nerve on the anterior thigh is the positive test result for L3 to L4 disc herniation.

(g) *Bilateral hip-knee flexion and rotation test* With the patient supine and both hips and knees fully flexed, use one hand to hold both knees and the other hand to push the feet, or hold up the patient's hips from below, and perform passive flexion of the lower waist and pelvic rotation. If it causes pain, the test is positive for lumbosacral soft tissue lesions or lower back strain. (See Figure 52.)

(h) *Pelvis separation and compression test* With the patient in a supine position; press both sides of the iliac crest concurrently, and squeeze in a lateral inferior direction. This is known as the pelvic separation test. The pelvic compression test is performed when you use both hands to push both iliac wings toward the center. If either of the tests induces pain, it is a positive test result, observed in pelvic ring fractures or sacroiliac joint pathology. (See Figure 53.)

(i) *Table-side/Gaenslen's test* The patient lies supine and slightly moves the affected side to the edge of the examination table with legs hanging.

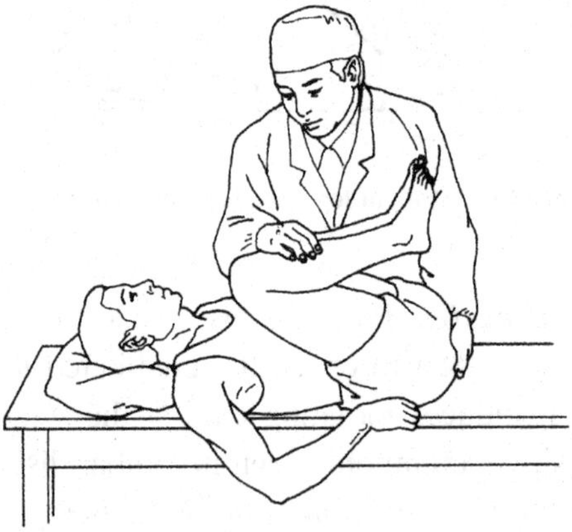

Figure 52 Bilateral hip-knee flexion and rotation test

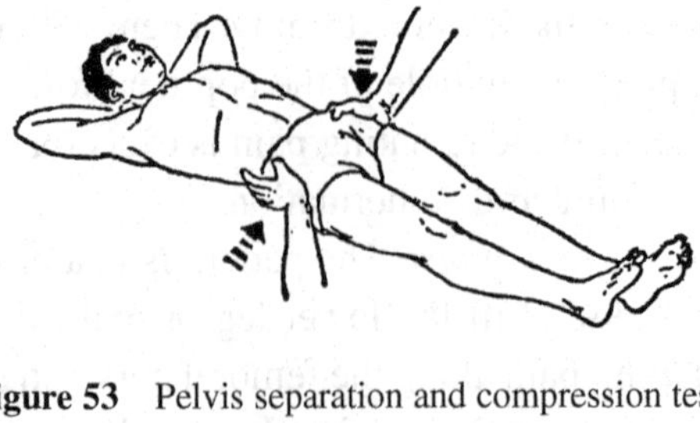

Figure 53 Pelvis separation and compression tests

The contralateral hip and knee should be flexed. Hold the contralateral knee on the anterior side with one hand, and with the other press down on the hanging thigh. If it induces sacroiliac joint pain, the test is positive, seen in sacroiliac joint pathology. (See Figure 54.)

(j) *Hip internal rotation test* With the patient supine, ask him or her to elevate and straighten the affected limb. When the existing sciatica appears, perform passive internal rotation to the hip with force, producing piriformis tension (also known as the piriformis tension test). If the sciatica increases, the test is positive for piriformis syndrome. (See Figure 55.)

Everyday Exercises

Try to memorize the physical examination and diagnostic methods of the neck and lumbar.

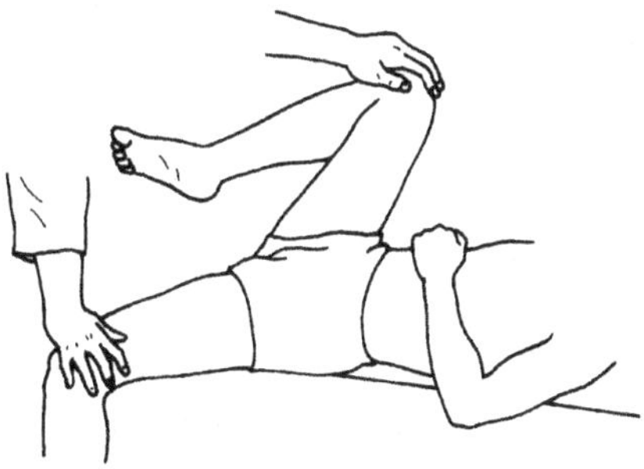

Figure 54 Table-side (Gaenslen's) test

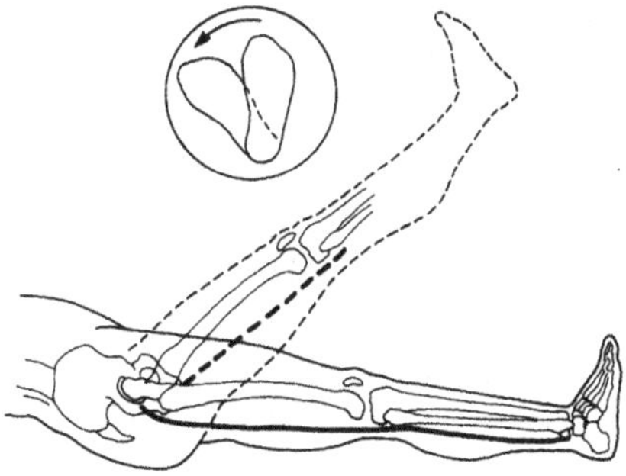

Figure 55 Internal hip rotation test

Day 5

EXAMINATION OF THE NEUROLOGICAL SYSTEM

A neurological examination is conducted to assess sensory responses and reflexes, and involves much more than this book can cover. In this book, we introduce only the main screening methods for neurological lesions and diseases associated with the neck, waist, legs, and peripheral nerves of the four limbs.

Sensory Responses

The test for sensory response is the pain sensation test. The tool used can be something with a sharp end, such as a pin. Use a new one for each patient. Start with gentle and slow jabs on the numb area or the area with no sensation identified by the patient. Jabs should be continuous, at moderate speed, and gradually moving to the normal area for a thorough check. The examination must be systematic, such as top-down, or lateral to medial, with both sides being compared. Once you find a sensory paralysis in an area, the site should be tested repetitively, moving from the area with reduced feeling to that with normal feeling. In this way, you will get more accurate results. Sensory testing relies tremendously on the patient's subjective response, so that it is essential for the patient to be fully cooperative, and for the examiner to be patient and careful.

In general, examination results for sensory responses can be classified into the following responses: normal, hypersensitivity (increased), dysesthesia (reduced), and loss of sensation (absent). The examiner must record the exact locations of paresthesia.

Myodynamia (Muscular Strength)

The examination method checks the muscle strength of a patient during active movement. The grading is shown the Table 18.

Table 18 Muscle strength grading table

Grade	Description of muscle strength grading
0	Complete paralysis of the muscle with no contraction
I – minute	Muscle shows slight contraction, but not capable of moving the joint
II – poor	Muscle can only complete joint activities without anti-gravity ability
III – mediocre	Muscle can drive the joint to perform activities with anti-gravity ability
IV – good	Muscle can complete joint activities against partial resistance with anti-gravity ability
V – normal	Muscle is able to complete joint activities against greater resistance with anti-gravity ability

Reflexes

1. *Superficial reflexes* These are reflexes obtained by stimulating the surface of the skin. Absence of superficial reflexes is of great clinical significance, indicating interruption of the reflex arc from the receptors on the body surface to the nerve center. Common superficial reflexes and their corresponding segment of the nerves are as follows.

   (a) *Abdominal reflex*

   Method and clinical significance With the patient supine and abdominal muscles relaxed, scratch the abdominal wall on both sides with a blunt object in the order of upper, middle, and lower area. This stimulation should lead to abdominal contraction. Each section is controlled by its corresponding nerve segment. Reflexes of the upper abdominal wall are controlled by T7 and T8, the middle abdominal wall by T9 and T10, and the lower abdominal wall by T11 and T12. If the abdominal reflex on one side is lost, it indicates pathologic changes in the corresponding nerve segment. (See Figure 56.)

   (b) *Cremasteric reflex*

   Method and clinical significance With the patient supine and the thigh slightly abducted and rotated externally, scrape the medial side of the skin of the thigh from the bottom up using a blunt object. This stimulation will normally cause the rapid contraction of the

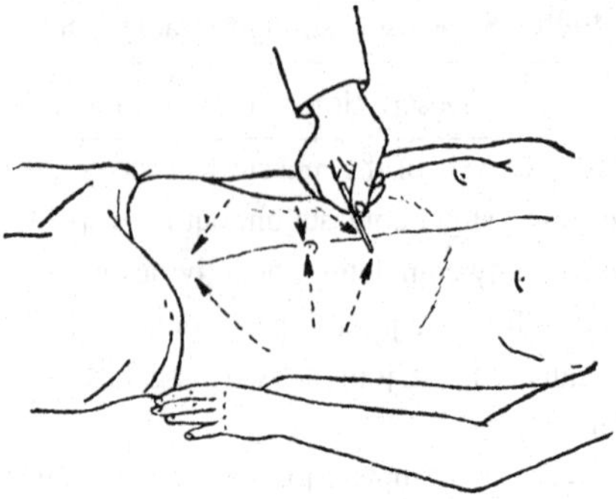

Figure 56 Abdominal reflex

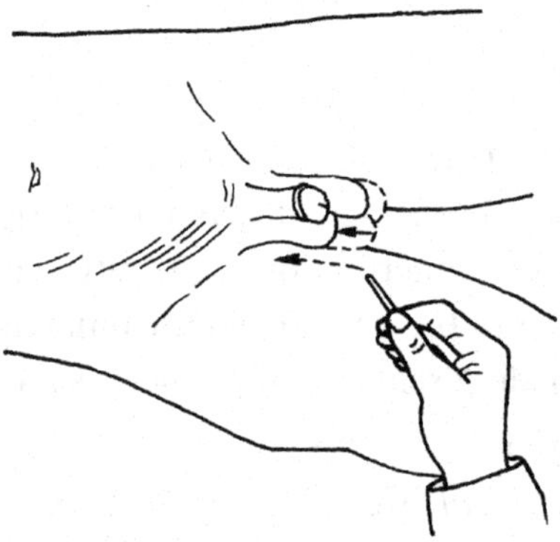

Figure 57 Cremasteric reflex test

ipsilateral cremaster muscle and move the testicles upwards. The nerve segment for the cremasteric reflex is L1 and L2. If this reflex is absent, it indicates pathologic changes of this nerve segment. (See Figure 57.)

(c) *Anal reflex*

Method and clinical significance With the patient lying laterally, scrape the skin around the anus with a blunt object to cause anal sphincter contraction. This reflex is controlled by the S5 nerve segment. The loss of this reflex is an indication of damage of the caudaequina nerve on both sides of the pyramidal tract. (See Figure 58.)

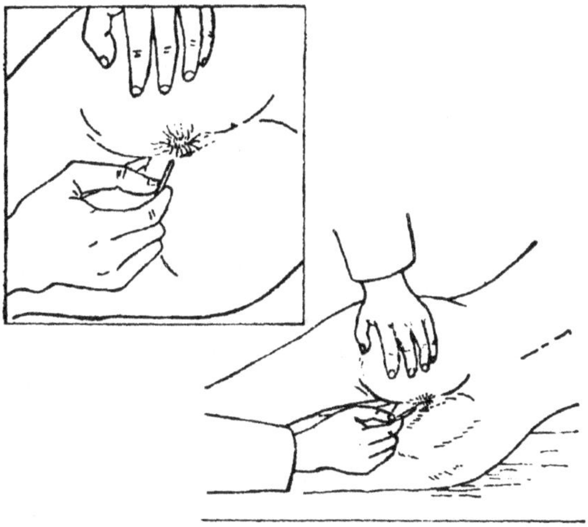

Figure 58 Anal reflex test

2. *Deep reflexes* Deep reflexes are induced by percussion on appropriate tendons or muscles with an examination hammer, resulting in reflexes with a short-term contraction. The inspection requires three things to be identical to ensure the accuracy and reliability of the result: both sides of the body's posture, location of the percussion, and intensity of the percussion. At the same time, both sides need to be compared thoroughly.

   Clinically, the active level of reflexion is usually classified and labeled as:

- Disappearance of the reflexion: (–)
- Hyporeflexia: (+)
- Normal: (++)
- Activereflexion: (+++)
- Hyperreflexia: (++++)

A weakened or disappeared reflexion is commonly seen in peripheral nerve or nerve root lesions, such as polio sequelae and progressive muscular dystrophy.

Hyperreflexia is common in conditions such as brain or spinal cord tumor, and spinitis.

Common deep reflexions include the following:

(a) *Biceps tendon reflex*

Method and clinical significance With the forearm of the patient rotated forward and semi-flexed, place one thumb on the biceps tendon of the patient, while with the other hand, hold a hammer and tap the patient's thumb. This stimulus normally leads to elbow flexion controlled by nervus musculocutaneusa. The brachial tendon reflex is a physiological reflex existing in healthy people. Hyperreflexia, hyporeflexia or dissappearence of the reflexion is pathological, often seen in lesions of C5. (See Figure 59.)

(b) *Radial periosteal reflex*

Method and clinical significance With the patient's elbow semi-flexed, tap the radial styloid process with a reflex hammer. This would normally lead to forearm flexion controlled by the radial nerve. Also a physiological reflex, the radial periosteal reflex exists in a normal individual. Alteration of this reflexion is mostly caused by C6 lesions. (See Figure 60.)

(c) *Triceps tendon reflex*

Method and clinical significance With the patient's forearm rotated and semi-flexed, hold the patient's forearm with one hand, and tap the triceps tendon with a hammer using the other hand. This would

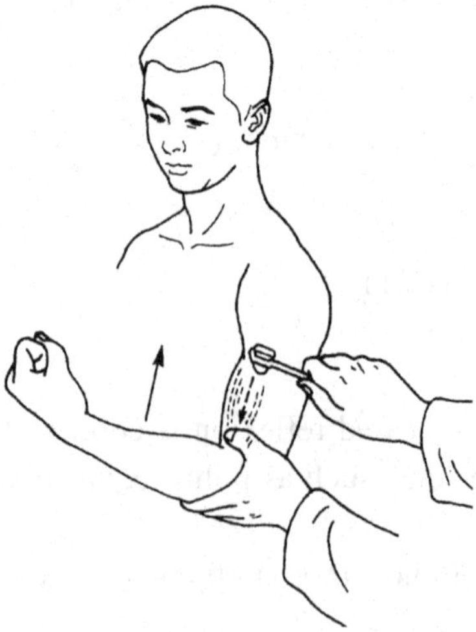

Figure 59 Biceps tendon reflex

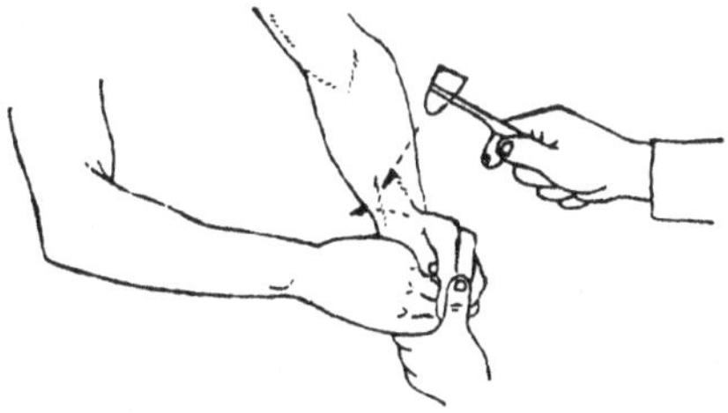

Figure 60 Radial periosteal reflex

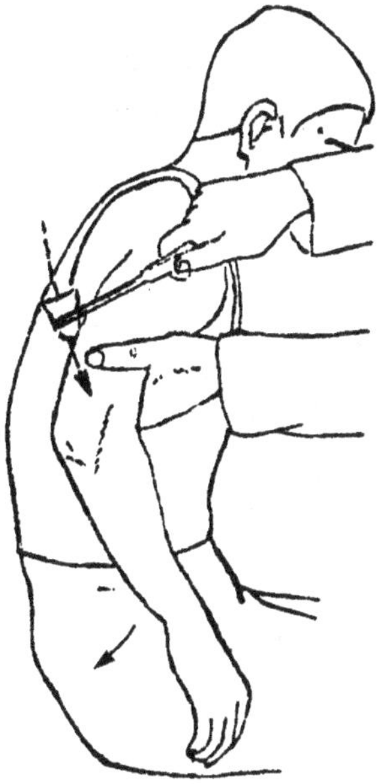

Figure 61 Triceps tendon reflex

normally lead to elbow extension controlled by the radial nerve. The triceps tendon reflex is also a physiological reflex existing in normal people. Abnormal reflexes are mostly caused by C7 diseases. (See Figure 61.)

(d) *Knee tendon reflex*

Method and clinical significance With the patient supine and both knees semi-flexed, hold the popliteal area of the patient using a hand or forearm to relax the muscle, while with the other hand, tap the patellar tendon with a reflex hammer. This would cause the calf to extend in a normal person. If an abnormal reflex appears, it is mainly related to L4 diseases. (See Figure 62.)

(e) *Ankle reflex*

Method and clinical significance The best way to perform this test is to have the patient kneeling on a chair with both feet unsupported. Hold the foot with one hand to make it slightly flexed dorsally, while with the other hand, tap the Achilles tendon with a reflex hammer. Or, with the patient sitting and both feet hanging, make the patient's foot slightly flexed dorsally, and tap the Achilles tendon. Either method will result in ankle plantar flexion in a normal person. Both methods have the advantage of easily relaxing the muscles and enabling the appearance of the reflexion. Abnormal reflexes are mostly due to S1 diseases. (See Figure 63.)

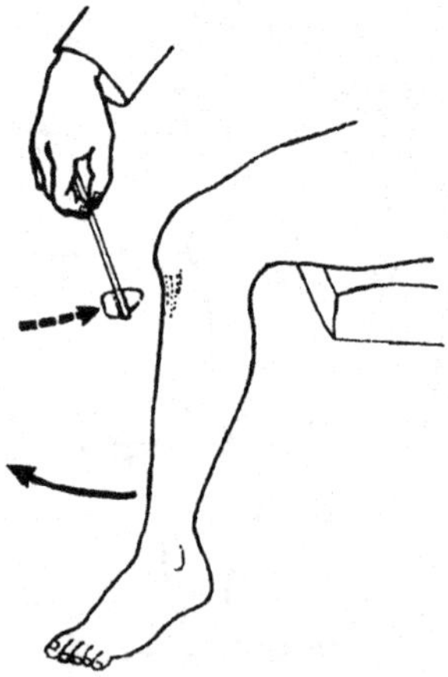

Figure 62 Knee tendon reflex

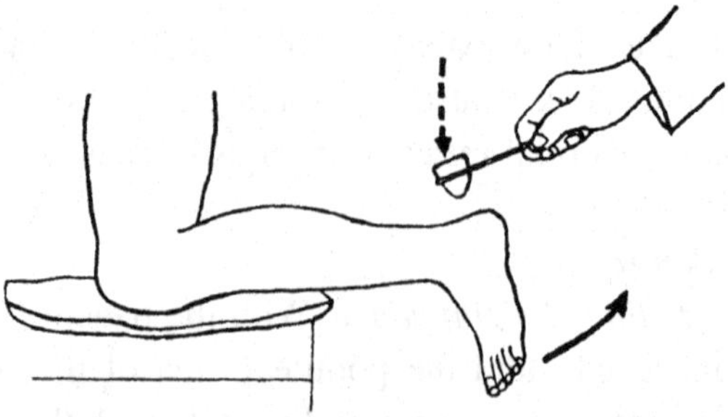

Figure 63 Ankle reflex (Achilles reflex)

3. *Pathological Reflexes*
   (a) *Hoffmann sign*
   Method and clinical significance Hold the patient's wrist with one hand, using your index and middle finger to fix the patient's middle finger, and make the wrist slightly dorsiflexed while allowing the rest of the fingers to be in a natural, relaxed state. Then, scrape the nail of the patient's middle finger with the thumb of your other hand. If this makes other fingers flex, the test result is positive, suggesting pyramidal tract damage. (See Figure 64.)
   (b) *Babinski sign*
   Method and clinical significance With the patient supine, use one hand to control the ankle of the patient, making the muscle relaxed. Then, with the other hand, use a blunt tool to scrape along the lateral side of the plantar, from the heel to the toe. If this leads to dorsiflexion of the big toe with the remaining four toes fanning out, the test result is positive, and is a reliable indication of pyramidal tract damage. (See Figure 65.)
   (c) *Chaddocksign*
   Method and clinical significance With the patient supine, scrape the lateral dorsal side of the patient's foot using a blunt object.

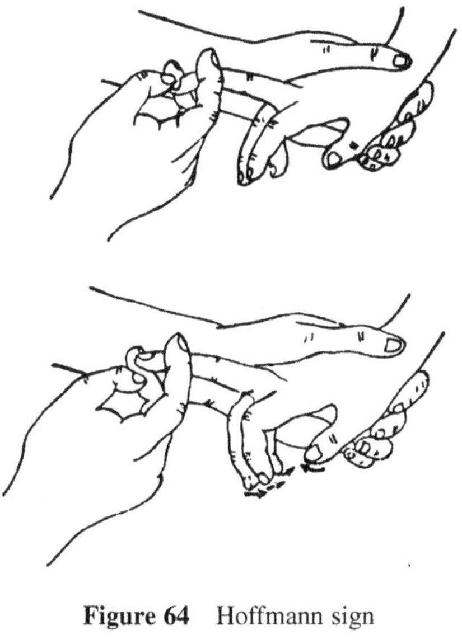

Figure 64 Hoffmann sign

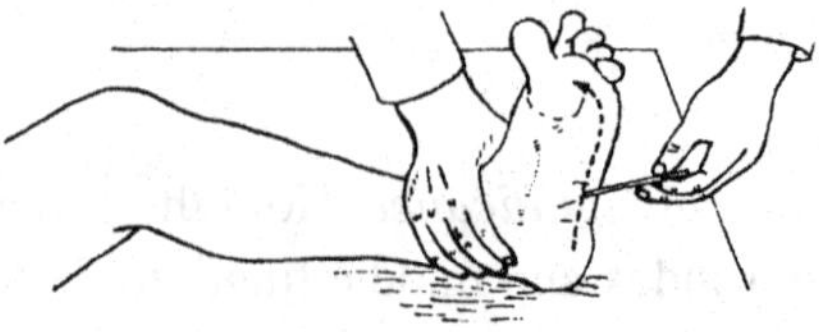

Figure 65 Babinski sign

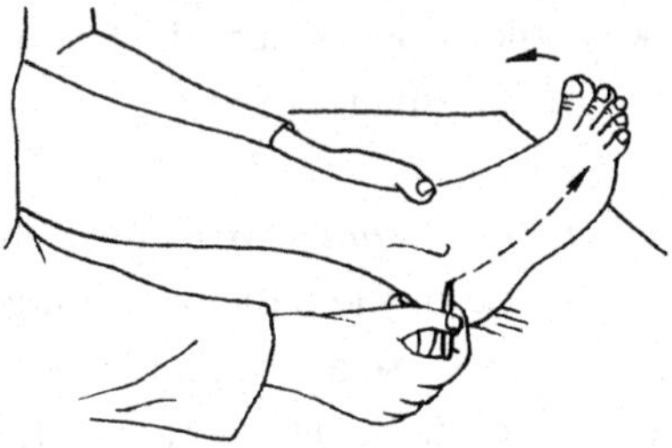

Figure 66 Chaddock sign

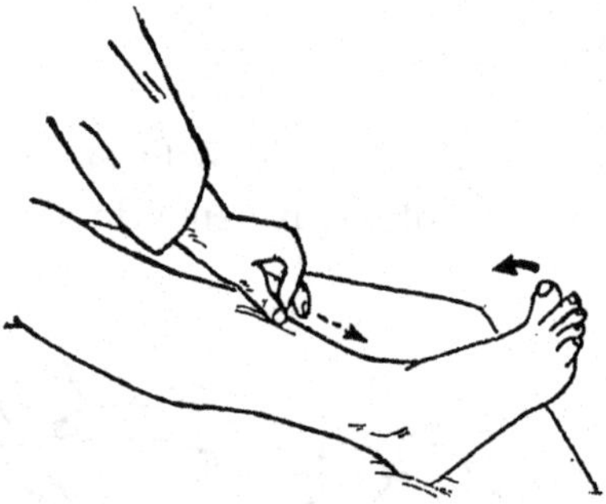

Figure 67 Oppenheim sign

A positive result indicates the same thing as the Babinski sign does. (See Figure 66.)

(d) *Oppenheim sign*

Method and clinical significance With the patient supine, push down along the anterior tibial side with the thumb and index finger. A positive result indicates the same thing as the Babinski sign does. (See Figure 67.)

(e) *Gordon sign*

Method and clinical significance With the patient supine, pinch the gastrocnemius of the patient firmly. A positive result indicates the same thing as the Babinski sign does. (See Figure 68.)

(f) *Patellar clonus*

Method and clinical significance With the patient supine, use the web between your thumb and index finger to hold on to the upper end of the patella, quickly moving your hand downwards, and then hold the patella tightly. If the patella contracts continuously and rhythmically, this condition is called patellar clonus, indicating upper motor neuron disease. (See Figure 69.)

(g) *Ankle clonus*

Method and clinical significance With the patient supine, use one hand to hold the popliteal fossa of the patient, and the other hand to hold the foot. Quickly perform passive dorsiflexion; then hold the foot in this position. If it leads to continuous rhythmic flexion and extension of the ankle, this condition is called ankle clonus, often indicating upper motor neuron lesions. (See Figure 70.)

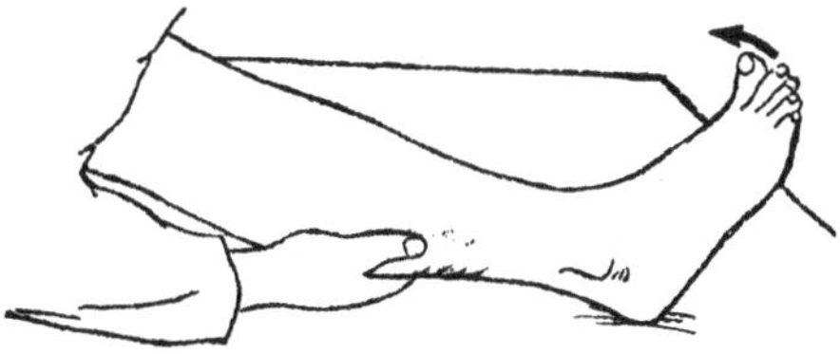

Figure 68 Gordon sign

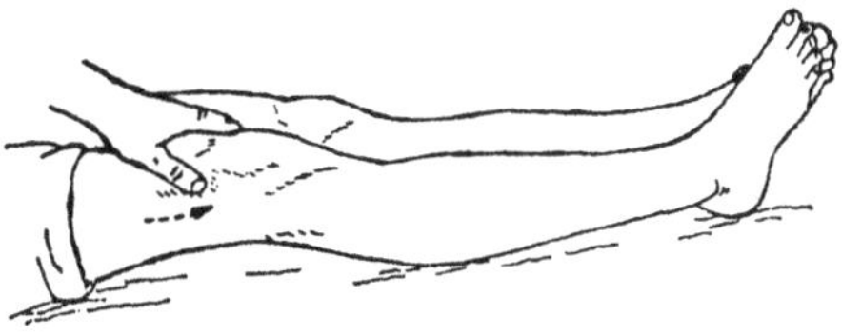

Figure 69 Patellar clonus

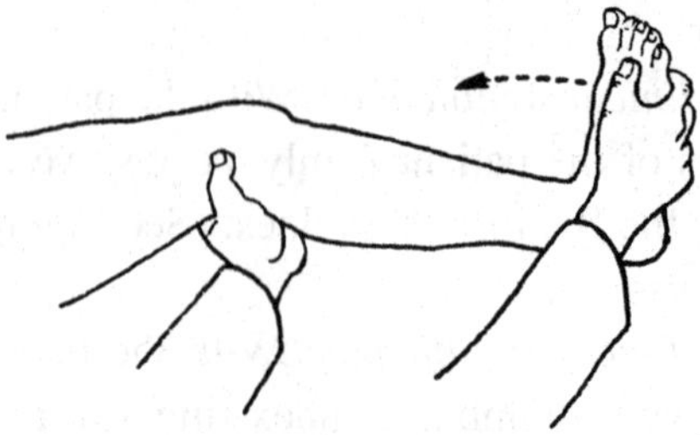

Figure 70 Ankle clonus

Everyday Exercises

Try to memorize the examination methods for, and the clinical significance of, superficial, deep, and pathological reflexes.

Day 6

ANATOMY OF NORMAL BONES AND JOINTS UNDER X-RAYS

Figure 71 shows what bones and joints look like under X-rays.

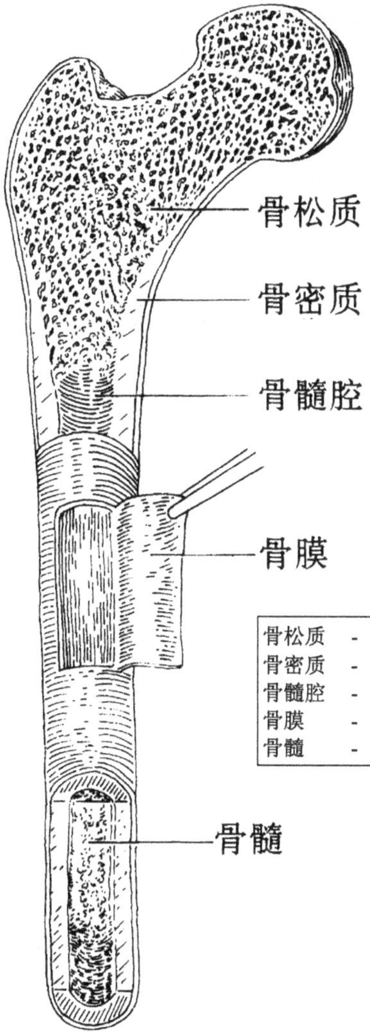

骨松质	-	cancellous bone
骨密质	-	dense bone
骨髓腔	-	bone marrow cavity
骨膜	-	periosteum
骨髓	-	bone marrow

Figure 71 Bone structure

1. *The periosteum* Normal periosteum will not appear in an X-ray image. If it looks like what is shown in Figure 71, it indicates pathological conditions, commonly found in trauma, cancer, inflammation, and other diseases of unknown cause.
2. *Cortex of bones* The density of the cortex of bones should be even, white in color, thickest in the middle of the diaphysis and gradually thinning toward both sides, and only a meager layer at its ends. The inner layer of the cortex connects with cancellous bone without obvious boundaries.

   Under pathological conditions, cortex bone can be sparse, delaminated, thinning, and damaged. When a tumor invades the bone cortex, tumorous new bone forms.
3. *Cancellous bone* Cancellous bone is formed with bone trabeculae and gaps of the bone marrow, and appears as fine and neat bone texture on an X-ray image. The structure and distribution of cancellous bone (also known as trabecular bone) are in accordance with the pressure and muscle traction they are bearing, as well as the special functions they perform.
4. *Bone marrow cavity* Bone marrow cavity under normal circumstances cannot be shown on an X-ray image owing to the covering and overlapping of cortex and cancellous bones.
5. *The epiphyseal line* Different widths of epiphyseal lines are visible at the end of the long bones during the growth and development period. Epiphyseal lines are usually equal in thickness and are symmetric bilaterally.

Figure 72 shows the anatomy of normal articulation under X-rays.

1. *Articular cavity* On an X-ray image, the joint space can be seen to comprise three components: the cartilage, fibrocartilage, and cavity of the articulation.
2. *Articular surface* Since the articular surface of the outer covering of the cartilage does not develop on an X-ray film, what we see is actually the cortex bone, formed by an extremely thin layer of dense bone with sharp-looking smooth edges.
3. *Synovial membrane* Thesis the inner tissue of the joint capsule that does not develop on an X-ray film. When there is intra-articular effusion, the image develops because of synovial swelling.

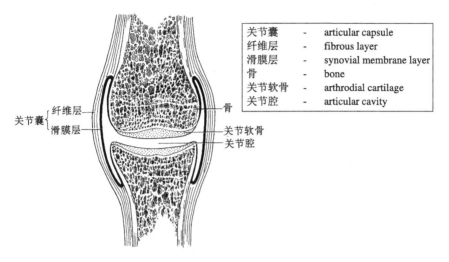

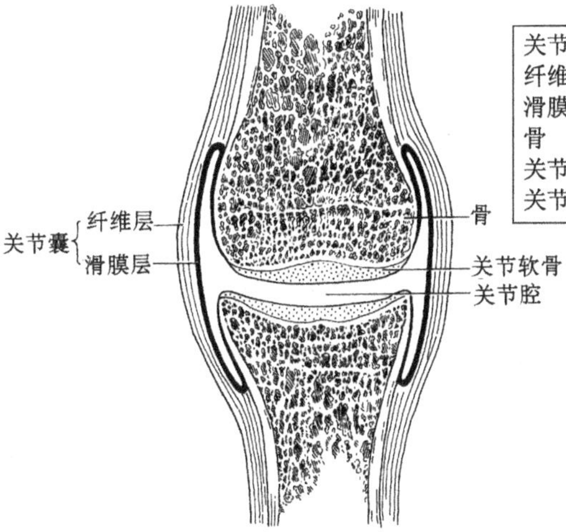

关节囊	-	articular capsule
纤维层	-	fibrous layer
滑膜层	-	synovial membrane layer
骨	-	bone
关节软骨	-	arthrodial cartilage
关节腔	-	articular cavity

Figure 72 Joint structure

Figures 73 to 80 show the X-Ray anatomy of the spine and joints of limbs.

Basic X-Ray Images of Bone and Joint Diseases

Basic X-Ray Findings of Bone Lesions

1. *Osteoporosis*

   Osteoporosis is the decreased unit volume of bone tissue within the bone. Osteoporosis in long bones of the four limbs can be shown on X-ray film as significantly reduced number of bone trabecular with widened gaps, sparse structure, and decreased density in cancellous substance. A typical image is one that looks like sketch lines drawn with a pencil.

   Spine osteoporosis on an X-ray image is indicated by cortical thinning and irregular longitudinal patterns on bone trabeculae. In serious situations, the bone pattern becomes blurred and even disappears, showing a flattened vertebral body with the upper and lower edge concaved, shaped like a fish spine. At the same time, the space between the vertebrae has double-convex deformation; therefore, a double concave and double convex change can be seen.

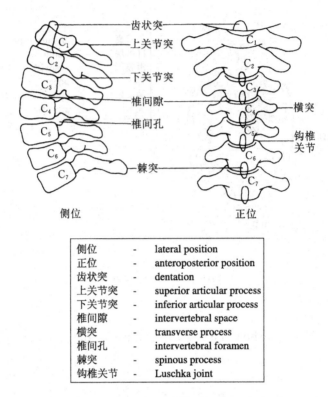

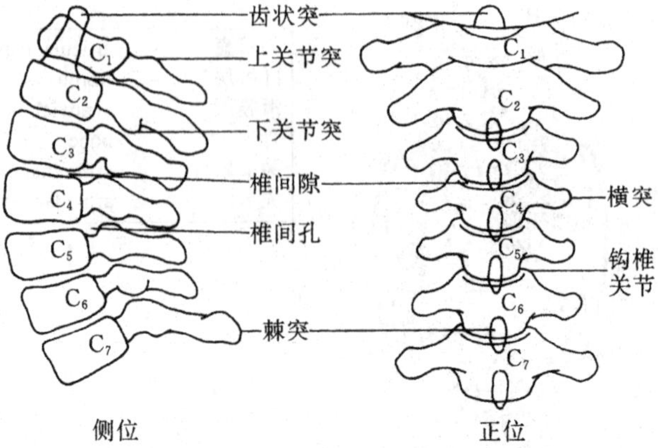

侧位	-	lateral position
正位	-	anteroposterior position
齿状突	-	dentation
上关节突	-	superior articular process
下关节突	-	inferior articular process
椎间隙	-	intervertebral space
横突	-	transverse process
椎间孔	-	intervertebral foramen
棘突	-	spinous process
钩椎关节	-	Luschka joint

Figure 73 X-Ray anatomy of normal cervical spine

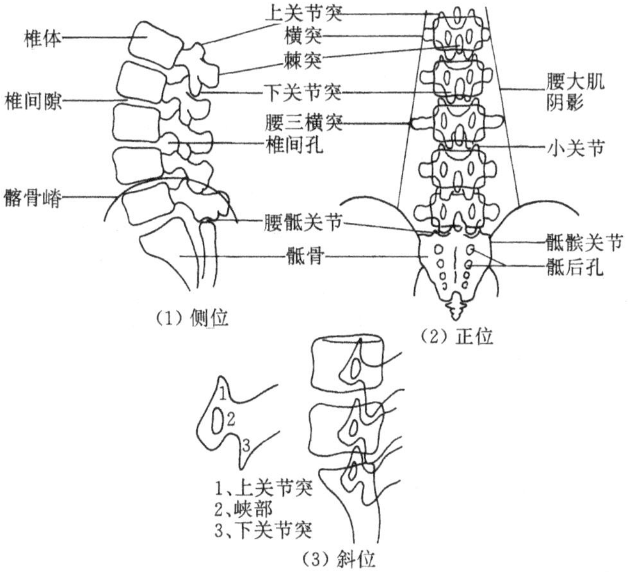

侧位	-	lateral position	椎间孔	-	intervertebral foramen
正位	-	anteroposterior position	腰骶关节	-	lumbosacral joint
斜位	-	oblique position	骶骨	-	sacrum
椎体	-	vertebral body	腰大肌阴影	-	shade of the greater psoas
椎间隙	-	intervertebral space	小关节	-	facet joint
髂骨脊	-	iliac crest	骶髌关节	-	sacral patellar joint
上关节突	-	superior articular process	骶后孔	-	posterior sacral foramen
横突	-	transverse process	1. 上关节突	-	superior articular process
棘突	-	spinous process	2. 峡部	-	pars interarticularis
下关节突	-	inferior articular process	3. 下关节突	-	inferior articular process
腰三横突	-	transverse process of L3			

Figure 74 Normal X-Ray anatomy of the lumbar spine

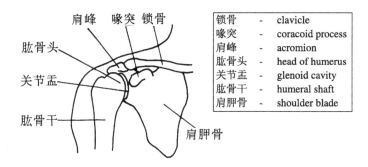

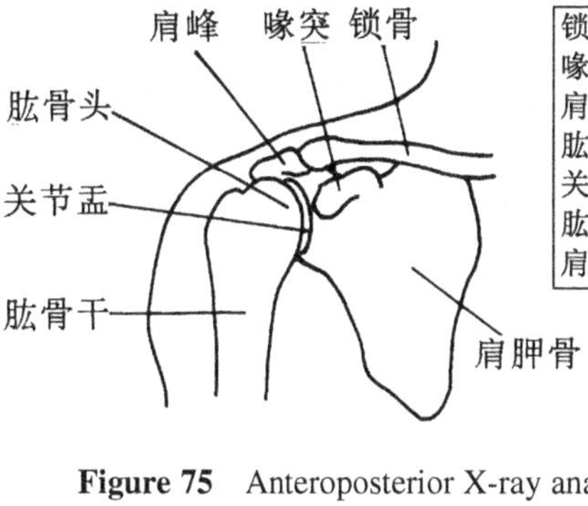

锁骨	-	clavicle
喙突	-	coracoid process
肩峰	-	acromion
肱骨头	-	head of humerus
关节盂	-	glenoid cavity
肱骨干	-	humeral shaft
肩胛骨	-	shoulder blade

Figure 75 Anteroposterior X-ray anatomy of the shoulder

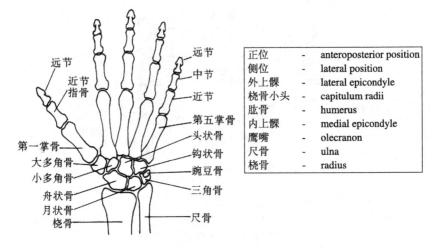

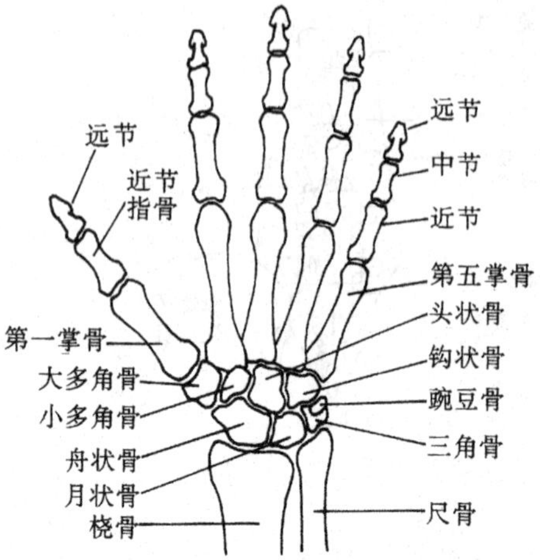

正位	-	anteroposterior position
侧位	-	lateral position
外上髁	-	lateral epicondyle
桡骨小头	-	capitulum radii
肱骨	-	humerus
内上髁	-	medial epicondyle
鹰嘴	-	olecranon
尺骨	-	ulna
桡骨	-	radius

Figure 76 X-Ray anatomy of the elbow joint

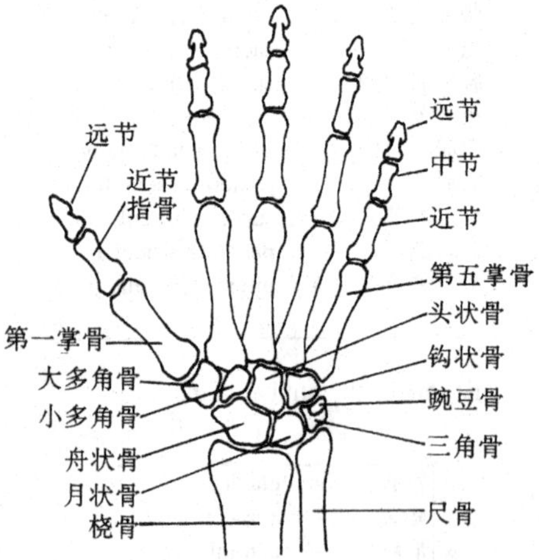

远节	-	distal phalanx
近节指骨	-	proximal phalanx
远节	-	distal phalanx
中节	-	middle phalanx
近节	-	proximal phalanx
第一掌骨	-	first metacarpal bone
大多角骨	-	trapezium
小多角骨	-	trapezoid
舟状骨	-	scaphoid
月状骨	-	lunate bone
第五掌骨	-	fifth metacarpal bone
头状骨	-	capitatum
钩状骨	-	unciform
豌豆骨	-	lentiform bone
三角骨	-	triangular bone
桡骨	-	radius
尺骨	-	ulna

Figure 77 X-Ray anatomy of the wrist and hand

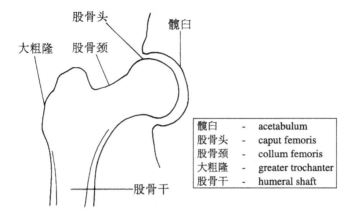

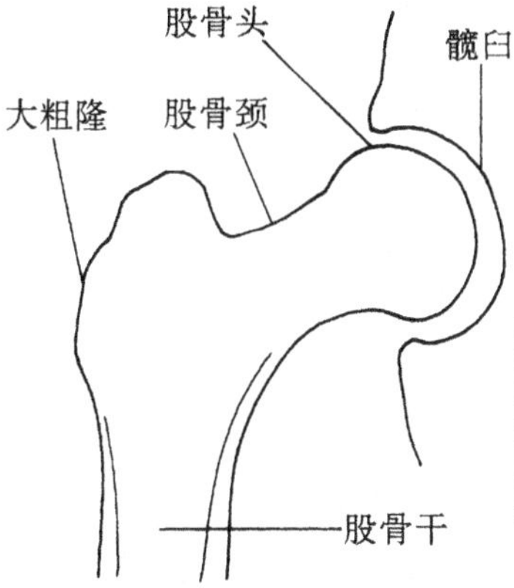

髋臼	-	acetabulum
股骨头	-	caput femoris
股骨颈	-	collum femoris
大粗隆	-	greater trochanter
股骨干	-	humeral shaft

Figure 78 X-Ray anatomy of the hip

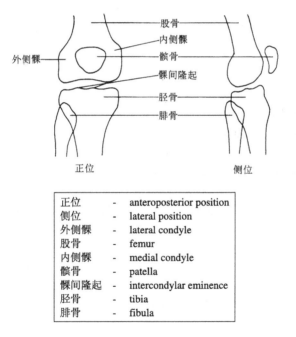

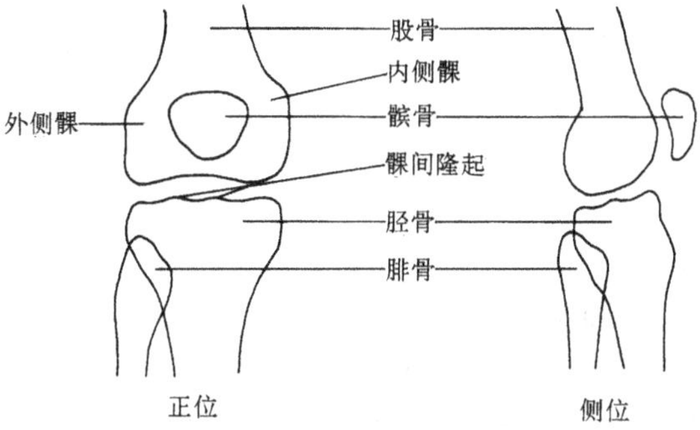

正位	-	anteroposterior position
侧位	-	lateral position
外侧髁	-	lateral condyle
股骨	-	femur
内侧髁	-	medial condyle
髌骨	-	patella
髁间隆起	-	intercondylar eminence
胫骨	-	tibia
腓骨	-	fibula

Figure 79 X-Ray anatomy of the knee

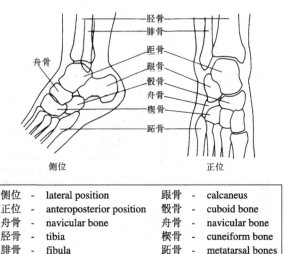

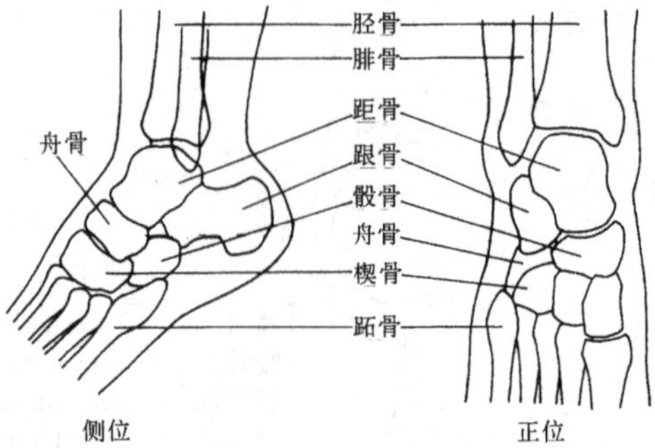

侧位	-	lateral position	跟骨	-	calcaneus
正位	-	anteroposterior position	骰骨	-	cuboid bone
舟骨	-	navicular bone	舟骨	-	navicular bone
胫骨	-	tibia	楔骨	-	cuneiform bone
腓骨	-	fibula	跖骨	-	metatarsal bones
距骨	-	talus			

Figure 80 X-Ray anatomy of a normal ankle

2. *Destruction of bone*
   Bone destruction is the result of bone tissue being dissolved and absorbed, and replaced by inflammation, tissue granulation, or tumor. Destruction owing to malignant tumors can be rapid, with bone tissue being totally destroyed and disappearing, leaving no marks.
3. *Hyperosteogeny or osteosclerosis*
   Hyperosteogeny or osteosclerosis is the opposite of osteoporosis. It is characterized by increased unit volume of bone content with a higher density compared to normal bone. It usually indicates a compensatory repair process of the body, often found in the repairing stage of injured bone, accompanied by chronic inflammation. It is also due to conditions such as bone tumor of osteogenesis type and metastases.
4. *Sequestrum of bone*
   Sequestrum of bone is the result of partial or complete blood supply disorder to the bone tissue, causing bone necrosis, which is common in osteomyelitis.

5. *Periosteal proliferation*
   Normal periosteum cannot be developed on X-ray film. It can be seen only in the event of ossification or hyperplasia, indicating a lesion. The visible change in periosteum varies: it can appear as monolayer parallel with the cortex bone, or an onion-peel-like multi-layer, or it can appear lace-like. It can also be perpendicular to the cortex, needle-shaped, or radiating. Most of the changes can be found in periosteal inflammation or tumors.
6. *Changes in surrounding soft tissues*
   Many bone diseases often cause changes of the surrounding soft tissues. At the same time, diseases originating in soft tissue lesions can also lead to bone changes. Therefore, bone photographs should include images of surrounding soft tissue in certain diseases to see the range and size of the swelling; whether there is swelling or shrinking; whether the boundaries are fuzzy or clear; whether the density is even; or whether there is calcification, any foreign bodies, or gas.

Basic X-Ray Findings of Joint Lesions

1. *Joint swelling* This includes joint effusion and swelling of intra-articular soft tissue. X-rays show widened joint spaces; increased and bulging joint soft tissue shadows; displaced, deformed, vague, or disappeared shadows of surrounding fat pads and fat layers between muscles. The changes are mostly seen in early arthritis.
2. *Joint destruction* Usually, early joint destruction involves only the articular cartilage, showing a narrowed joint space. If the lesions continue to develop, partial or one side of the bone will have damages and defects. In severe cases, the whole joint is damaged, resulting in subluxation and deformity.

   The site and progress of joint destruction may vary due to the nature of the disease. The damage in acute suppurative joint starts from the weight bearing area, followed by rapid progression, and soon involves the sclerotin under the articular cartilage. The bone destruction of synovial tuberculosis, on the other hand, starts from both sides of the non-weight bearing joints, and it progresses at as low rate (a matter of months), involving the bone sclerotin at a much later time. Lastly, joint sclerotin destruction in rheumatoid arthritis progresses very slowly at the late stages, often in years.

3. *Early joint degeneration* This is limited to the articular cartilage, which is gradually replaced by fibrous tissue, resulting in varying degrees of joint space narrowing. Later, the lesion gradually involves the bone, with secondary osteoarthritis on the edge of the joint. This phenomenon is common seen in the elderly, and is most obvious on greater weightbearing joints such as the spine, hip, and knee.
4. *Joint ankylosis* Joint ankylosis is a common consequence of arthritis, and is classified as bony ankylosis and fibrous ankylosis. Bony ankylosis is the result of massive destruction of cartilage and bone, causing convergence of rough articular surface, and is more common in acute septic arthritis. On X-ray film, it shows up as significant space narrowing or the complete disappearance of the original joint, with trabecular bone throughout the joint space between the two bones, making them look like one.

   Fibrous ankylosis, clinically, is the disappearance of part or most of the joint, but the narrow joint space can still be observed on X-ray film. There is no coherent or crossing of trabeculae, generally appearing to be sparse and with lower bone density, which is common in rheumatoid arthritis.
5. *Articular dislocation* Articular dislocation results in a relative position change at the two ends of the bones that form the joint. It can be classified as either subluxation or complete dislocation. It is mostly found in external trauma cases. In addition, severe joint damage such as purulent or tuberculous lesions, and rheumatoid arthritis also can cause different degrees of dislocation.
6. *Articular soft tissue changes* This is the swelling, thickening, and density increase of the soft tissue external to the joint capsule, causing the fatty tissue around the joint to disappear.

Everyday Exercises

Try to memorize the X-ray anatomy of the normal bones and joints.

WEEK 3

Day 1

TUI NA FOR ADULTS

Subject 1 — Tui Na Maneuvers

Tui na maneuvers or manipulations are an integral part of tui na, and form a set of specialized foundational skills that practitioners need to acquire to treat diseases. Tui na maneuvers are by no means ordinary, simple, or arbitrary actions. The effect of tui na in treating diseases is realized using skillful manipulations rather than brute force. As the lines in *Golden Mirror of the Medical Tradition — Key Points to the Hearty Methods of Bone Alignment*, written in the Qing Dynasty, read: "only manipulations without making the patient miserable can be referred as maneuvers." However, there is no easy way or shortcut to achieve this goal, so practitioners must obtain the skill via a rigorous training process.

Training of tui na maneuvers, especially that of the major manipulation techniques, can be divided into three stages. The first stage is to practice each maneuver until it closely resembles the requirements of the instructor or the instructions in a professional book. It is very important to do this, because if you cannot reproduce the maneuver correctly, it is very difficult to improve your skills moving forward. The second stage is to increase the frequency of the maneuver while ensuring it is still correct. The third stage is to gradually increase the intensity of the manipulations based on correct actions and appropriate frequency. This last stage integrates the physical power, skills and techniques required in tui na.

Basic requirements of tui na manipulations in clinical application must include the following five components: durability, power, evenness, gentleness, and in-depth penetration. "Durability" means the maneuver must be in accordance with the essential norm for a certain period of time; the continuity of the maneuver must be maintained for a specified time period. "Power" means that the implementation of stimulus must have certain intensity. This is a specific skill, but by no means a brute force. More importantly, the force applied should be in accordance with the tolerance level of the patient, whether the disease is of deficient or excess pattern, the location of the body, and the kind of the maneuver by nature."Evenness" refers to a certain rhythm and stability of the action that needs to be maintained, not sometimes faster and sometimes slower, or sometimes forceful and sometimes powerless. "Gentleness" means that the manipulation must be stable, gentle, and with moderate power, so that it is light but not superficial, intense but not rigid. "Gentle" should not be misinterpreted as soft and weak. "In-depth penetration" refers to the fact that the stimulation can make the patient reach the sensation of *de-qi* (arrival of qi), in order to ensure the treatment effect. When a maneuver has in-depth penetration, it appears to be acting on the surface, but the power should actually be deep enough to reach the deep subcutaneous tissue, and even organs.

The five components are closely related, complementary to each other, and form a mutual blend. In clinical applications, manipulation skill is the key, and the intensity serves as the foundation for the skill to be carried out thoroughly, so that both are indispensable. The practitioner must have sufficient physical strength before his or skills can be realized fully. On the other hand, if the practitioner lacks physical strength, even with a good grasp of the maneuvers, his or her efforts will be inadequate to reach the expected clinical outcome.

Rome was not built in one day. Every tui na professional needs to exercise and enhance physical strength in addition to acquiring techniques. Practice makes perfect. Only after a certain period of sustained training, can one apply the techniques proficiently.

Pressing

Pressing is the manipulation using a finger or the palm to apply a gradual and downward force on certain body areas or acupoints. Clinically, it is further divided into finger pressing and palm pressing methods. Pressing can also be used in conjunction with other maneuvers. When it is combined with kneading, it is known as pressure kneading.

Finger pressing This technique uses the pulp or tip of the thumb to press a certain body surface area. When the force of one thumb is insufficient, the therapist can overlap the other thumb to apply pressure. Clinically, it is often used in conjunction with rubbing. (See Figure 81.)

1. *Essentials of the maneuver*

   a. Apply the pressure downward and perpendicularly.
   b. The force should be from gentle to intensive, steady, and sustained, so that stimulation can reach the deeper tissues. Avoid using rapid and violent force.
   c. At the end of the pressing session, the clinician should not suddenly stop, but gradually decrease the degree of the pressure.

2. *Applicable locations*: points along the meridians all over the body.
3. *Actions*: releasing spasms, relieving pain, warming the meridian, and dissipating cold.
4. *Indications*: pain, difficulty in urination.
5. *Examples*

   a. *Epigastric pain*: press *píshū* (BL 20), *wèishū* (BL 21), or para spinal sensitive spots; one to two minutes for each point.
   b. *Abdominal pain*: press *zúsānlǐ* (ST 36) and *nèiguān* (PC 6).

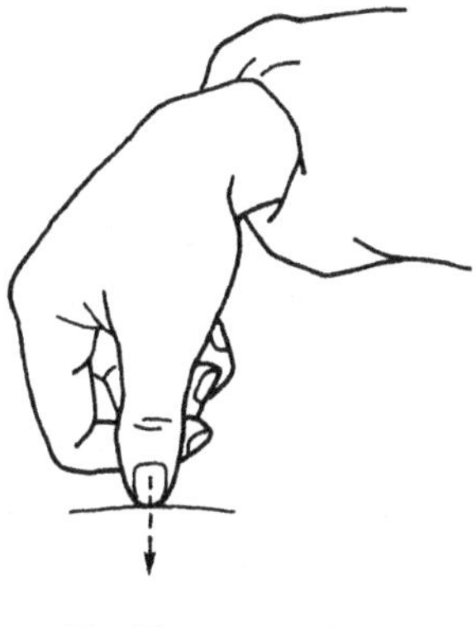

Figure 81 Finger pressing maneuver

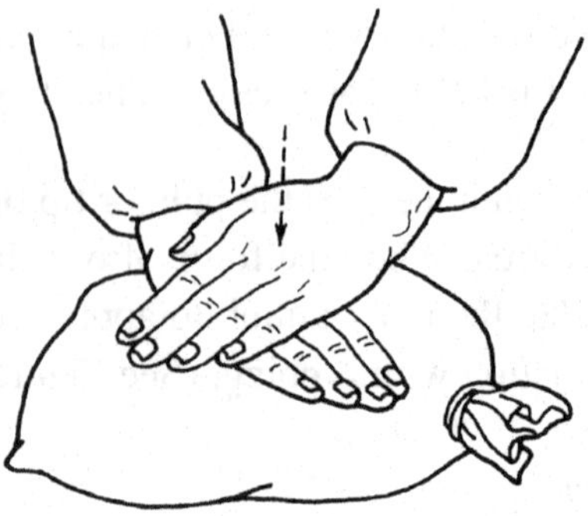

Figure 82 Palm pressing maneuver

c. *Neck stiffness and pain*: press *lièquē* (LU 7) and *hòuxī* (SI 3).
d. *Toothache*: pressure kneading on *hégŭ* (LI 4).
e. *Dysmenorrhea*: pressure kneading on *sānyīnjiāo* (SP 6).
f. *Urinaryretention*: press *zhōngjí* (RN 3).

Palm pressing This method uses the heel of the palm or the whole palm to press the surface of the body. It can be with one palm or both palms overlapped. It can be used in conjunction with kneading.(See Figure 82.)

1. *Essentials of the maneuver*

   a. Stop for a brief moment after a previous pressing prior to another press.
   b. To increase the compression force, extend both elbows straight, with body slightly forward, pressing down with some body weight.

2. *Applicable locations*: back, waist, abdomen, and body surfaces with a relatively bigger area and are relatively flat.
3. *Actions*: loosing up tendons and vessels, warming the center, dissipating coldness, invigorating blood, and dissolving stasis.
4. *Indications*: backpain, scoliosis, abdominal pain.
5. *Examples*

   a. Low back pain: palm pressing sacral spine muscles.
   b. Cold stomach pain: palm pressing on the abdomen with mild to moderate force; let the palm go up and down following the breathing of the patient.

Point Pressing (Acupressure)

This method requires a flexed inter phalangeal knuckle as the point of force on the acupoints. It is derived from the pressing maneuver. With the force focused on one point at a time, its stimulation is strong. There are three forms of acupoint pressing maneuver: thumb-end pressing, flexed thumb point pressing and flexed index finger point pressing.

1. *Essentials of the maneuver* (*Fig. 83*)

   a. *Thumb-end acupressure* Make a loose fist with the thumb straight and tightly touching the radial side of the index finger between the 1st and 2nd knuckle, and use the tip of the thumb to apply pressure on a treatment point.

   b. *Flexed thumb acupressure* Make a fist with the flexed thumb against the radial side of index finger between the 1st and 2nd knuckles, and apply pressure to the treatment point with the radial side of the inter phalangeal joint of the thumb.

   c. *Flexed index finger acupressure* Make a fist with the index finger protruded, and use its proximal inter phalangeal joint to apply pressure on the treatment site.

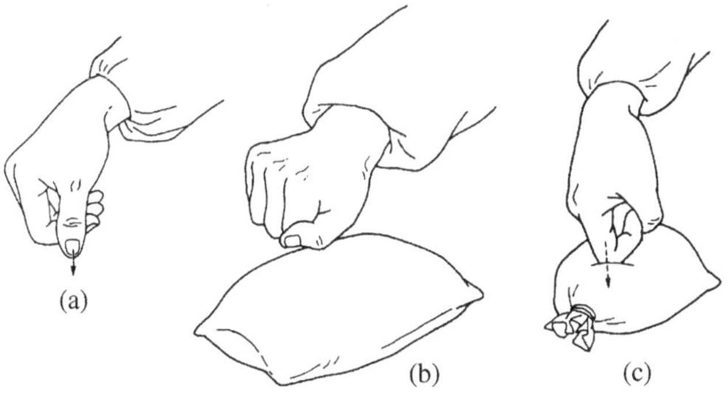

a. 拇指端点法	-	Thumb-end point pressing
b. 屈拇指点法	-	Flexed thumb point pressing
c. 屈食指点法	-	Flexed index

Figure 83 Point Pressing

(a) Thumb-end point pressing (b) Flexed thumb point pressing (c) Flexed index finger point pressing

2. *Applicable locations*: all parts of the body, especially the limbs and distal joint tender points.

See the finger pressing maneuver section for the actions and indications of the acupoint pressing maneuver.

Intense Pressing

This maneuver uses the surface of the thumb, palm or ulnar olecranon to apply pressure on the surface treatment site. In clinical practice, it includes intense finger pressing (acupressure), intense palm pressing and elbow pressing with intense pressure and strong stimulation. Compared to the pressing maneuver, intense pressing applies more force. In current clinical practice, the maneuver is often limited to elbow pressing with the following characteristics:

1. *Essentials of the maneuver*

   a. Have the elbow flexed and use the tip, i.e., the ulnar olecranon (see Figure 84) as the point to apply pressure in the treatment site on the body surface.

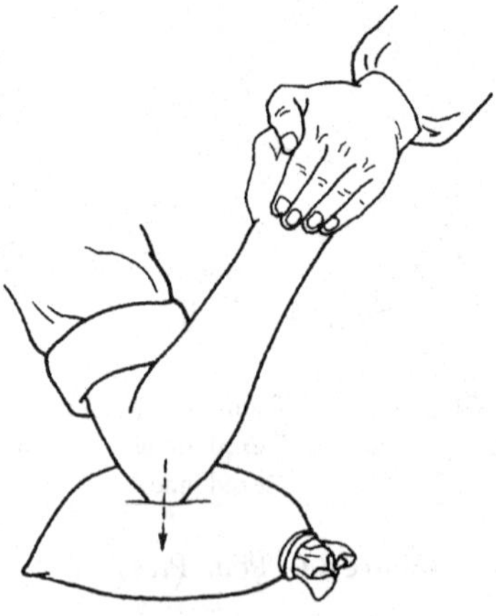

Figure 84 Elbow pressing

   b. The pressure should be applied in an even, stable, slow, and gentle manner without sudden and violent force.
   c. Consider the how much force the patient can endure

2. *Applicable locations*: applies only to muscular body ares a such as the buttocks.
3. *Actions*: relaxing tendons, unblocking the vessels, resolving spasms, and relieving pain.
4. *Indications*: intractable low back pain of *bì* pattern, stiffness and pain on the waist muscles.
5. *Examples*: *stiff pain of the lumbar muscles*: use the elbow pressing maneuver to work on both sides of the lumbar muscle.

Everyday Exercises

1. What is the definition of tui na maneuvers? What are the fundamental requirements?
2. Master the clinical application of pressing, acupoint pressing, and intense pressing maneuvers.

DAY 2

RUBBING

This maneuver uses the pulp of the index, middle and ring fingers, or the palm to rub certain body surfaces in a rhythmic and circular motion. The maneuver using a finger is called finger rubbing, while it is called palm rubbing if the palm is used. In ancient times, the method was often supplemented with medicinal creams to enhance the therapeutic effect; this was known as cream rubbing.

The action of rubbing is similar to that of kneading, but rubbing is lighter and only applied on the body surface, while kneading is a little more intense and affects the subcutaneous tissues.

1. *Essentials of the maneuver*

   a. *Finger rubbing* With the wrist slightly flexed, metacarpophalangeal and interphalangeal joints naturally straightened, use the fingerprint side of the index, middle, and ring fingers to touch the treatment site, and perform clockwise or counter-clockwise circular movements with the coordination of the wrist and forearm. (See Figure 85a).
   b. *Palm rubbing maneuver* With the wrist slightly dorsiflexed, fingers naturally straight, lay the whole palm flat on the surface treatment site. Coordinate movements of your fore arm and wrist to have the palm perform clockwise or counterclockwise movement on the treatment site. (See Fig. 85b.)

The maneuvers need to be gentle, with even pressure. Finger rubbing needs a lighter and faster motion with 120 strokes per minute, while palm rubbing is a little heavier and slower with 80 to 100 strokes per minute.

2. *Applicable locations*: the whole body; especially common in the chest, abdomen, and hypochondria.

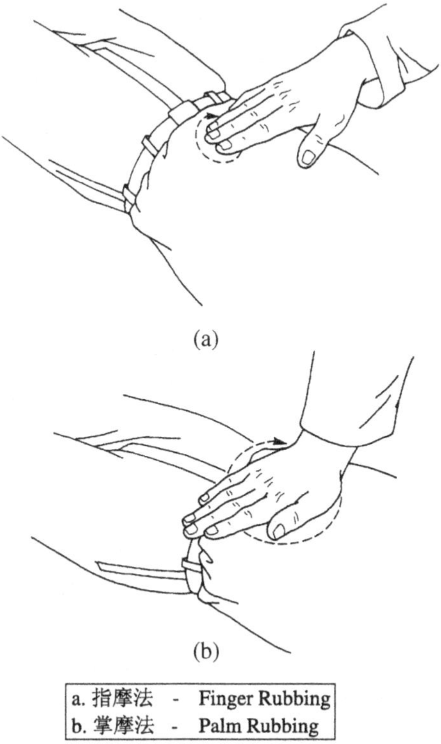

Figure 85 Rubbing

3. *Actions*: soothing the chest, rectifying qi, strengthening the spleen and harmonizing the stomach, invigorating blood, and dissipating stasis.
4. *Indications*: cough, chest tightness, abdominal distention and pain, and swelling and pain due to trauma.
5. *Examples*
   a. *Hypochondriac pain*: apply finger rubbing to *dànzhōng* (RN 17) and the flanks.
   b. *Indigestion*: apply palm rubbing to *zhōng wǎn* (RN 12).
   c. *Irregular menstruation*: apply palm rubbing on lower abdomen.

Kneading

Use the thenar, heel of the palm, or finger pulp for a mild, gentle, and slow circular motion on the treatment area, with the desired effect of reaching the subcutaneous tissues. The method of kneading with the thenar is called thenar kneading; kneading with the palm is called palm-heel kneading, and kneading with the finger tip is referred to as finger kneading. Among the three types of kneading, thenar kneading requires the most skill.

Thenar Kneading

1. *Essentials of the maneuver*

   a. The point to apply force is the thenar eminence. The maneuver requires moderate downward pressure with the thumb slightly adducted and the interphalangeal joints naturally flexed. The wrist needs to be relaxed, so that you can coordinate a swinging motion with the wrist and forearm, and drive the thenar to perform a circular kneading movement on the treatment site (see Figure 86). If the practitioner performs the same activity using the heel of the palm, it is known as the palm-heel kneading maneuver.
   b. The action should be flexible with moderate and gentle strength. Avoid causing friction or intensive pressure on the treated area.
   c. The action should follow a certain rhythm with the frequency of 120 to 160 strokes per minute.

2. *Applicable locations*: the whole body, most commonly the head, face, chest, abdomen, limbs, and joints.
3. *Actions*: soothing tendons, unblocking the meridians, dissolving swelling, relieving pain, invigorating blood, dissipating stasis, fortifying the spleen, harmonizing the stomach, comforting the chest, and rectifying qi.

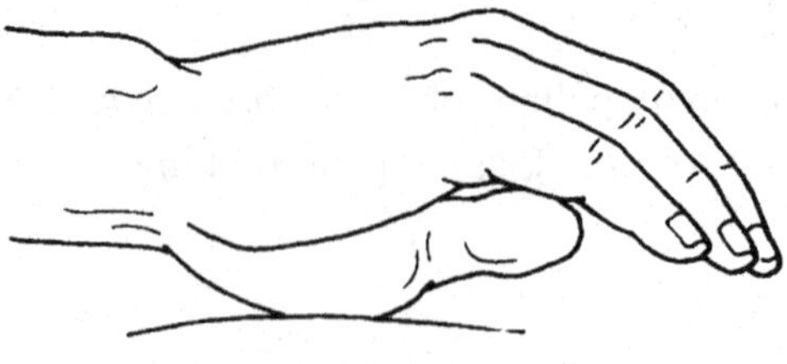

Figure 86 Thenar kneading

4. *Indications*: headache, facial paralysis, chest and abdominal distention and pain, and soft tissue injuries of the four limbs.
5. *Examples*
   a. *Headache and facial paralysis*: apply thenar kneading on the forehead and face.
   b. *Hypochondriac pain*: palm kneading on *zhāngmén* (LR 13), *qīmén* (LR 14), and the affected area.
   c. *Acute soft tissue injury*: apply kneading maneuver surrounding the affected area. At the same time, perform ice *anmo* on the affected site and restrict its movement.

Finger Kneading (*Fig. 87*) The maneuver uses the palm side of the thumb or one finger tip;, the index and middle finger tips together; or the index, middle, and fourth finger tips together to perform gentle massage in a small circular motion. Therefore, finger kneading can be divided into single finger kneading, double finger kneading, and triple finger kneading maneuvers.

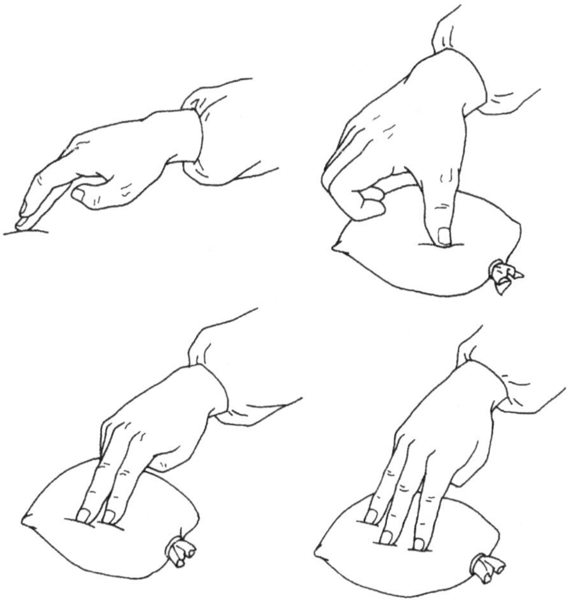

Figure 87 Finger kneading

Clinically, finger kneading is often combined with pressing to form a compound technique named pressure kneading. Single finger kneading can be applied to various parts of the body, while double finger kneading can be used on back *shu* points, in pediatric tui na applying on the lateral side of the chest, the acupoint *rǔgēn* (ST 18), or bilateral *tiānshū* (ST 25). Lastly, triple finger kneading can be used on back *shu* points, or in children with congenital muscular torticollis.

Foulage

Foulage requires the practitioner to use both palms holding a limb or a part of the patient's body, and apply symmetric and opposite force to either twist it quickly back and forth, or perform clockwise circular kneading movements.

It is an auxiliary manipulation in tui na practice, often as an ending maneuver on four limbs, flanks, waist or lower back, with the desired actions of dredging the meridians, regulating qi and blood, and relaxing the muscles. It also varies according to specific body locations.

1. *Foulage on a shoulder* The patient sits in an upright position, with both shoulders and arms relaxed and naturally hanging down. Hold the affected shoulder of the patient with both palms, similar to holding an imaginary ball, and perform foulage with force clockwise for ten to 20 times. It is used to treat frozen shoulder.
2. *Foulage on an upper limb* Have the patient assume the same posture as in (1) above. Use both hands to hold the ipsilateral upper arm of the patient to perform forward-and-backward foulage. Gradually move down from the forearm to the wrist, then quickly go up to start from the axilla again (see Figure 88). Repeat the manipulation three to five times. This maneuver treats *bì* pattern pain of the upper limbs.

   Foulage applied on shoulders and upper limbs can be seen as one maneuver starting from the shoulder and ending at the wrist, or as two separate manipulations. The choice can be made based on clinical need.

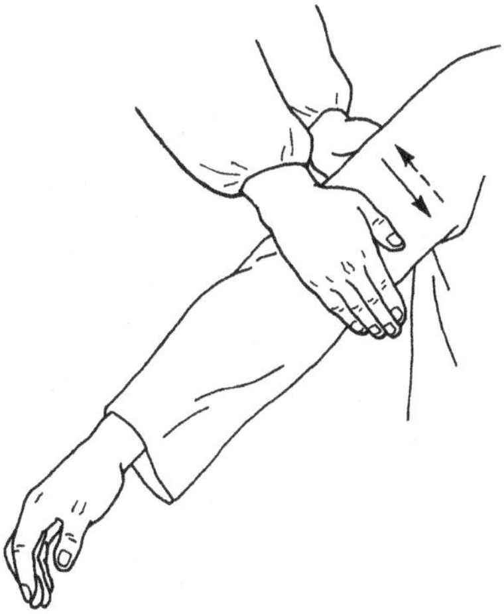

Figure 88 Foulage on an upper limb

3. *Foulage on hypochondria* Have the patient sit upright. Standing at the patient's back, hold the ribcage of the patient from both sides, applying a relatively strong force to perform concurrent front-and-back foulage maneuver along the lateral side, from the ribs to the iliac crests. Repeat three to five times. This maneuver treats sudden hypochondriac burst injury and liver qi stagnation.
4. *Foulage on a lower limb* Have the patient lie supine with the lower limbs slightly bent. Use both your hands to grip the medial and lateral sides, or the anterior and posterior sides of the thigh. Then, apply foulage with a certain level of force, along the leg to gradually reach the knee, calf, and ankle. Continue the operation backwards until the starting point is reached. The maneuver needs to be performed three to five times. It is often used to treat lower extremity pain of *bì* pattern.
5. *Foulage on the lower back* With the patient sitting or prone, stand at his or her back. Place both hands on the back and perform horizontal foulage, top-down from the upper to lower back. Repeat the action three to five times. This maneuver is meant to treat lower back pain.

Essentials of the Maneuver

a. The movement extent of both hands should be equal and even with symmetrical forces.
b. The frequency of foulage can be fast, but the transition on the body surface should be gradual.
c. The strength applied when gripping the limb or other parts of the body using both hands should be appropriate. Foulage would be difficult to perform if you grip too tight or too loose.

Everyday Exercises

1. What are the similarities and differences between the rubbing and kneading maneuvers?
2. Memorize the clinical application of rubbing, kneading, and foulage.

DAY 3

TWIDDLING

Use the palmar side of the tips of thumb and index finger to grasp the treatment area, and twist it quickly with moderate strength, similar to twiddling threads.

1. *Essentials of the maneuver*
   a. The action should be agile, gentle, flexible, and persistent at the speed of about 200 times per minute.
   b. The force should be symmetrical and even, and not rigid and sluggish.
2. *Applicable locations*: small distal joints on four limbs.
3. *Actions*: moving qi, invigorating blood, resolving swelling, dissolving blood stasis, and benefiting the joints.
4. *Indications*: rheumatoid arthritis, inter phalangeal joint injury.
5. *Examples*

Rheumatoid hand: twiddle the troubled inter phalangeal joint with alternating clockwise and counter-clockwise motion. It can be combined with spreading and passive joint flexion and extension.

Pushing

Pushing is one of the main tui na manipulation techniques. However, a number of movements with different names were developed because of historical reasons and various academic schools. According to its original meaning, "pushing [is the action of using], one finger to push without returning..." In other words, the technique uses the thumb, the palm, or other parts of the body to apply force on certain acupoints or an area of the body, pushing along a straight or curved line in one direction.

In adult tui na, the flat pushing maneuver is dominant, while there are many kinds of pushing maneuvers in pediatric tui na, such as straight, bilateral, and rotating pushing. Pediatric pushing manipulations will be dealt with in a separate unit in this book.

In the adult pushing method, flat pushing with the thumb is named flat thumb pushing; pushing with the palm is called flat palm pushing; and pushing with the fist is called flat fist pushing; pushing with the tip of the elbow is known as flat elbow pushing. Flat pushing is the maneuver that pushes in a straight line in one direction, allowing a bigger surface area to absorb the force, in relative slow motion. The intent is to promote the circulation of qi and blood.

Flat thumb pushing With the thumb pulp as the force-applying point in the site receiving the treatment, and the remaining fingers close to each other to enhance the force of the thumb, the clinician pushes from point A to point B along a meridian line or parallel to the muscle fiber. Generally, it can be repeated five to ten times or even more. (See Figure 89.)

1. *Essentials of the maneuver*
   a. The force and speed used in pushing from points A to B should be even.
   b. Along the path from points A to B with the pushing maneuver, if there is a need to increase the stimulation on a given acupoint, you can combine it with other maneuvers such as pressure kneading or pressing.
   c. Apply a small amount of ointment such as wintergreen cream on areas to be treated; the ointment should lubricate the skin, facilitate

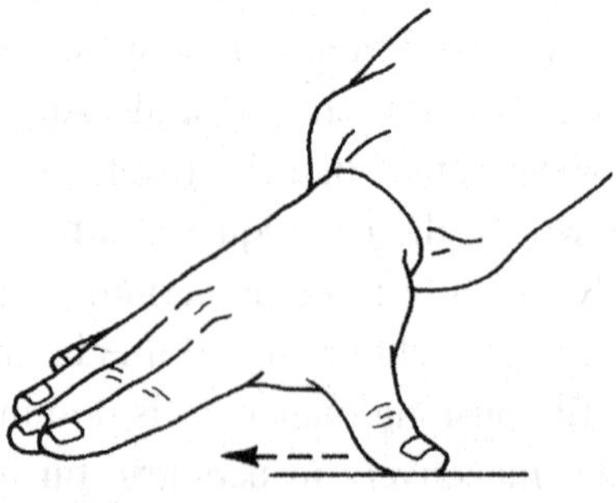

Figure 89 Flat thumb pushing

the operation, and prevent the skin from breaking owing to the friction of pushing.

2. *Applicable locations*: limbs, shoulder, back, waist, hip, chest, and abdomen.
3. *Actions*: unblocking meridians and collaterals, adjusting tendons, dissipating nodules, invigorating blood, resolving stasis.
4. *Indications*: pain in the neck, shoulder, waist and legs, abdominal distention and pain.
5. *Examples*

   a. *Làozhěn (acute stiff neck)*: apply flat thumb pushing on the spasmodic trapezius.
   b. *Abdominal distention and fullness*: apply flat thumb pushing at *zhōngwǎn* (RN 12), a common technique in pediatric tui na.

Flat palm pushing Use the heel of the palm to apply force on areas receiving the treatment, and push from points A to B. If you need to increase the pressure, put the other hand on top of the original palm and slowly progress. Generally the operation needs to be repeated five to ten times. (See Figure 90.)

1. *Essentials of the maneuver*: same as for flat thumb pushing.
2. *Applicable locations*: back, waist, chest, abdomen, lower extremities, and more.
3. *Actions*: soothing tendons, unblocking the collaterals, dissolving food accumulations, and regulating the center.
4. *Indications*: back and waist pain, food retention, and constipation.
5. *Examples*

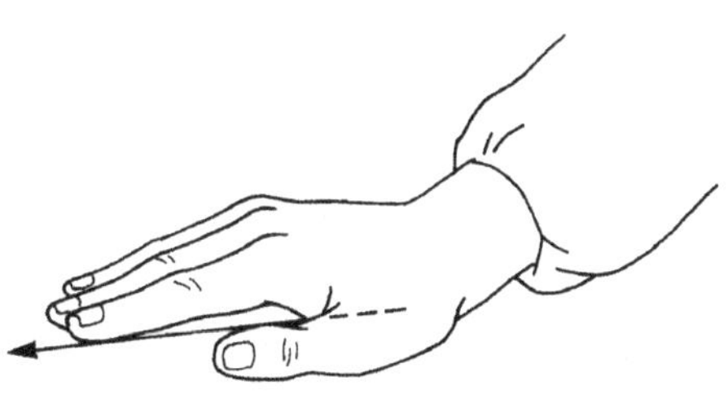

Figure 90 Flat palm pushing maneuver

a. *Lower back soreness and pain*: apply flat palm pushing over fascia on the back.
b. *Food accumulation*: apply flat palm pushing on the upper abdominal area.

Flat fist pushing Make a fist with the proximal interphalangeal joints of the index, middle, ring and little fingers to apply forces on areas to be treated, and push from point A to B. Due to the intensity of stimulation caused by this maneuver, generally, it only needs to be operated three to five times or less.(See Figure 91.)

1. *Essentials of the maneuver*: same as for flat thumb pushing.
2. *Applicable locations*: lower back, buttocks, and four limbs.
3. *Actions*: rectifying tendons, relieving spasms, invigorating blood, and stopping pain.
4. *Indications*: pain of wind-damp *bì* pattern, and muscle strain.
5. *Examples*

Pain of wind-damp bì pattern: use flat fist pushing technique to stimulate the affected area.

Flat elbow pushing Use the olecranon of the ulna to apply pressure on the treatment site and push from point A to B. It should only be performed one to two times owing to its extremely strong stimulation. (See Figure 92.)

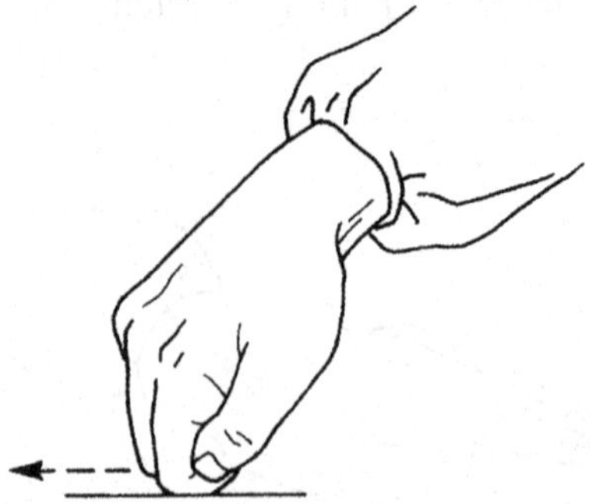

Figure 91 Flat fist pushing maneuver

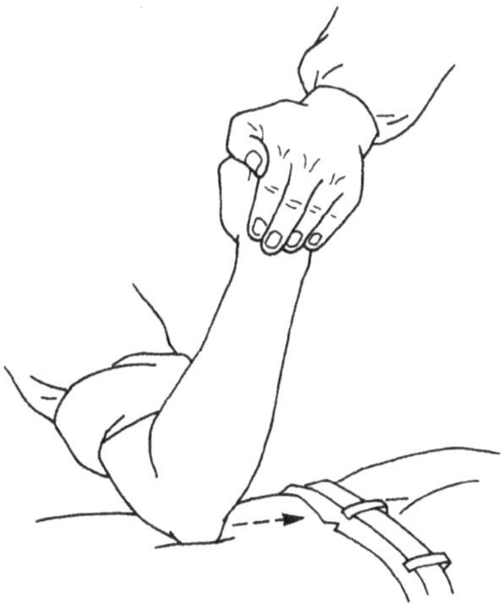

Figure 92 Flat elbow pushing maneuver

1. *Essentials of the maneuver*: same as for flat thumb pushing.
2. *Applicable locations*: along the bladder meridian on the back.
3. *Actions*: rectifying tendons, invigorating blood, dispelling wind, and dissipating cold.
4. *Indications*: back rheumatism with decreased sensitivity, and ankylosing spondy litis.
5. *Examples*

A*nkylosing spondylitis*: gently apply the flat elbow pushing maneuver bilaterally on the sacro spinalis along the spine.

Scrubbing

The scrubbing maneuver involves the palm being placed firmly on the skin, and pressure applied downwards, with repetitive top-down or left-to-right scrubbing movements performed in a straight line. This maneuver is stopped once it generates a warm sensation on the skin. The technique can be divided into palm scrubbing, thenar scrubbing, and lateral scrubbing (see Figure 93).

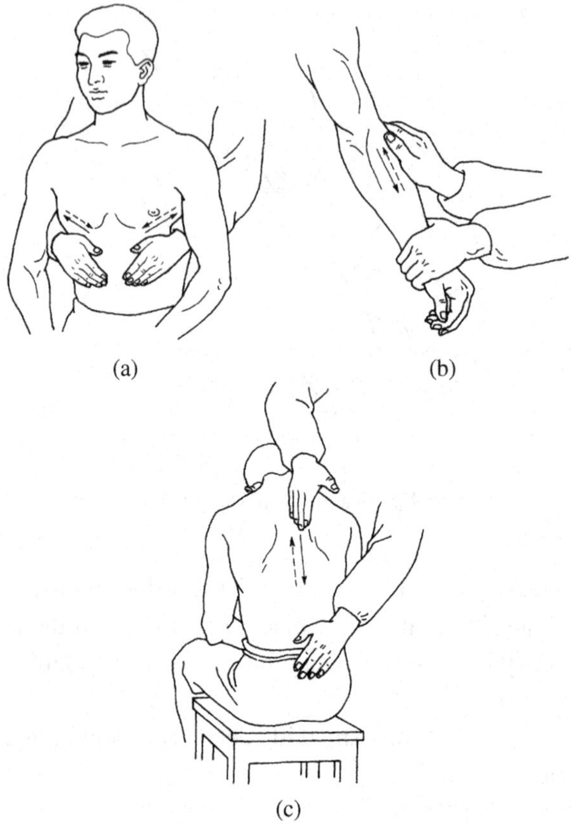

a. 掌擦法	-	Palm Scrubbing
b. 鱼际擦法	-	Thenar Scrubbing
c. 侧擦法	-	Lateral Scrubbing

Figure 93 Scrubbing

1. *Essentials of the maneuver*

   a. Ask the patient to relax the upper limbs and extend the wrist naturally. Use your palm, thenar, or hypothenar as the focal point to work on the treatment area. The active movement of the upper arm should lead the hand to perform up-and-down or left-to-right scrubs back and forth. The action should not be skewed, and the movement of the hand should not be driven by swinging the body.

b. The distance of the scrubbing should be great enough, with the strokes being similar to dragging a saw back and forth without pause. If the operating distance is too short, there is the danger of scrubbing the skin off; on the other hand, too many intermittent pauses will affect heat generation and penetration, thus, discounting the therapeutic effects.
c. The pressure should be even and moderate; make sure that the skin does not fold as a result of too much friction.
d. Do not rush through the maneuver. Breathe evenly, making sure you do not hold your breath, as sudden inhaling or exhaling may damage the internal qi movement.
e. The frequency is generally about 100 times per minute.

2. *Applicable locations*: the whole body. Palm scrubbing is mostly applied to the chest, abdomen, and hypochondriac area. Thenar scrubbing is mainly used on limbs, especially the upper limbs. Lateral scrubbing is used for the back and lumbo sacral areas.
3. *Actions*: fortifying the spleen, harmonizing the stomach, warming yang qi, enhancing kidney yang, expelling wind, invigorating blood, dissipating stasis, and relieving pain.
4. *Indications*: feebleness, weakness, abdominal distention and pain, irregular menstruation, pain of wind-damp *bì* pattern on the lower back.
5. *Examples*

   a. *Feebleness and powerlessness*: scrubbing *dumai*, *shènshū* (BL 23), and *yǒngquán* (KI 1).
   b. *Irregular menstruation*: scrubbing the *bāliào* (BL 31 to 34) and lower abdomen.

Precautions

1. Keep the treatment room warm to prevent the patient from catching cold.
2. Apply a small amount of oil-based lubricant to protect the skin against abrasions prior to the treatment, since the scrubbing maneuver creates friction on the body surface

3. Scrubbing in clinical practice is often the last maneuver. Usually, there will not be another maneuver used on the same area after the completion of scrubbing, so as to avoid skin damage. However, moist heat patches, i.e., fomentation, can be applied after scrubbing to enhance the efficacy.

Everyday Exercises

1. How many pushing maneuvers are introduced in this section? What are the essentials of the pushing maneuver?
2. What are the essentials of the scrubbing maneuver?

DAY 4

SMEARING

Use the surface of the thumb pulp to cast up-and-down, left-and-right, or curvy movements, either one-way or back and forth.

1. *Essentials of the maneuver*
   a. The pulp of the thumb or both thumbs should attach to the surface of the treatment area tightly. The other four fingers should support the thumb pulp for firm strokes.
   b. The action of both hands should be coordinated and flexible with even strength.
2. *Applicable locations*: head, face, chest, abdomen, dorsum of hands and feet.
3. *Actions*: opening sensory orifices, calming the *shén* (spirit), improving vision, unblocking the meridians and collaterals.
4. *Indications*: headache, insomnia, myopia, colds, chest tightness and fullness, numbness in the hands.
5. *Examples*
   a. *Headache*: apply the smearing maneuver on the forehead, pressing *lièquē* (LU 7) and kneading *bǎihuì* (DU 20);
   b. *Numbness of the hand and palm*: apply the smearing maneuver on the dorsum of the hand, while twiddling the fingers of various joints.

Scattering Sweeping

This maneuver uses back-and-forth strokes with the fingers to create some level of friction on the temporal area of the patient.

1. *Essentials of the maneuver*
   a. The posture of the hand: the thumb should be extended outwards, and the four fingers are close together and slightly flexed (see Figure 94a).

b. Use the radial side of the thumb as a focal point to apply the force, at about the location of *shàoshāng* (LU 11). Push back and forth along the straight line from the front hairline to *tàiyáng*(EX-HN 5) with the four finger tips rubbing back-and-forth along the curvy path of the gallbladder meridian, i.e., between the auricular edge and the mastoid process of the ear.

c. During the operation, the wrist should be slightly dorsiflexed, with a small range of swinging from side to side, and the elbow performing mild flexion and extension. The patient usually sits while the therapist stands facing the patient and holding one side of the head of the patient to maintain the stability, so that the scattering sweeping maneuver can be applied with the other hand on the ipsilateral temporal area. The treatment can be applied on both sides, each with 30 to 50 back-and-forth manipulations. (See Figure 94b.)

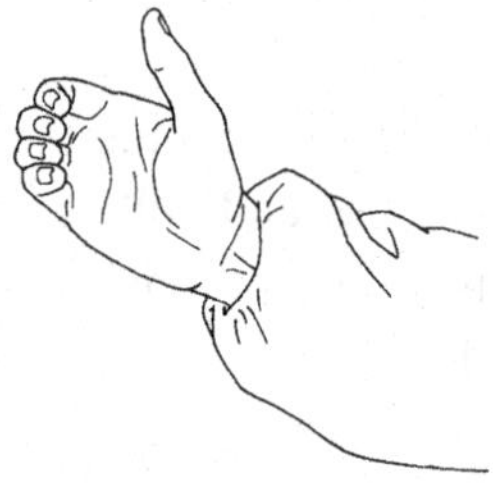

(a)

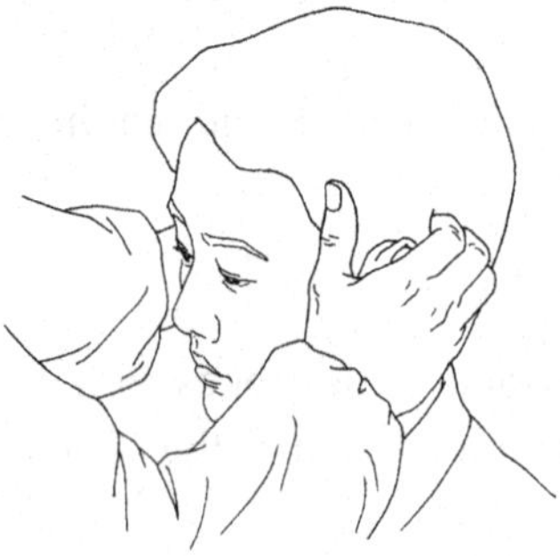

(b)

a. 手势	-	The Hand Posture
b. 动作	-	Manipulations

Figure 94 Scattering sweeping

d. The action should be stable enough to prevent the patient's head from swinging when applying the maneuver.
e. The thumb and fingers should cling to the scalp to avoid pulling the hair roots and causing pain.

2. *Applicable locations*: tempora.
3. *Actions*: calming liver yang and sending it downward, refreshing the brain, calming the *shén*, expeling wind, and scattering cold.
4. *Indications*: headache, dizziness, high blood pressure, insomnia.
5. *Examples*

a. *Hypertension*: scattering sweeping maneuver on the tempora, pressure kneading *bǎihuì* (DU 20), and pushing *qiáogōng* (bridge arch), the area from *yìfēng* (SI 17) to *quēpén* (ST 12).
b. *Migraine*: scattering sweeping on the tempora, finger kneading *lièquē* (LU 7).

Grasping

The maneuver requires the thumb to apply opposing forces against the index and middle fingers, or all other fingers, then lift and pinch, or knead and pinch a certain area or acupoint. Grasping is a common technique in tui na. Clinically, there are three kinds of grasping. Three-finger grasping uses the thumb, index finger and middle finger while five-finger grasping uses the thumb to act against there maining fingers.

1. *Essentials of the maneuver*

a. The power has to come from the grasp with the opposing forces of the thumb and other fingers; then the power of the lifting pinch or kneading pinch of the muscle should be gradually increased and decreased alternately and continuously in a consistent rhythm.
b. The wrist should be relaxed to allow flexibility of the fingers to work in a coordinated manner while applying forces on the area being treated.
c. Start gently, then gradually increase the intensity to provide a balanced stimulation. Nipping with finger tips should be avoided.

d. The stimulation of grasping is relatively strong. In especially the three-finger grasping maneuver, it is often followed by kneading to mitigate the stimulation.

2. *Applicable locations*

   a. *Three-finger grasping*: mainly in neck and *jiānjǐng* (GB 21);
   b. *Five-finger grasping*: mainly used for the head and limbs.

3. *Actions*: dredging the meridians and collaterals, releasing the exterior, promoting sweating, tranquilizing and relieving pain, opening the orifices, and refreshing the *shén*.
4. *Indications*: neck stiffness and pain, muscle aches, headache, nasal congestion.
6. *Examples*

   a. *Exogenous headaches*: grasping the five meridians on the head, grasping *fēngchí* (GB 20), scattering sweeping maneuver.
   b. *Làozhěn* (*acute stiff neck*): grasping *fēngchí*, pressure kneading spasmodic trapezius, finger kneading *lièquē* (LU 7);
   c. *Abdominal pain*: grasping *zúsānlǐ* (ST 36), pressing *píshū* (BL 20) and *wèishū* (BL 21), rubbing abdomen.

Five-finger grasping When applying the maneuver to the head, it is called grasping the five head *jīng*. First of all, have the patient sit in an upright position. Stand on the rear side of the patient, one hand holding his or her forehead, and the fingers of your other hand fanning out. Use the pulp of the fingers to apply force on the surface of the head. The middle finger works on *du mai*, index and ring finger on both sides of foot *taiyang* bladder meridian, the thumb and the little finger on both sides of foot *shaoyang* gallbladder meridians. That is how it gets the name of "grasping the five meridians". All five fingers should apply pressure at the same time, starting from the front hairline, grasping the scalp and releasing it right away. Repeat the grasping and releasing actions and gradually move the fingers toward the posterior side of the head. When the hand reaches the occipital area, the fingers should gradually transition and get close together. Then, the maneuver is shifted to three-finger grasping, and finally ends at *fēngchí*. It can be repeated three to five times, and performed with the right and left hand alternately.

Shaking

Shaking is the maneuver of holding the distal aspect of the ipsilateral limb with a single hand or both hands, and using slight forces to shake it up and down continuously with a small amplitude, making the joints and muscles of the affected limb have the sense of loosening up. Clinically, shaking is often used as an adjunct or ending maneuver. It can be applied to either the upper or lower limbs.

Shaking an upper limb With the patient sitting and upper limbs relaxed, stand at the anterolateral side of the patient with your upper body slightly forward, holding the patient's wrist — not too tightly — with both hands. Then, slowly lift the affected limb anterolaterally to about 60° to 70°, and shake it up and down continuously with a mild amplitude, so the wave-like shape of the arm is transitioned from the distal wrist gradually to the proximal shoulder (see Figure 95). Alternatively, use a palm to hold the ipsilateral shoulder, with the other palm holding the distal wrist, and shake in an up-and-down direction continuously with a small amplitude.

Shaking a lower extremity Have the patient supine and the lower limbs relaxed. Stand on the rear side of the patient's feet, each hand holding one side of the ankles. The next step is to lift the patient's legs slowly off the treatment table a distance of 20 to 30 cm, then shake both legs concurrently with a small amplitude in an up-and-down motion, creating a comforting feeling to the entire lower extremities. The maneuver can also be coordinated with internal or external rotation. For tall and heavy individuals, shaking may be performed on one leg at a time.

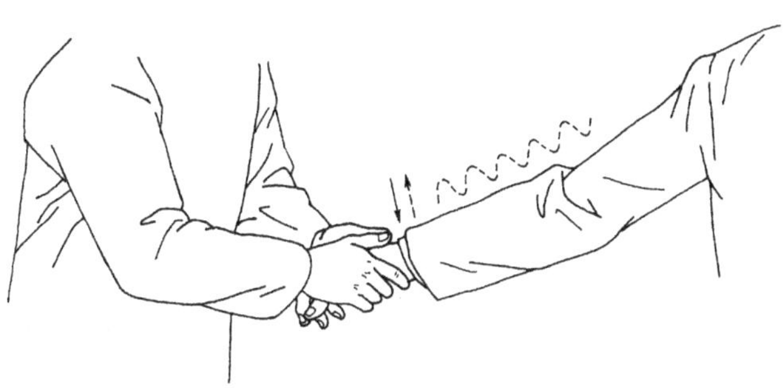

Figure 95 Shaking an upper limb

1. *Essentials of the maneuver*

   a. The force should be applied naturally at a high frequency with a small amplitude, generally about three to five centimeters. The frequency for the upper limbs is 200 times per minute while the frequency for the lower limbs is 100 times per minute.
   b. Ask the patient to relax the limbs to accommodate a successful treatment.

2. *Applicable locations*: four limbs.
3. *Actions*: dredging the vessels and collaterals, benefiting the joints.
4. *Indications*: shoulder, arm, and leg pain.
5. *Examples*

Shoulder periarthritis (frozen shoulder): foulage on the shoulder, shaking the upper limb, and other maneuvers on the shoulder.

Everyday Exercises

1. What is the scattering sweeping maneuver? What are the essentials to master it? What diseases can it treat?
2. Try to memorize the clinical applications of the smearing, grasping, and shaking maneuvers.

DAY 5

LATERAL STRIKING WITH PALMS CLASPED

With the palms clasped and fingers natural separated, this maneuver uses the radial aspect of the hypothenars and little fingers to strike the treatment site, and is often used as a muscle relaxing or ending manipulation.

1. *Essentials of the maneuver*

With the palms clasped, both forearms should rotate to create the driving force for the hypothenar ulnar little fingers to strike the treatment area. Because the fingers are naturally apart, they will make a rhythmic sound while hitting each other.

2. *Applicable locations*: the back, waist, and four limbs.
3. *Actions*: soothing tendons, unblocking the collaterals, and dissolving fatigue.
4. *Indications*: spasms and pain of the back muscles, wind-damp pain of *bì* pattern.
5. *Examples*

Lower back pain: at the end of the tui na session, use clasped palms striking on the back from the top to the lumbo sacral area to loosen up spasmodic muscles.

Pecking

This manipulation needs to have the fingers flexed and separated from each other, so it can use the flexion and extension of the wrist as the source of power, and the tips as focal points. Following a certain rhythm, make brisk strikes at the site being treated, as if your fingers are birds pecking at grains (see Figure 96). This maneuver may be performed with a single hand or both hands; usually, it is performed with both hands.

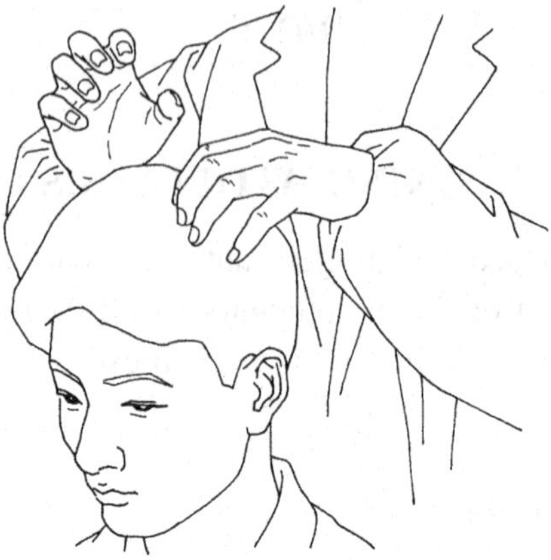

Figure 96 Pecking

1. *Essentials of the maneuver*

    a. Your wrist and fingers need to be relaxed. The main operating power should be from the wrist.
    b. The technique should be agile, flexible, and rhythmic with both hands in coordination.

2. *Applicable locations*: the head.
3. *Actions*: calming the *shén*, refreshing the brain, promoting the circulation of qi and blood.
4. *Indications*: headache, insomnia, neurasthenia.
5. *Examples*

Headache with insomnia: often, after applying other maneuvers such as grasping the five meridians on the head, scattering sweeping, and pressure kneading *lièquē* (LU 7) and *shénmén* (HT 7), it may be used as a supplemental maneuver to the whole head from the front to the back, and from the top to the sides.

Patting

This maneuver requires fingers naturally close together, and metacarpophalangeal joints slightly flexed to make the palm concaved. Then, use the palm to slap the treatment site following a certain rhythm (see Figure 97).

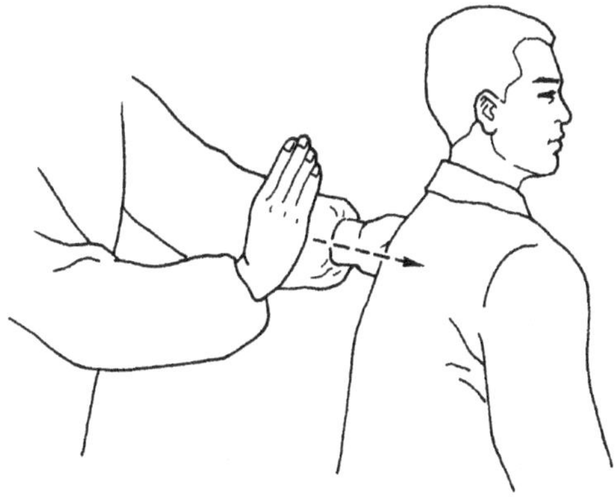

Figure 97 Patting

1. *Essentials of the maneuver*

    a. With fingers close together and palm concaved, the maneuver takes advantage of air vibration, so that a rhythmic and brisk patting sound can be heard.
    b. With the main force coming from the wrist, patting should be flexible and smooth.
    c. Generally, this manipulation can be repeated three to five times. For those with decreased skin sensation, you can perform the maneuver until the skin turns pinky red.

2. *Applicable locations*: shoulder, back, lumbo sacral area, lateral side of the vastus and legs.
3. *Actions*: moving qi, invigorating blood, relaxing tendons, and unblocking the meridians.
4. *Indications*: rheumatism, heaviness sensation with numbness, muscle spasms.
5. *Examples*

Rheumatic pain of the lower back: after applying local tui na and pressure kneading on *wěizhōng* (BL 40), smear a small amount of wintergreen oil on the lower back, then perform top-down patting until the skin turns pinky red.

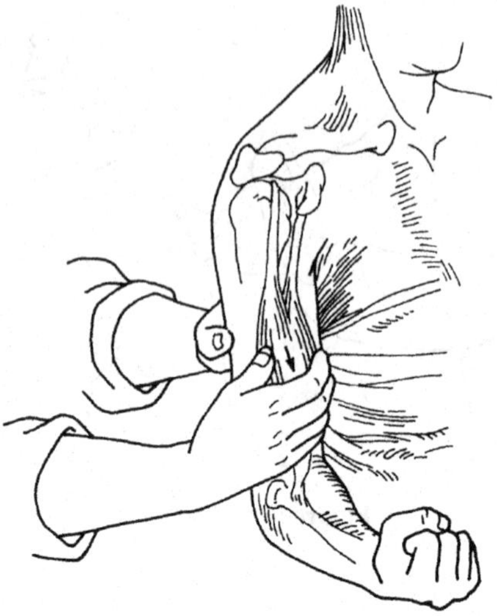

Figure 98 Plucking

Plucking

This maneuver uses the thumb to deeply press the treatment site and pluck the subcutaneous tissues back and forth, as if plucking a string (see Figure 98).The maneuver has a wide range of uses and can treat all kinds of pain if we have a good grasp of it.

1. *Essentials of the maneuver*
   a. The depth of pressure from the thumb should be in accordance with the depth of the affected tissue, such as the muscle, tendon or ligament. The direction of the plucking should be perpendicular to the diseased tissue. Continue to perform the maneuver even when the patient feels adistended soreness or ache, as the pressure of the thumb is getting to the spot. If the force of one thumb is insufficient, overlap the other thumb on top of it to perform the plucking maneuver.
   b. This manipulation is a strong stimulus to deep tissues, so brisk kneading and rubbing techniques need to be applied afterwards to alleviate the painful response.
2. *Applicable locations*: limbs, neck, back, and waist.

3. *Actions*: releasing spasms, relieving pain, and loosening adhesions.
4. *Indications*: chronic soft tissue damage and pain, abnormal joint range of motion.
5. *Examples*

   a. *Lào zhěn*: plucking at the tender point, supplemented with passive movements of the neck such as flexion and extension, rotation, and lateral flexion.
   b. *Tennis elbow*: in addition to local manipulations, plucking can be applied at the tendon of the tender point.

Everyday Exercises

1. Try to memorize the clinical applications of lateral striking with palms clasped, pecking and patting maneuvers.
2. What is the definition of the plucking maneuver? What are the essentials of the maneuver? What diseases can it be used to treat?

DAY 6

ROTATING

This manipulation uses one hand to hold or support the proximal joint of the limb to be treated, and the other hand to hold the distal joint of the same limb and rotate it gently in slow motion, either clockwise or counter-clockwise. (See Figure 99.)

The rotating maneuver is one of the common tui na techniques; it also can be seen as a passive activity. It is used to prevent and treat illnesses such as joint pain and soreness, or motor dysfunction.

Since the method can be widely used on various joints of the spine and limbs, it is necessary to address some important key points for improving the accuracy of the manipulation and avoid iatrogenic trauma owing to passive movements.

First, make sure the direction and range are in accordance with the physiological characteristics while the rotating manipulation is performed. At the same time, it should be in the range of what the patient can tolerate. Start with mild movements and gradually increase the range.

Second, the forces should be gentle and steady with even and slow speed, while the action need to be suitable for the given circumstance. Different parts of the body has different requirements regarding how rotating manipulation needs to be operated, which is described in the following paragraphs.

1. *Neck rotating* The patient sits with neck relaxed. Stand on the posterior lateral side of the patient, supporting the head of the patient with one hand, and with the other hand, lift up the lower jaw. With the hands coordinated, slowly rotate the head in the opposite direction, either clockwise or counter-clockwise for three to five times.

   The maneuver is often used to treat *laozhen* (acute stiff neck), cervical spondylosis, pain or soft tissue strain of the neck, and restricted movements.
2. *Shoulder rotating* From a safety perspective, we are introducing an elbow-supported shoulder rotating method. Have the patient in a

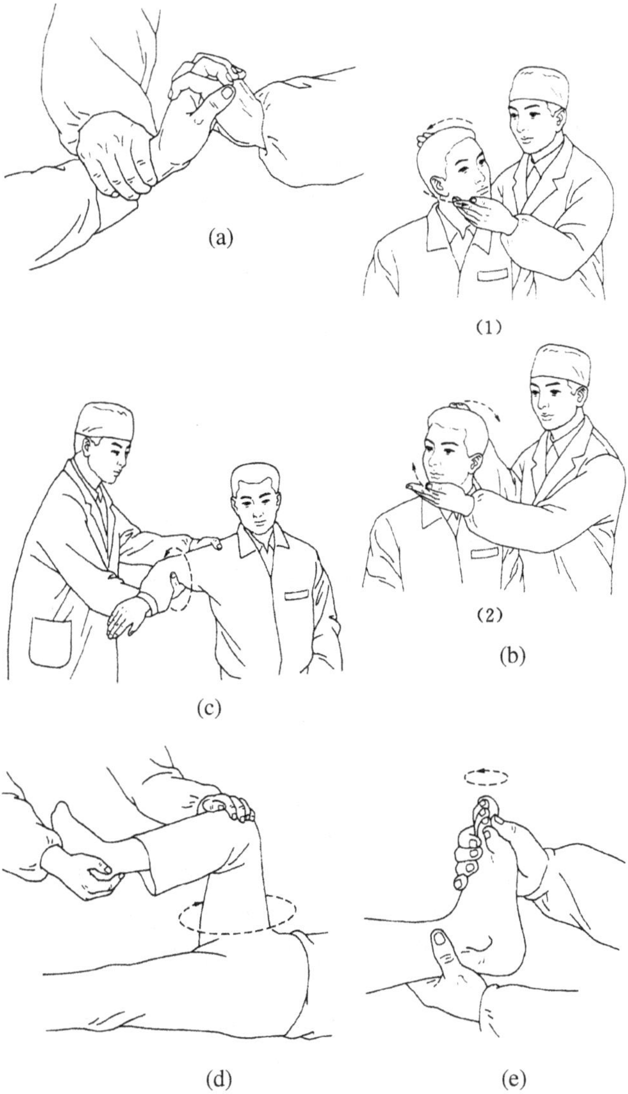

a. 腕关节摇法	-	Wrist Rotating Maneuver
b. 颈项部摇法	-	Neck Rotating Maneuver
c. 肩关节摇法	-	Shoulder Rotating Maneuver
d. 髋关节摇法	-	Hip Rotating Maneuver
e. 踝关节摇法	-	Ankle Rotating Maneuver

Figure 99 Rotating Maneuver

sitting position with shoulders relaxed and ipsilateral elbow flexed. Stand on the lateral side of the patient, with middle stand position and upper body slightly leaning forward. Hold the upper shoulder of the patient with one hand, and support the ipsilateral elbow with your other hand, so that the arm of the patient rests on the forearm of the practitioner. Then, slowly rotate the shoulder clockwise or counter-clockwise.

This manipulation is often used for conditions like shoulder periarthritis, injury of the shoulder tendons, and shoulder fracture sequelae.

3. *Elbow rotating* The patient sits with elbow semi-flexed. Using one hand to support the elbow, and your other hand to hold the wrist of the affected limb, rotate the elbow clockwise or counter-clockwise. This maneuver is often used to treat tennis elbow and elbow fracture sequelae.
4. *Wrist rotating* Ask the patient to sit up or lie supine. Stand on the affected side, and with one hand holding the proximal wrist of the ipsilateral limb, and the other hand holding the palm, rotate the wrist clockwise or counter-clockwise. This maneuver is commonly used to treat soft tissue injury and fracture sequelae of the wrist.
5. *Rotating of the metacarpophalangeal joint* Ask the patient to sit up or lie supine. With one hand holding the ipsilateral palm, and the other hand holding the ipsilateral finger, rotate the metacarpophalangeal joint clockwise or counter-clockwise. This maneuver is commonly used to treat finger tenosynovitis and rheumatoid arthritis.
6. *Waist rotating* With the patient sitting and waist relaxed, sit posterior to the patient, one hand holding one side of the patient's waist, thumb pressing at the middle of the waist, and four fingers on the hypochondriac area. At the same time, support the opposite shoulder with the other hand. Then, use both hands in coordination to slowly rotate the waist.

Another waist rotating maneuver is to ask the patient to lie in a prone position with the lower limbs straight and relaxed. Use one hand to hold the waist, and, using your other forearm to support the distal anterior aspect of both thighs, lift up the thighs. Then, perform clockwise or counter-clockwise rotation to the hyperextended waist. This method requires a fair amount of physical power, and is only used in the recovering stage of waist movement disorders. Generally, waist rotating can be performed in a sitting position as previously described. This maneuver is commonly used to treat lower back soreness, pain, stiffness, and restricted range of motion.

7. *Hip rotating* Have the patient lie supine with the lower extremities naturally relaxed. Stand on the ipsilateral side of the patient with a hand supporting the anterior aspect of the patient's knee, while your other hand holds the heel or ankle. First, make the hip and knee flexed to about 90°. Then, rotate the patient's hip clockwise or counter-clockwise by coordinating both hands.
   Another way of hip rotating is to have the patient lie in the prone position, with lower extremities naturally relaxed. Stand on the affected side, with one hand pressing down the buttocks. Place your other hand at the distal end anterior to the thigh and lift up the lower limb, then rotate the hyperextended hip clockwise or counter-clockwise.
   Hip rotating is often performed to treat conditions like low back and leg pain and restricted range of motion of the hip.
8. *Ankle rotating* The patient is supine with the lower limbs naturally straightened. Stand at the feet of the patient, holding the heel with one hand, and the toes with the other hand. Then, coordinate both hands and rotate the affected ankle clockwise or counterclockwise.

Ankle rotating is commonly used to treat conditions such as pain caused by injury and fracture sequelae of the ankle.

Back Carrying

Carry the patient back-to-back. The feet of the patient should be off the ground, so the lumbar spine can be stretched and extended. This maneuver is also known as the back-to-back carrying method (see Figure 100).

Essentials of the Maneuver

Your patient and you should stand back to back. Spread your feet apart, about a shoulder width, and, using your elbows to hook on to the patient's elbow fossa, tightly hook on to the patient's arms. Then, bend your knees

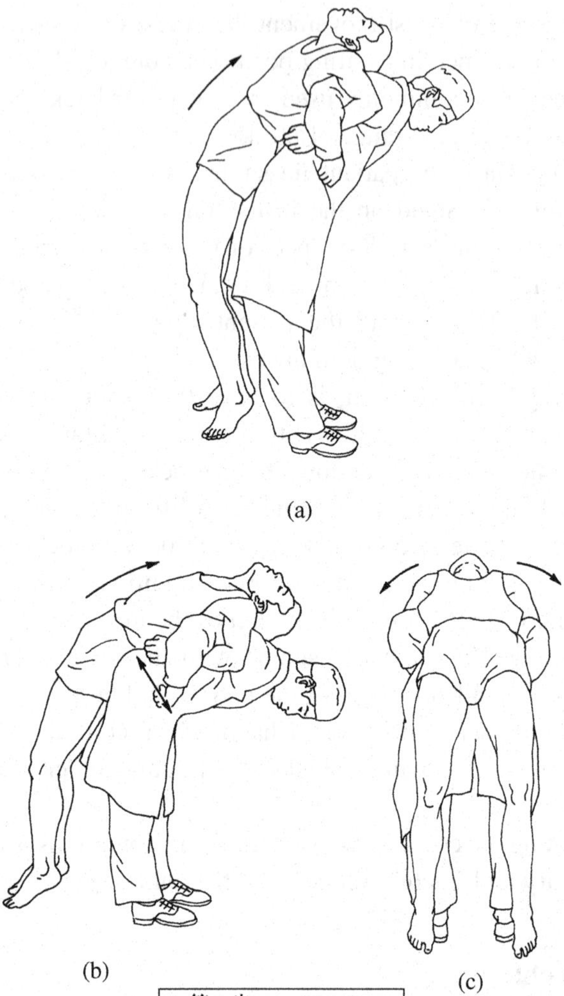

a. 第一步	-	Step One
b. 第二步	-	Step Two
c. 第三步	-	Step Three

Figure 100 Back carrying

and lean forward, flexing your hips, and carrying the patient on your back till his feet is lifted off the ground. At this moment, the patients should raise his head and back, and lean on your back. Throughout this maneuver, the patient should keep his arms hooked tightly and relax. What you are doing is using the patient's own weight to stretch the patient's lumbar spine. Finally, shake your body side to side or straighten up your hips to correct dislocations of small joints.

This maneuver can ease lumbar muscle spasms and restore dislocation of the lumbar joints. It is commonly used to treat functional disorders of the lumbar joints, acute lumbar sprain, and a herniated lumbar disc.

Rolling

Rolling is the main maneuver of the rolling tui na school. It is characterized by a large contact area on the body surface, and strong, yet fairly gentle, stimulation. It is mainly used to treat diseases of the locomotor and peripheral nervous systems.

Beginners and self-learners may find a certain degree of difficulty in trying to master the rolling maneuver. However, because of its dramatic treatment effect, it is necessary to cover it in this book. The manipulation requires a great deal of coordination and is composed of two parts: rotation of the forearm, and flexion and extension of the wrist. The parts of the body applying the forces include the hypothenar muscle and the dorsal part of the fourth and fifth metacarpal area.

1. *Essentials of the maneuver*

   a. Forearm rotation should be concordant with wrist flexion and extension. In other words, upon the pronation of the forearm, the wrist must be extended with the hypothenar muscle as the focal site. Upon the supination of the forearm, the wrist should be flexed with the dorsal aspect of the fourth and fifth metacarpal joints as the focal point. Therefore, the maneuver creates a continuous back-and-forth movement on the body surface with a frequency of 120 to 160 repetitions per minute. (See Figure 101.)
   b. Your body should be straight. Do not bend the back or the waist, or shake your body.
   c. The shoulder should hang naturally, and the upper arm and the chest should maintain a distance of 10 cm. Do not swing the upper arms.
   d. The wrist has to relax, and its flexion and extension should total up to about 120° (about 80° for flexion, and 40° for extension).

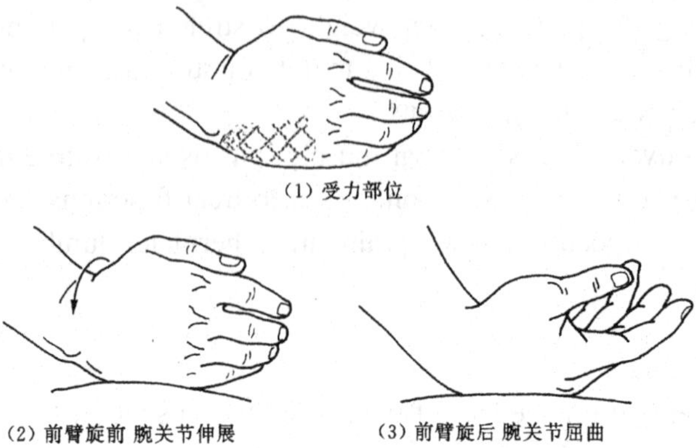

Figure 101 Rolling

  e. The key to the rolling maneuver is the word "rolling."Avoid dragging the hand back and forth.
  f. All fingers need to be naturally relaxed; they should never be intentionally separated nor clenched.

2. *Applicable locations*: muscular areas on the body such as the nape of the neck, shoulders, back, waist, hips and limbs.
3. *Actions*: soothing tendons, invigorating blood, releasing spasmodic pain, loosening adhesions, and benefiting the joints.
4. *Indications*: soreness and pain owing to rheumatism, skin numbness, paralysis, and motor dysfunction.
5. *Examples*

  a. *Lower back pain*: mainly apply rolling on the sacrospinalis.
  b. *Frozen shoulder*: mainly use the rolling maneuver with focus on the deltoid, supplemented by the passive movement of various joints.
  c. *Sciatica*: apply the rolling method along the bladder meridian from hips to the femoral and popliteal area, posterior lateral aspect of the leg, then all the way down to the heel and dorsum of the feet, and supplemented by the pressing of the acupoints and passive movements.

Everyday Exercises

1. Try to memorize the technique of the rotating maneuver on shoulders, elbows, wrists, hips, knees, and ankles.
2. What is the rolling maneuver and what are its essentials? What are the actions and indications of this maneuver?

WEEK 4

Day 1

Subject 2 —Tui Na Treatment for Adults

Headache

One of the chief complaints the patient may have as a subjective symptom is headache, which can be the result of many diseases. The etiology of headache is fairly complex; therefore, we must take the symptom of headache very seriously, and be clear about the priorities in order to avoid misdiagnosis.

Tui na is inappropriate for the following conditions: cerebral abscess, brain tumor, acute stage of cerebrovascular accident, cerebral contusion, and acute period of intracranial hematoma. On the other hand, it has obvious treatment effects for vascular headaches such as migraine, muscle tension headache, and headache due to the common cold.

Migraine

Migraine headache is a type of vascular headache where the patient suffers periodic attacks on the temporal aspect of the head. There are three characteristics: sudden onset of pain on the lateral side of the head, automatic remission or without sequelae after being treated, and customary recurrence accompanied by painless intermittent periods.

It has been proven that the onset of migraine is related to intracranial and extracranial vascular contraction and relaxation. The biphasic change in blood vessels begins within tracranial vasoconstriction causing clinical prodrome, followed by extracranial vascular relaxation, accompanied by unbearable pulsating pain on the lateral side of the head.

Migraine is closely related with the endocrine system, often starting in adolescence, and gradually becomes less severe or stops after menopause. Migraine disappears in the majority of women of childbearing age after three months of pregnancy, and recurs after the delivery. Migraine can be triggered by factors such as environmental changes, external stimulation, physical fatigue, mental stress, anxiety, and lack of sleep.

Clinical Manifestations

1. *Prodromal symptoms* About ten minutes or half an hour before the attack of the migraine headache, a series of symptoms may appear. The most common one is visual disorder: flares of dark spots like sparks, auras, color rings, and bright objects; hemianopia; unequal pupil size; or disappearance of light reflex. In addition, the patient may have other symptoms such as general malaise, lassitude, language disorder, numbness of the fingers and lips, dizziness, vertigo, pallor, and polyuria.
2. *Headache* There is a sudden onset of unilateral pain on the forehead or parietal area, which spreads to the orbit and parietal regions, and also may affect the back of the eyeball. The intensity of the pain, mostly pulsating, gradually increases and extends to one entire side of the head. Patients may have nausea, vomiting, facial flushing, photophobia, lacrimation and other symptoms for two to three hours, or even one to two days. Then, the pain gradually subsides, and transitions to a dormant or post dromal period.

Typical migraines often have the first onset in puberty. Some patients may have a family history of migranes. The frequency of migraine attacks is uncertain, ranging from a few times a day to once in a few months.

Diagnosis and Differentiation

Key Diagnostic Criteria

1. The onset of migraine occurs usually at adolescence.
2. There is sudden unilateral head pain accompanied by nausea and vomiting.
3. Response to ergotamine caffeine.

Differential Diagnosis

1. *Headache due to hypertension* Mostly intermittent dull pain of the entire head; rarely is the headache severe; headache is usually experienced in the early morning.
2. *Temporal arteritis* This is a condition often seen in elderly. It starts with a pulsating pain, and becomes persistent as the disease progresses. The headache is exacerbated when the patient is supine, and it gets even worse with the head lowing down. Pressing the carotid artery can alleviate the pain.
3. *Others* These include intracranial space-occupying lesions, epileptic headache, and cerebral vascular malformations. Tests using modern medical equipment may be necessary to identify the problem, for example the use of plain skull X-rays, brain ultra sonography, electroencephalogram (EEG), and brain CT.

Treatment

1. *Commonly used maneuvers* grasping, kneading, smearing, and scattering sweeping.
2. *Commonly used acupoints and areas yìntáng* (EX-HN 3), *jīngmíng* (BL 1), *yángbái* (GB 14), *tàiyáng* (EX-HN 5), *bǎihuì* (DU 20), *fēngchí* (GB 20), *hégǔ* (LI 4), *yǒngquán* (KI 1), sites on the lateral aspect of the head and foot *shaoyang* gallbladder meridian.

3. *Operational methods*

   Basic operations

   a. The patient is supine with the head tilting to the unaffected side. Using the finger kneading maneuver, begin from *fēngchí* (GB 20), follow the splenius down along the neck to the collar area, and start over again, totaling up to about three to five minutes.
   b. Perform grasping on *fēngchí* and neck splenius three to five times.
   c. Apply pressure kneading with fingers on *yìntáng* (EX-HN 3), *jīngmíng* (BL 1), *yángbái* (GB 14), *tàiyáng* (EX-HN 5), *bǎihuì* (DU 20), and *shuàigǔ* (GB 8), 20 to 30 times on each point.
   d. Use the smearing maneuver on the forehead and on the upper and lower orbit, three to five times on each area.

e. Perform finger kneading on *hégŭ* (LI 4) 30 to 50 times.
f. Apply the scattering sweeping method at the lateral cephalic area and along the path of the gallbladder meridian on the head from the anterior-superior location to the posterior-inferior site 30 to 50 times.
g. With the patient sitting at the edge of the examination table, use five-finger grasping maneuver (i.e., grasping the five meridians on the head), starting from the front hairline and passing the parietal area. Then, switch to three-finger grasping when you reaching the occipital area. Lastly, apply grasping on *fēngchí*. Repeat the procedure three to five times.
h. The last step at the end of the treatment session is to perform pressure kneading technique on both sides of *yǒngquán* (KI 1).

Treatment Based on Pattern Differentiation

For those with symptoms such as facial flushing, nausea and vomiting, add the finger kneading maneuver on points such as *nèiguān* (PC 6), *fēnglóng* (ST 40), and *wèishū* (BL 21). For those who have obvious visual disorders, enhance the smearing operation on acupoints around the eyes, and apply the finger kneading maneuver on *guāngmíng* (GB 37).

Self-Preventional Methods

1. *Smearing on the forehead* With fingers of both hands flexed to form the shape of bows, and using the proximal in terphalan geal joints of the radial side as the focal points, apply smearing maneuver starting from the middle of the forehead to both temples (*tàiyáng*). The operation may be repeated 20 to 30 times. (See Figure 102.)
2. *Pressure kneading on fēngchí* Use the thumb pulps on both sides of *fēngchí* (GB 20), and apply force to perform pressure kneading 20 to 30 times. (See Figure 103.)
3. *Combing the head* With the ten fingers as the "comb", proceed from the front hairline to the occipital area, 30 to 50 times on each side.
4. *Pressure kneading onyǒng quán* Use the left hand to apply pressure kneading on the right side of *yǒngquán*(KI 1), and use the right hand to apply pressure on the left side of *yǒngquán*, 50 to 100 times each side.

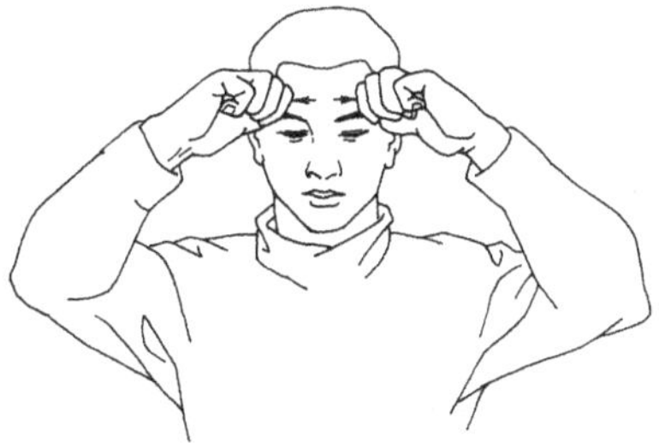

Figure 102 Smearing on the Forehead

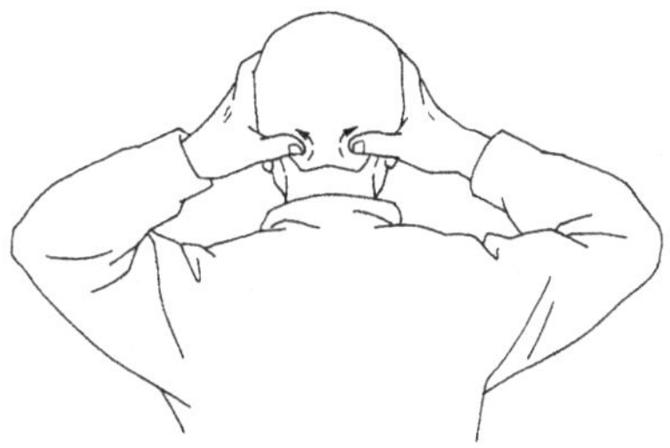

Figure 103 Rubbing the *FēngChí*

Precautions

1. Avoid adverse external stimuli and mental stress.
2. Ensure adequate sleep, a balanced lifestyle and a moderate diet.

Muscle Tension Headache

Muscle tension headache is also known as muscle contraction headache. It is the most common form of chronic headache, and occurs mostly in young adults, especially women. The primary conditions causing muscle tension headache include cervical spondylosis, visual fatigue, and head trauma.

Muscle tension headaches often occur on the occipital area, sometimes on one or both sides of the temporal area. Patients often complain of having an oppressive and heavy feeling, or a sense of "tightness." Tender spots can be found on the nape of the neck and shoulder muscles. Sometimes one or multiple hard knots can be felt, causing pain. The knots indicate tension and contraction of cervical muscles.

Treatment

Apply finger kneading on painful nodules and tender points, or plucking on tensed muscles, supplemented by five-finger grasping and scattering sweeping.

Headache Due to the Common Cold

Headache can be an associated symptoms of common cold.

Treatment

First, perform pressure kneading of the Bladder meridian on the back, followed by finger kneading on *fèishū* (BL 13) and *dàzhuī* (DU 14). Then, apply grasping on *jiānjǐng* (GB 21), *fēngchí* (GB 20), *qǔchí* (LI 11), and *hégǔ* (LI 4) with enough power resulting in a "swelling soreness" sensation, a sign of *de*-qi, on the patient. Afterwards, use the patting maneuver along the Bladder meridian on the upper back, and end the session with five-finger grasping and scattering sweeping.

Everyday Exercises

1. What is migraine? How is tui na therapy done for migraine?
2. How does one perform self-preventative tui na for migraine?

Day 2

HYPERTENSION

Hypertension (also known as high blood pressure) is a condition with increased systemic arterial blood pressure as the main clinical manifestation. Clinically, it is generally believed that if the systolic blood pressure (peak pressure in the arteries) measures over 18.7 kPa (140 mm Hg), and the diastolic pressure (minimum pressure in the arteries) measures over 12 kPa (90 mm Hg) when one is at rest, one can be diagnosed as suffering from hypertension. Diastolic pressure, which does not vary with age, is the major factor in determining hypertension. Systolic pressure, however, could increase with age.

There are two kinds of hypertension by clinical definition: primary hypertension (or simply, hypertension) and secondary hypertension (or symptomatic hypertension). Primary hypertension accounts for the vast majority of hypertension cases. Primary hypertension has no obvious underlying medical cause, and can be due to excessive mental stress, or some intense and repeated stimulation over an extended period of time. Secondary hypertension has a known direct cause, such as kidney disease or tumors.

A broad range of small-artery spasms can cause visceral ischemia, especially renal ischemia, that would cause a series of metabolic changes, speeding up the hardening of small arteries, so that the blood pressure is further increased. In consequence, in addition to the characteristics of arterial blood pressure, hypertension may be accompanied by lesions of the blood vessels, heart, brain, kidney, eye, and other organs.

Hypertension occurs most often in people more than 40 years of age, with a higher prevalence among obese individuals, white collar workers, and urban residents. Also, the condition runs in the family to a certain extent.

Clinical Manifestations

1. *Blood pressure* The arterial blood pressure of someone suffering from hypertension is consistently higher than 18.7 kPa/12.0 kPa (140 mm Hg/90 mm Hg).
2. *Common symptoms* These include headache that is commonly experienced on temporal, occipital, and frontal areas in the morning or daytime; dizziness, vertigo, distension of the head, palpitations, forgetfulness, insomnia, and irritability.

A "hypertensive crisis" occurs when the condition becomes suddenly aggravated, accompanied with symptoms such as a sharp rise in blood pressure, severe headache, blurred vision, increased heart rate, palpitations, and pale or flushing face. Sometimes the dramatically increased blood pressure may cause circulation disorder of the brain, resulting in severe headache, vomiting, stiff neck, breathing difficulties. In extreme cases, the sufferer may enter into a coma. This condition is known as "hypertensive encephalopathy." Most patients who survive this condition would have sequelae such as hemiplegia and impaired language skills.

Diagnosis and Differentiation

1. *Blood pressure measures*
    - *Normal blood pressure*: systolic pressure ≤16 kPa (120 mmHg), diastolic pressure ≤10.7 kPa (80 mmHg)
    - *Hypertension*: systolic pressure ≥18.7 kPa (140 mmHg) and/or diastolic pressure ≥12 kPa (90 mmHg)
    - *Pre-hypertension*: systolic pressure 16–18.5 kPa (120–139 mmHg) and/or diastolic pressure 10.7–11.9 kPa (80–89 mmHg).
2. *Medical examination* Left ventricular enlargement can be found with hyperactivity of the second heart sound, and fundus examination may detect retinal artery spasm, sclerosis, hemorrhage, and papilledema.
3. *Laboratory tests*
    - *Urine tests*: protein uria, red blood cells (RBCs), and casts.
    - *Blood tests*: increased level of cholesterol, triglyceride, β lipoprotein, glucose, creatinine and urea nitrogen levels.

- In addition, EEG, chest X-rays, and other tests may be helpful in diagnosing hypertension.

4. *Differentiation between hypertension and symptomatic hypertension*

   - *Chronic glomerulonephritis*: history of kidney disease, often accompanied by anemia, edema, facial character of kidney disease, and renal inadequacy.
   - *Gestosis*: in gestosis, high blood pressure generally occurs in the third trimester of pregnancy, and gradually increases, accompanied by edema and proteinuria.

Treatment

Tui na therapy is applicable in chronic hypertension, and stage I and II hypertensive patients. However, it is not recommended for accelerated hypertension and stage III hypertensive patients, especially among patients showing hypertensive crisis.

1. *Treatment principles* calming the liver, suppressing yang, calming the nerves, and descending the turbid.
2. *Commonly used maneuvers* pressing, kneading, smearing, grasping, scattering sweeping, and scrubbing.
3. *Commonly used acupoints and areas* *bǎihuì* (DU 20), *yìntáng* (EX-HN 3), *fēngchí* (GB 20), *qiáogōng* (bridge arch), *shuàigǔ* (GB 8), *qǔchí* (LI 11), *fēnglóng* (ST 40), *tàichōng* (LR 3), *yǒngquán* (KI 1), lower abdomen, lumbosacral.

4. *Operational methods*

   - *Basic operations:* with the patient sitting, stand at his or her side. First, perform the crucial portion (steps *a* through *d*) of the treatment:

     a. The healer uses the pulp of the thumb to apply the pushing maneuver along the straight line of *qiáogōng* for 20 to 30 times. Then, apply the maneuver with the same frequency on *qiáogōng* on the other side. (See Figure 104.)
     b. Next, use both thumbs alternately to apply the smearing maneuver on the forehead from *yìntáng* (EX-HN 3) to the front

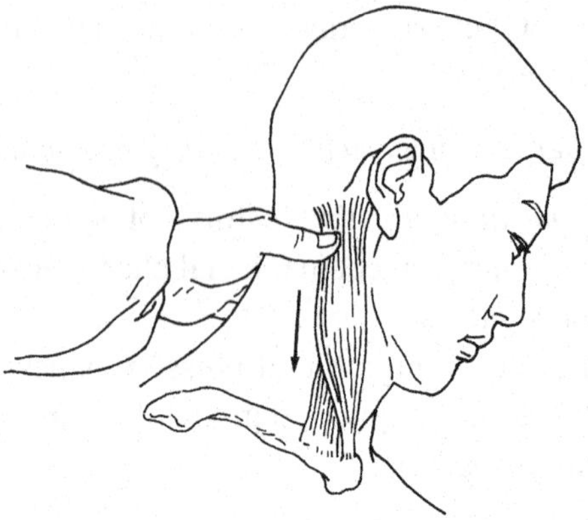

Figure 104 Pushing *Qiáo Gōng*

hair-line; then from *yìntáng* to both sides of *tàiyáng* (EX-HN 5) along the supra orbital arch, and lastly from the forehead to temporal area bilaterally both ways, five to ten times for each section.

c. Then, use the pulp of the finger to perform kneading on *yìntáng*, *jīngmíng*(BL 1), *tóuwéi* (ST 8) and *tàiyáng*; apply five-finger grasping on the parietal area and gradually altering to three-finger grasping on the occipital area, grasping the splenius bilateral to the nape of the neck until reaching *dàzhuī* (DU 14) on both sides. Repeat the step three to five times.
d. Perform scattering sweeping on the temporal areas bilaterally for a half to one minute, and end with pressure kneading on *bǎihuì*, *shuàigǔ* and *qǔchí*, 50 times for each point.
e. Have the patient in a prone position. Sit to the right of the patient and perform the finger-kneading maneuver on *mìngmén* (DU 4) and *shènshū* (BL 23), each for a minute; then apply horizontal scrubbing on the lumbosacral area until the area senses the heat from the friction. Lastly, scrub straight on *yǒngquán* (KI 1) until it feels the heat.

- *Treatment based on pattern differentiation*

a. Hypertension accompanied by palpitation and insomnia: add kneading on *nèiguān* (PC 6), *shénmén* (HT 7), *xīnshū* (BL 15), and *sānyīnjiāo* (SP 6), each for a minute.

b. Hypertension accompanied by shortness of breath and mental sluggishness: perform kneading on the lower abdomen, and finger kneading on *qìhăi* (RN 6) and *guānyuán* (RN 4) for five to ten minutes.

Self-Preventional Methods

The patient can perform the self tui na manipulations for lowering blood pressure two to three times daily, each time repeating an eight-beat set four to eight times.

1. *Preparation* Sit quietly and empty your mind, breathing evenly and naturally.
2. *Operations*
    a. *Improving the eyesight* Have the pulps of the two index fingers pressing on *cuánzhú* (BL 2) bilaterally, and the pulps of the thumbs pressing on both sides of *tàiyáng* (EX-HN 5). Next, with both hands, start kneading on the acupoints with a circular motion.
    b. *Calming the liver* Overlap the middle fingers of both hands, and have the pulps touching *băihuì* (DU 20), putting both the thumb pulps on *shuàigŭ* (GB 8) bilaterally. Then, both hands should start kneading on the acupoints with a circular motion.
    c. *Relieving vertigo* Place the middle finger pulps on both sides of *fēngchí* (GB 20), and the pulps of the index fingers on *tiānzhù* (BL 10). Start kneading on the acupoints with both hands con currently in a circular motion.
    d. *Refreshing the brain* Use the fingers of both hands as a comb, and start combing from the front hairline to the occipital area with the left and right hands alternately.
    e. *Lowering the blood pressure* Place the right the nar on the upper border of the left *qiáogōng*, slowly and gently smearing down to the supraclavicular fossa. Then, put the left thenar at the top edge of the right *qiáogōng*, and repeat the previous operation. The direction of this maneuver can only be from the superior posterior to the inferior anterior, and the force should be the gentle, and never reckless.

f. *Clearing heat* Use the pulp of the right thumb to perform kneading on left *qǔchí* (LI 11); then, the pulp of the left thumb to perform kneading on the right *qǔchí*.
g. *Nourishing the heart* Knead on the left *nèiguan* (PC 6) with the right thumb pulp first; then, do it the other way around.
h. *Regulating qi* With the elbows slightly bending and both wrists hanging naturally, lift up both the upper limbs slowly to eye level, inhaling at the same time. Next, slowly lower down the arms, exhaling at the same time.

Precautions

1. Stay on a diet low in salt. Avoid animal organs and fat in the meal. Stop smoking and consuming alcohol.
2. Live to a regular schedule. Avoid emotional turmoil and over-exhaustion. Maintain bowels open. Exercise properly under the guidance of a physician.

Everyday Exercises

1. What is hypertension? How is the tui na treatment done for hypertension?
2. Master the self tui na manipulations for lowering blood pressure.

Day 3

STOMACHACHE

Stomachache, commonly known as the "pain below the heart", is a condition of the digestive tract where pain is manifested in the epigastric area. Stomachache is a common clinical symptom. It is mostly seen in acute or chronic gastritis, gastric or duodenal ulcer, and gastric nerve psychosis.

Acute gastritis is usually caused by chemical or physical factors, microbial infection and bacterial toxins, and other stimulants causing damage to the surface of gastric cells, which leads to a specific gastric mucosal inflammation.

Chronic gastritis and its incidence ranks first place among a variety of stomach diseases. The older the individual, the higher the incidence. It is mainly due to acute gastritis being persistent and unhealed for an extended period of time. In chronic gastritis, the gastric mucosa is subjected to repeated damage, resulting in various chronic inflammatory changes of the mucosa.

Ulcers can be divided into chronic ulcers of the stomach and chronic ulcers of the duodenum. The formation of ulcers is due to a variety of factors, chief among which is the corrosive action of stomach acid and pepsin on the mucosa. As the ulcer further develops, it can involve the muscular layer or serosa, causing gastric perforation. When the ulcer leads to stomach vascular erosion, bleeding occurs. Gastric ulcers often occur in the lesser curvature of the stomach, while duodenal ulcers often occur in the bulb of the duodenum.

Stomach nerve disorder or stomach nervous sensory disorder is closely related to mental factors. When the normal activity of the hypothalamus and the central nervous system is interfered with by overwhelming psychological stress or trauma, resulting in these systems not being capable of effectively regulating autonomic nerve functions, gastric secretion and motor dysfunction can occur.

Clinical Manifestations

The main symptom is upper abdominal pain.

1. *Acute gastritis* The acute onset of gastritis is often due to the intake of drugs or food that is a negative stimulus to the stomach. Symptoms include upper abdominal pain, nausea, vomiting, and diarrhea.
2. *Chronic gastritis* It is characterized by a slow onset, persistent upper abdominal pain that feels distended and dull, loss of appetite, indigestion, and epigastric discomfort after eating. For patients having an trum gastritis, there is a burning sensation under the xiphoid, or recurrent gastrointestinal bleeding mainly featured by melena, which most often automatically stops.
3. *Ulcers* There is rhythmic upper abdominal pain. Gastric ulcer pain usually strikes a half hour to two hours after a meal, and is mostly felt in the upper left abdomen. In contrast, duodenal ulcer pain often has a postprandial onset of three to four hours, which can lessen or completely disappear after a meal, and is mostly located in the upper right abdomen. The nature of the pain may be insidious, distended, dull, burning, or sharp, and is often accompanied by gastrointestinal symptoms such as belching, acid regurgitation, a feeling of hunger, nausea, and vomiting. If it is complicated by upper gastrointestinal bleeding, hematemesis and melena may occur. If it is complicated by perforation, severe abdominal pain, tabulate venter, and shock may result.
4. *Gastroneurosis* The main symptoms include epigastric pain and discomfort associated with acid reflux, burning sensation under the xiphoid, a feeling of fullness after meals, and indigestion. It is often accompanied by the following:

   a. *Nervous vomiting* This is characterized by vomiting after eating, and the ability to eat right after vomiting.
   b. *Nervous belching* This is characterized by persistent belching with emotions, mostly occurs while there are people around.
   c. *Anorexia nervosa* This is an eating disorder mostly among young women, characterized by an irrational fear of gaining weight.
   d. Gastroneurosis can also have accompanying symptoms such as amnesia, dreaminess, insomnia, fatigue, anxiety, inability to

concentrate, headache, palpitations, chest tightness, irritability, and other nerve (sensory) symptoms. Female patients may have irregular menstruation, while nocturnal emission and decreased sexual function can be observed in male patients.

Diagnosis and Differentiation

1. *Acute gastritis* There is mild tenderness on the upper abdomen, and around the navel. Auscultation may detect hyperactive intestinal gurgling. There might be a slightly elevated white blood cell (WBC) count. Acute gastritis can be diagnosed based on the above symptoms in conjunction with the history of the patient and clinical manifestations. It is required to differentiate the diagnosis from acute appendicitis and acute cholecystitis:

    a. *Acute appendicitis* There is metastatic lower right abdominal pain, tenderness, rebound tenderness, and a significantly increased blood leukocyte count.

    b. *Acute cholecystitis* There is persistent pain on the upper right quadrant of the abdomen radiating to the right shoulder. If there are stones, paroxysmal colic would occur, and is often induced by eating high fat food. Other symptoms include upper right quadrant abdominal tension, gallbladder tenderness with deep breathing and significantly increased WBCs.

2. *Chronic gastritis* Endoscopy is the main method for diagnosing chronic gastritis, by determining its location and nature. Similarly, the use of stomach or duodenum fiber endoscopy can be used to differentiate chronic gastritis from other gastrointestinal diseases such as ulcers.
3. *Ulcers* Gastric ulcers are mostly evidenced by a tenderness in the upper left quadrant of the abdomen, while tenderness caused by duodenal ulcers is felt in the upper right quadrant of the abdomen. The occult blood test for patients is positive when there is bleeding. A gastrointestinal barium meal X-ray examination serves as one method to confirm ulcers. Stomach and duodenum fiber endoscopies are the most reliable methods in diagnosing ulcers.

4. *Gastric psychoneurosis* The diagnosis should be based on family history, and requires a close follow-up session, as well as a longer period of observation and clinical examination, with all other organic diseases being excluded.

Treatment

Tui na massage has a certain degree of therapeutic effect in treating chronic superficial gastritis, and superficial stomach or duodenum ulcers with small affected areas. Tui na is a good method to relieve pain when no drug or medical assistance is available.

1. *Commonly used maneuvers* pressing, point pressing, kneading, grasping, rubbing, scrubbing, and foulage.
2. *Commonly used acupoints and areas* *zhōngwǎn* (RN 12), *liángmén* (ST 21), *píshū* (BL 20), *wèishū* (BL 21), *nèiguān* (PC 6), *zúsānlǐ* (ST 36), and lower abdomen.

3. *Operational methods*
   Basic operations

   a. The patient lies supine with the practitioner sitting at the right side. First, gently apply rubbing maneuver on the epigastric area for one to two minutes. Then, perform thenar kneading for about 15 minutes, coordinating with finger kneading on *zhōngwǎn* and *liángmén*. For gastric ulcers, focus on the upper left abdomen while for duodenal ulcers, work more on the upper right abdomen. For those with a longer disease history or weak constitution, add kneading and rubbing in the lower abdomen for about five minutes.
   b. At the end, use both thumbs to perform pushing along the costal arch on both sides for three to five times.
   c. After operating on the abdominal area, apply finger kneading on *zúsānlǐ*, *nèiguān* and *nèitíng* (ST 44) for 30 to 50 times on each point.
   d. The patient can then change to prone or sitting position. Use the kneading maneuver on back-*shu* points, especially *píshū* and *wèishū*, each for one to two minutes. Next, apply hypothenar

scrubbing on the two acupoints until the patient feels the heat as a result of the friction.

e. Lastly, end the operation with grasping *jiānjǐng* (GB 21) and scrubbing the back.

Treatment Based on Pattern Differentiation

For those with obvious stomachache, change the operational procedure. Start with acupressure analgesic maneuver using point pressing. First, press on distal acupoints of the limb, such as *nèiguān*, *nèitíng* and *zúsānlǐ* to relieve pain. Following that, apply point pressing or pressing on *huàtuójiájǐ* (also known as *jiájǐ*, EX-B 2), *píshū*, *wèishū*, or nearby tender spots to alleviate pain. Work until the stomachache of the patient eases, then treat the abdominal area. For patients suffering from gastric psychoneurosis, focus the operation on the forehead by using pressure kneading on *bǎihuì* (DU 20) and *sìshéncōng* (EX-HN 1).

Self-Preventional Methods

1. *Harmonizing the stomach* Lie supine and with your body relaxed. With palms overlapped with *zhōngwǎn* on the epigastric area as the center, start kneading and rubbing clockwise for ten minutes until the belly feels unblocked, comfortable, and warm.
2. *Strengthening the stomach* Sit up. Use both thumbs to pressure knead on both sides of *zúsānlǐ* for two to three minutes. Next, use the thumb pulp of the left hand to apply pressure kneading on the right *nèiguān* for two to three minutes, and switch to the left *nèiguān* with the right thumb pulp for another two to three minutes. The effect is considered good if you get soreness and a distended *de*-qi sensation.

Precautions

1. For patients at the bleeding stage of stomach or duodenal ulcer, tui na therapy should be temporarily prohibited.
2. Live to a regular schedule. Avoid excessive mental stress and fatigue.

3. Avoid hard liquor, thick tea, coffee, and spicy food that may stimulates the gastric mucosa. Stop smoking tobacco.
4. Avoid or be careful of drugs like aspirin that may induce and aggravate stomach ache or cause complications.

For those with gastric psychoneurosis, the main focus should be on psychiatric treatment to improve their mental well-being.

Everyday Exercises

1. Try to memorize the clinical manifestations of chronic gastritis, gastric ulcers, and duodenal ulcers.
2. Describe the basic tui na operation in treating stomachache.

Day 4

GASTROPTOSIS

Gastroptosis refers to the prolapse or downward displacement of the stomach. The condition is caused by such factors as decreased muscle tensility of the lower abdomen, insufficient fat layer on the abdominal wall, decreased diaphragmatic position, and deficient suspension force of the diaphragm or that of the associated ligaments of the stomach and adjacent organs. These may result in the lesser curvature of the stomach descending to a point below the line connecting the iliac crests, or the duodenal bulb shifting to the left. Usually, people who suffer from this condition are of frail constitution and have a feeble physique. They are mostly women who have had multiple child births or people who have suffered a significant sudden weight-loss.

In traditional Chinese medicine, it is believed that gastroptosis is due to deficient spleen and stomach, causing the center qi to sink. The spleen is the foundation of postnatal constitution. The stomach governs the intake of food and fluids, while the spleen governs the transportation, transformation, and muscles. When the spleen weakens, the center qi fails to raise and lift, so that prolapse of the organ occurs.

Clinical Manifestations

1. Wasting, fatigue, and reduced food intake.
2. Abdominal swelling and distention that worsens after eating.
3. A sensation of heaviness in the epigastric area, and borborygmus (intestinal rumbling) after eating.
4. Vomiting, belching, diarrhea, constipation, or alternating constipation and diarrhea with flat and short stool.
5. Vertigo, dizziness, palpitations, insomnia, and orthostatic hypotension.
6. May have complications such as the ptosis of kidney and uterus.

Diagnosis and Differentiation

1. The patient may have an overly slim body and a feeble appearance. His or her upper abdomen is flat or even sunken, while the lower abdomen is distended with loosened muscles and reduced myodynamia. When the upper abdomen is palpated, there is strong aortic pulsation, and the lower abdomen often has the vibrating sound of fluids.
2. The result of an X-ray barium meal examination provides a major diagnostic evidence of the disease. The stomach is loppy, and the lowest point of the lesser curvature arc is below the level of the iliac crest. The duodenal bulb is affected by the gastroptosis and pulled towards left.
3. The X-ray barium meal examination can differentiate gastroptosis from other stomach diseases.

Treatment

Rehabilitation is possible if the patient suffering from gastroptosis is persistent with tui na treatment, and proactively supplements the treatment with functional exercises.

1. *Commonly used maneuvers* kneading, rubbing, pressing, lift-kneading, slotting, and grasping.
2. *Commonly used acupoints and areas zhōngwǎn* (RN 12), *qìhǎi* (RN 6), *guānyuán* (RN 4), *zúsānlǐ* (ST 36), *píshū* (BL 20), *wèishū* (BL 21), and the lower abdominal area.

3. *Operational methods*
   Basic operations

   a. The patient is supine, with the practitioner sitting to the right side of the patient. First, apply kneading and rubbing on *zhōngwǎn* for three to five minutes, gradually transitioning to *qìhǎi* and *guānyuán,* focusing on these two points with the pressure kneading maneuver for about ten minutes.
   b. Next, place the palm on the lower abdomen with four fingers closed and the thumb fanning out. Use the hypo thenar and the ulnar aspect

of the palm as the focal site to form an arc, and hold the area where the lower end of the stomach is located to perform the supported kneading. This method is called lift-kneading (see Figure 105). The kneading should follow the rise and fall of the abdomen. After the lower end of the stomach has been held, gradually move the hand toward the center, then the upper abdomen. Repeat the procedure for three to five minutes.

c. The patient changes to a prone position, and the practitioner remains seated. Use the pulps of the index and middle fingers as focal points and place them on both sides of the Bladder meridian. Apply top-down and back-and-forth pressure kneading along the meridian three to five times, with the focus on pressure kneading *píshū* and *wèishū*, each point for one or two minutes.
d. The patient changes to a sitting position with his left arm relaxed and elbow flexed backwards over the lower back. The practitioner stands on the patient's left. Place your left palm on the patient's anterior left shoulder, and with the right hand fingers closed, use the fingertips as the focal area and "slot" the finger tips in a superior lateral direction from the lower corner of scapula, equivalent to *yìxī* (BL 45) and *géguān* (BL 46), two to three finger cun between the scapula and the ribs. Hold the position for one to two minutes. This maneuver is called slotting (see Figure 106). Very often, the patient

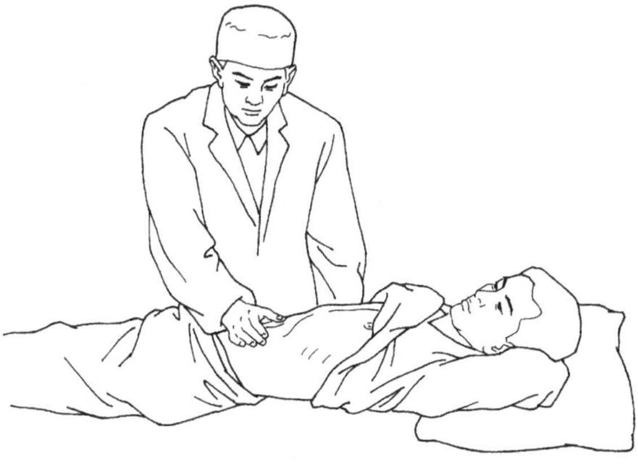

Figure 105 Lift-kneading Maneuver

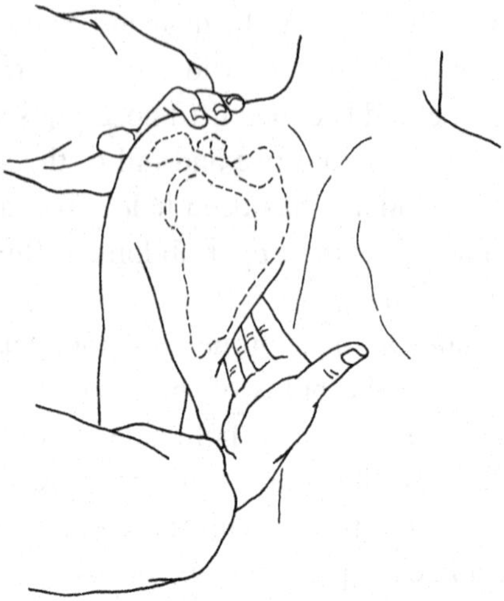

Figure 106 Slotting Maneuver

would have the feeling as if the stomach has been lifted up. Repeat the operation two or three times. The same method can be done on the right side.

Treatment Based on Pattern Differentiation

a. For patients with weight loss, fatigue, and poor appetite: focus more on pressure kneading on *zhōngwǎn*, and add a spine-pinching maneuver.
b. For dizziness and insomnia: add head tui na, pressure kneading *nèiguān* (PC 6) and *shénmén* (HT 7).
c. For patients with visceral ptosis: focus more on *qìhǎi* and *guānyuán* with pressure kneading, and lift-kneading on the lower abdomen.

Self-Preventional Methods

1. *Lift-kneading of the lower abdomen* Overlap the palms and place them on the lower abdomen. Use the lift-kneading maneuver in slow motion and move the palms upwards. Do this three to five minutes at a time, two or three times a day.

2. *Lift grasping* Use both hands alternately and apply lift grasping to the skin and subcutaneous tissue of the whole abdomen for 20 to 30 times.
3. *Abdominal exercises* Gradually increase the strength of the abdominal muscles by doing the following physical exercises:

    a. *Supine leg lifting* Lie supine with both legs straight. Raise the legs alternately for two to four sets, each set lasting for eight beats.
    b. *Leg lifting with abdomen drawn in* Lie supine with both legs straight. Raise both legs together, drawing in the abdomen, for two to four sets of eight beats per set.
    c. *Supine biking* Lie supine with lower limbs elevated, and perform bike riding moves for two to four sets of eight beats per set.
    d. *Sit-ups* Lie supine. Hold the head with both hands, perform sit-ups for two to four sets of eight beats per set.
    e. *Inverted shoulder and back stand* Lie supine, with both hands supporting the back. Gradually lift up the legs with them close together, and stretch upwards to make the body upside down with the back, shoulders, and head supporting it. This is a great exercise for patients with visceral ptosis. However, there is a certain level of difficulty. Therefore, it may require a friend's help or the need of using the wall. Do what is possible in accordance with your physical ability and ensure individual safety.

Precautions

1. Eat easy-to-digest food and avoid cold, raw, or spicy food. Eat multiple meals in smaller quantities, and consume a certain amount of fat.
2. Exercise regularly to improve the abdominal muscles.
3. Those who have severe gastroptosis should use a stomacher.

Everyday Exercises

1. What is gastroptosis?
2. How do you perform the lift-kneading and slotting maneuvers in a tui na operation?

Day 5

THE COMMON COLD

The common cold is upper respiratory tract inflammation caused by bacteria or viruses. The incidence of the common cold is high and it may occur throughout the year, but is more common in the cold seasons of winter and early spring. It can be divided into the common cold and epidemic influenza.

Chinese medical practice believes that the common cold is usually caused by pathogenic wind attacking the exterior of the body, resulting in the failure of the lung to diffuse and descend its qi. In fact, the Chinese folk term for the common cold is "wind damage." Lung governs qi with the nose as its external opening, and relates to the skin and pores. When the exterior pathogen attacks, the lung is the front-line target, which usually leads to illnesses of wind-cold or wind-heat pattern, depending on the overall clinical manifestations.

Clinical Manifestations

1. *Wind-cold pattern* Symptoms may include headache, fever, absence of sweating, aversion to cold, soreness and lassitude of the four limbs, nasal congestion, clear runny nose, thin white tongue coating, and floating tight pulse.
2. *Wind-heat pattern* Symptoms may include fever, distended head pain, slight sweating, dry mouth, mild aversion to cold, sore throat, thick nasal discharge, coughing with yellow sputum, constipation, dark yellow urine, thin yellow tongue coating, floating rapid pulse.
3. *Secondary respiratory infections with coughs* When secondary bronchitis and lung infection occur, there may be coughs, chest pain, detection of rales with lung auscultation, and increased total number of WBCs and neutrophils. It can also be complicated by otitis media and sinusitis.

Diagnosis and Differentiation

It is relatively easy to diagnose the common cold based on the medical history and clinical manifestations of the patient. In general, the common cold has a slow onset, relatively mild symptoms, and moderate fever without significant complications or secondary infections. On the other hand, influenza can spread rapidly, has more severe symptoms, and is often accompanied by secondary infections of the respiratory system.

Treatment

The common cold usually lasts for three to seven days after its onset. Tui na therapy is designed to relieve symptoms, shorten the natural recovery time, and reduce other body systems from secondary infections.

1. *Treatment principles* dispersing and releasing the exterior.
2. *Commonly used maneuvers* kneading, pressing, grasping, smearing, scattering sweeping, and scrubbing.
3. *Commonly used acupoints and areas yìntáng* (EX-HN 3), *tàiyáng* (EX-HN 5), *yíngxiāng* (LI 20), *fēngchí* (GB 20), *qŭchí* (LI 11), *hégŭ* (LI 4), *jiānjǐng*(GB 21), *fèishū* (BL 13), and forehead, temporal Bladder meridian points, and back *shu* points.

4. *Operational methods*
   Basic operations

   a. The patient sits with the clinician standing in front of the patient. Use the thenar kneading maneuver on the whole forehead up and down, and left to right for about three to five minutes.
   b. Next, use disjoining and joining maneuvers on the forehead (see Figure 107).
   c. Apply smearing maneuver on the upper and lower orbitals for five to ten times each side.
   d. Apply pressure kneading using the thumb pulps on both sides of *tàiyáng* and *yíngxiāng* 30 to 50 times each.
   e. Keeping the same body position, apply scattering sweeping on the temporal area for 30 to 50 times each side.

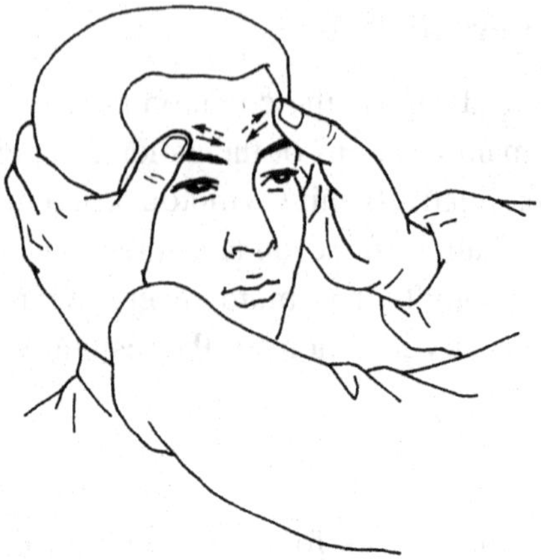

Figure 107 Disjoining and joining on the forehead

f. Then, perform five-finger grasping, alternating between the left and the right for five to ten times. When the fingers reach *fēngchí*, apply the grasping maneuver until the patient has soreness *de*-qi sensation.
g. Slowly move down with the grasping maneuver along the splenius bilaterally until the root of the neck. Return and repeat the same procedure for five to ten times.
h. Now perform grasping or pressure kneading on bilateral *hégŭ* for 30 to 50 times.
i. Ask the patient change to a sitting position while you stand at the patient's side. Apply hypothenar scrubbing maneuver along the bladder meridian on the back until the patient feels warm.
j. Lastly, stand posterior to the patient and end the treatment with the grasping maneuver on *jiānjǐng*.

Treatment Based on Pattern Differentiation

a. Accompanied with headache: add kneading on *bǎihuì* (DU 20).
b. Sore throat: add pressure kneading on *tiāntū* (RN 22) and *yújì* (LU 10).

c. Fever: add pressure kneading on *qŭchí*.
d. Gastrointestinal symptoms: add pressure kneading on *zhōngwăn* (RN 12) and *zúsānlĭ* (ST 36).

Self-Preventional Methods

1. *Rubbing the nose* Use the radial side or the tips of both index fingers to rub the bridge of the nose on both sides up and down until it feels warm. Do this for two to three minutes daily (see Figure 108).
2. *Kneading on tàiyang and yíngxiāng* With both middle fingers or thumbs, apply kneading on both sides for *tàiyáng* and *yíngxiāng*, for one to two minutes each (see Figure 109).
3. *Smearing on the forehead and orbits* With both index fingers slightly flexed, apply smearing with the radial side of the fingers on the forehead and upper and lower orbits of the eyes for two to three minutes each (see Figure 110).
4. *Pressure kneading on fēngchí* Use both thumb pulps to apply pressure kneading on both sides of *fēngchí* for about a minute each.
5. *Face-wash with cold water* Wash the face with cold water every morning and night.

The above methods not only treat common cold, but also prevent it from happening. It is particularly effective for those with frail physique and easy to catch cold.

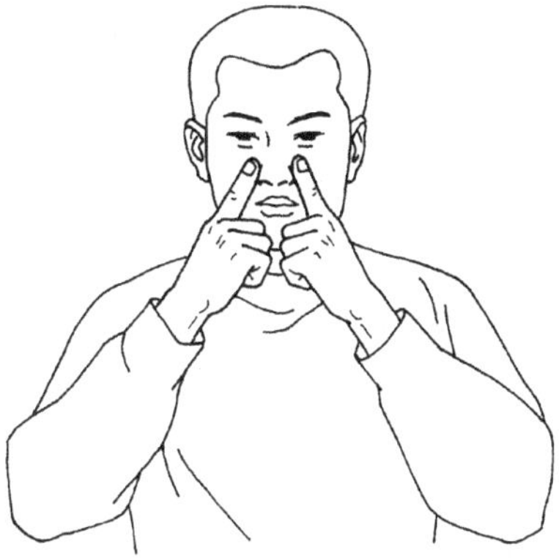

Figure 108 Rubbing the Nose

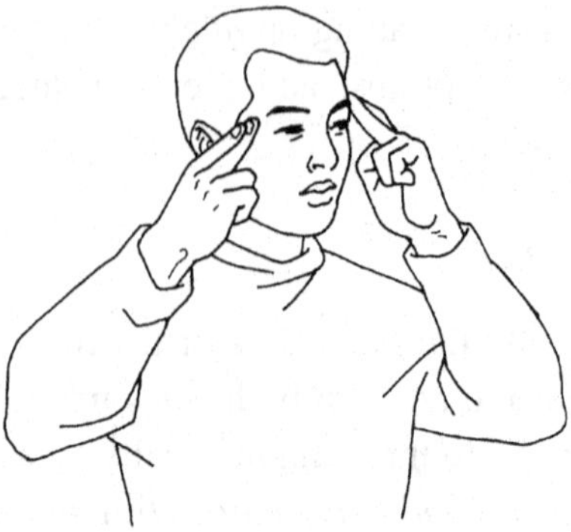

Figure 109 Kneading on *TàiYáng*

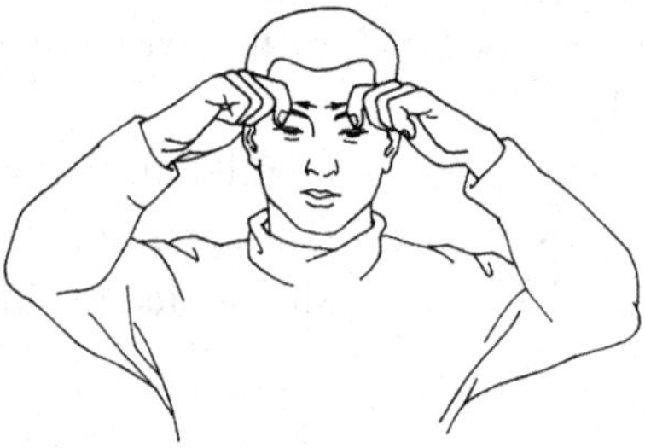

Figure 110 Smearing on forehead and orbits

Precautions

1. Avoid crowded public places during the common cold and influenza seasons.
2. Seek timely treatment if you succumb to the common cold, rest well, and drink adequate boiled water.
3. The use of antibiotics must follow the professional orders of a physician when there is secondary infection.

Everyday Exercises

1. What is the definition of the common cold?
2. How would you treat the common cold using tui na?

Day 6

CHRONIC BRONCHITIS

Chronic bronchitis is a condition where there is chronic inflammatory changes of the bronchial passages. Chronic bronchitis can result from under-treated acute bronchitis, or from long-term smoking, air pollution, and other physical and chemical stimuli. In addition, allergies and climate changes often lead to the recurrence of the disease. The pathology is characterized hyperplasia of glandular tissue on the bronchial wall, causing the increase of bronchial mucus secretion and poor drainage. The pathological progress is slow, but acute attack happens quite frequently.

Clinical Manifestations

1. Middle-aged or older people contribute to the majority of the incidences of the disease. The course of the disease is fairly long, often with a recurrent tendency. The occurrence rate is higher in the cold seasons such as late fall and winter.
2. Chronic bronchitis is characterized by persistent coughing, and is often accompanied by shortness of breath in severe cases. The coughing worsens significantly in the early morning or at bedtime. The phlegm is white, sticky, and profuse. Thick and purulent phlegm with scattered traces of blood may be associated with infection.
3. If the disease persists for a long time, it may be complicated by obstructive emphysema and chronic pulmonary heart disease, showing various degrees of symptoms such as dyspnea, wheezing, and cyanosis.
4. In general, there is no abnormal signs in the early periods of the disease. When disease has run its course for some time, dry moist rales may be discovered by auscultation, and thickened and disordered striae of the lung shows up under chest X-rays. If it is associated with emphysema, there may be barrel chest, clubbing fingers, increased photo permeability of the lung on chest X-rays, widened inter costal spaces, and lowered diaphragm. When it is accompanied by secondary infection, there will be increase in total blood leukocytes and neutrophils.

Diagnosis and Differentiation

Based on the medical history, clinical manifestations, and chest X-ray of the patient, the diagnosis of the disease should not be difficult. Chest X-rays should be taken to exclude other lung diseases.

Treatment

1. *Treatment principles* diffusing and unblocking lung qi, relieving coughing and transforming phlegm, supplemented with fortifying the spleen and kidney.
2. *Commonly used maneuvers* pressure kneading, rubbing, disjoining, scrubbing, and spinal pinching.
3. *Commonly used acupoints and areas* *zhōngfŭ* (LU 1), *yúnmén* (LU 2), *dànzhōng* (RN 17), *zhōngwăn* (RN 12), *chĭzé* (LU 5), *yújì* (LU 10), *fèishū* (BL 13), *píshū* (BL 20), *shènshū* (BL 23), *fēnglóng* (ST 40), and the midline on the back.

4. *Operational methods*
   Basic operations

   a. The patient is supine, with the practitioner sitting to the right of the patient. First, apply finger rubbing on *zhōngfŭ*, *yúnmén*, and *dànzhōng*, two to three minutes for each point.
   b. Next, use pressure kneading on *zhōngwăn* with the heel of the palm for two to three minutes, followed by disjoining from the center to both sides along the inter costals spaced with a gradual top-down order using both thumbs. Do it two to three times.
   c. Use the thumb to perform pressure kneading on *chĭzé* and *fēnglóng*, one to two minutes for each point.
   d. The patient should then take the prone position, with the practitioner sitting on the side of the patient. Place the pulps of the index and middle fingers on *fèishū*, *píshū*, and *shènshū* in turn to perform the double-finger kneading maneuver on each acupoint for one to two minutes (see Figure 111).
   e. Finally, scrub along *du mai* and the Bladder meridian on the back using the hypothenar until the patient feels the heat from the friction.

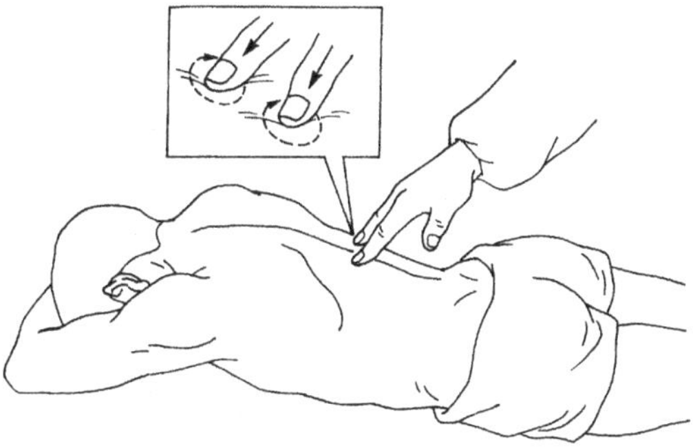

Figure 111 Double-finger kneading on back *shu*-points.

Treatment Based on Pattern Differentiation

a. For chronic patients with weak constitution: add spinal pinching for three to five times, and pressure kneading on *zúsānlǐ* (ST 36) for one to two minutes.
b. For patients with severe coughs and labored breathing: add double-finger kneading on *dìngchuǎn* (EX-B 1), 0.5 cun lateral to *dàzhuī* (DU 14), and finger kneading on *yújì* for one to two minutes.

Self-Preventional Methods

1. *Push-rubbing the thoracic area* Use the full left palm to apply push-rubbing on the right thoracic area, from the center to both sides, in a top-down order; then, use the full right palm to work on the left side. Operate on each side for about two to three minutes.(See Figure 112.)
2. *Kneading and rubbing zhōngwǎn* With the full palm placed around the area where *zhōngwǎn* is located on the upper abdomen, apply clock-wise kneading and rubbing for two to three minutes.
3. *Kneading and rubbing zhōngfǔ* Apply thenar kneading and rubbing on *zhōngfǔ* for a minute, with the left hand working on the right side, and vise versa.
4. *Breathing exercise* This can be done in any body position. The key is to be natural with all muscles relaxed, and with the mind focused. The inhalation should be slow and deep, while the exhalation should be slow. A breath in and a breath out count as one breath; complete 30 to 50 breaths.

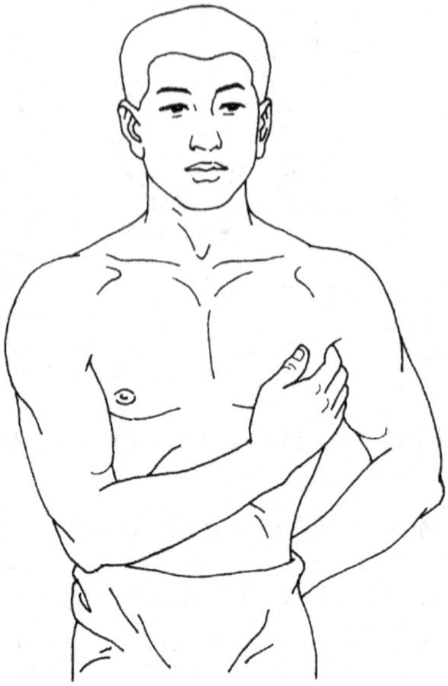

Figure 112. Push-rubbing the Thoracic Area

(1) to (4) above can be done daily, one set in the morning and another one in the evening.

Precautions

1. Stay warm with sufficient clothing, and try to avoid catching a cold or other respiratory diseases.
2. Increase physical wellness training, such as walking, jogging, and taiji-quan.
3. Quit smoking.
4. Rest well and follow the doctor's instructions on taking the medicine during the onset period.

Everyday Exercises

1. What is chronic bronchitis?
2. What are the main clinical manifestations of chronic bronchitis? What are the procedures in self-preventative care for chronic bronchitis?

WEEK 5

Day 1

CORONARY HEART DISEASE

Coronary heart disease (CHD) is the short name for coronary atherosclerotic heart disease, the most common cardiovascular disease in the elderly. The coronary artery is the main artery supplying blood to the heart. Coronary artery stenosis and infarction are the results of atherosclerosis, a condition in which the artery wall thickens because of the accumulation of fatty substances. As a result, the arteries become narrowed and blood circulation is impeded, resulting in myocardial ischemia and hypoxia, further leading to myocardial damage. Other conditions such as high cholesterol, hypertension, and endocrine disease can cause CHD. In addition, the disease is related to psychological factors and family history.

Chinese medical practice classifies CHD as "chest *bì*" pattern, which pertains to the disease category of "real heart pain." Chinese medical practice believes that the disease is due to poor chest yang, causing qi occlusion that leads to chest distension and pain. Since yang qi fails to warm the organs inside the chest, it causes excessive internal yin cold. At the same time, since the sluggish yang qi is not able to transform and transport body fluid, it is easy for turbid phlegm to form. The turbid phlegm combines with cold qi to further lead to blockage of blood vessels and forming of blood stasis. The formation of blood stasis will exacerbate chest pain, so severe as if it penetrates the whole back.

Clinical Manifestations

The patient often has precordial fullness, discomfort, and shortness of breath especially while moving. After extensive work or on a rainy day with low air pressure, there will be compressive, pricking, or stabbing pain in the sternum area.

In severe cases, there may be a sudden onset of angina pectoris with the pain radiating to the left shoulder and left upper extremity. Severe pain can be accompanied by sweating, pallor, extremely cold limbs, and decreased blood pressure. In extreme cases, shock and heart failure may result in sudden death.

In an ECG of a patient suffering from CHD, visible ST segment depressions and T-wave inversions can be detected.

Diagnosis and Differentiation

1. *Key diagnostic criteria of CHD*
   a. Existent angina or myocardial infarction without severe aortic valve disease or other coronary diseases.
   b. Patients over 40 years of age with cardiac enlargement, heart failure, or severe arrhythmia, and no obvious high blood pressure or other lesions. Severe arrhythmia means frequent or multiple-borne premature ventricular contractions, atrial fibrillation or flutter, ventricular tachycardia, left bundle branch block, Type II and III conduction block.

2. *Main differential diagnosis*
   a. *Acute pancreatitis* There is persistent upper abdominal pain; there maybe paroxysmal aggravation, often accompanied by nausea and vomiting, moderate fever, upper abdominal tenderness, and increased serum amylase.
   b. *Acute cholecystitis* There is colic in the right upper quadrant of the abdomen that radiates to the right scapular or right shoulder (often induced by a rich or high-fat diet), accompanied by nausea and vomiting, mild jaundice, and fever after the onset of pain; right upper quadrant tenderness and obvious muscle tension; increased WBCs. X-rays and ultrasonic scans can help in the diagnosis of this disease.

Treatment

Chronic myocardial insufficiency and stable angina can be treated by tui na therapy. Clinical research shows that tuina can reduce myocardial oxygen consumption and improve myocardial blood volume. Therefore, it can be used as a complementary treatment.

1. *Treatment principles* invigorating blood, dissolving stasis, warming and unblocking heart yang, supplementing qi, and nourishing the heart to improve cardiac blood supply.
2. *Commonly used maneuvers* kneading, rubbing, and scrubbing.
3. *Commonly used acupoints and areas dànzhōng* (RN 17), left *qīmén* (LR 14), *xīmén* (PC 4), *nèiguān* (PC 6), *yīnxī* (HT 6), *shénmén* (HT 7), *xīnshū* (BL 15), *géshū* (BL 17), *juéyīnshū* (BL 14), *zhìyáng* (DU 9), *tàixī* (KI 3), and the left anterior chest.

4. *Operational methods*
   *Basic operation*s

   a. The patient is supine, with the practitioner sitting at the right side of the patient. Apply finger rubbing on *dànzhōng* and left *qīmén* to unblock and rectify the chest qi, relieve depressed qi, and resolve restlessness. Then perform the same maneuver on the left thoracic area. Work on each area for five to eight minutes. The manipulation should be agile and gentle.
   b. Then, use the finger kneading maneuveron the upper limbs, *xīmén* and *shénmén*, or *nèiguān* and *yīnxī*, and *tàixī*, one to two minutes for each location or acupoint.
   c. Next, ask the patient to take a sitting position with his arms flat and facing down at the table. Stand at the patient's back. Apply double-finger kneading on back *shu* points such as *xīnshū*, *géshū,* and *juéyīnshū*, then *zhìyang*. Work on each acupoint for one to two minutes.
   d. Finally, perform horizontal scrubbing on *zhìyáng* and *xīnshū* to warm the heart yang until the patient feels the heat from the friction.

   Treatment based on pattern differentiation
   If the patient suffers an acute coronary attack, the first thing you should do is to get him or her to a doctor practicing either Western or Chinese medicine. At the same time, find the most sensitive points where the soreness is the most obvious, often near back *shu* points along the

Bladder meridian. Apply finger kneading on them. When the pain is relieved, switch to basic operational methods. For those who have severe palpitations or chest tightness, apply finger kneading on *xīmén*, *yīnxī* and *dàn zhōng*, one to two minutes for each point.

Self-preventional Methods

1. *Push-rubbing at thoracic area* Place the entire right palm on the precordial area, and perform clockwise pushing and rubbing for one to three minutes.
2. *Finger kneading acupoints of the hand* Use a finger on the left hand to knead *nèiguān* and *shénmén* of the right hand, and do the same the other way around. Work on each acupoint for one minute. It is preferable but not mandatory to have *de*-qi sensation such as soreness and distension.

Precautions

1. Do not overwork.
2. Eat moderately and refrain from smoking and consuming alcohol.
3. Engage in appropriate physical exercises but do not over do it.

Everyday Exercises

1. What is coronary heart disease?
2. What are the categories of coronary heart disease that can be treated with tui na therapy? How would you perform the treatment?

Day 2

DIARRHEA

Diarrhea is marked by frequent bowel movements with loose or watery stool. Diarrhea can be due to a number of factors, including insufficient treatment of dysentery, acute enteritis and food poisoning, or overeating of greasy food. Tui na is excellent for treating functional diarrhea, a chronic condition for which no cause can be found.

Clinical Manifestations

1. *Abdominal pain* There is irregular pain around the navel or on the left lower quadrant of the abdomen. The pain ranges from distended abdominal pain to spasmodic colic. The pain often occurs after a meal, with the patient having a strong desire to pass motion. The pain then eases after passing gas or defecation.
2. *Abnormal bowel movements* Diarrhea is often associated with eating and mood swings, and sometimes may also alternate with constipation. The feces is loose without pus and blood, but often with mucus.
3. *Digestive symptoms* These include anorexia, nausea, vomiting, belching; bloating, farting that eases after bowel movement.
4. *Systemic symptoms* These include anxiety, depression, fatigue, insomnia, cold and sweaty extremities, loss of appetite, general weakness, and weight loss.
5. *Stool examination* There should be no other abnormal findings other than mucus in the stool.

Diagnosis and Differentiation

The diagnosis of diarrhea may be made based on the following: chronic abdominal pain, abnormal bowel movements, mucus detected in the stool under microscopy, and negative results for pus or red blood cells (RBCs). A barium enema shows colonic spasms and a bag-shaped increase, with normal mucosal pattern. Except for sigmoid spasms, sigmoidoscopy does not show any other positive findings.

The differential diagnosis is mainly one of colon cancer and chronic dysentery.

1. *Colon cancer* This is mostly found in middle-aged or older people with ingravescent symptoms. Stool examination often detects RBCs and the occult blood test is positive. Whenever necessary, rectal sigmoidoscopy or barium enema examination should be done to confirm the condition.
2. *Chronic dysentery* Pus or RBCs can be found in repeated stool microscopic examinations, often with amebic cysts or trophozoites. In addition, a germiculture result is positive for bacillus dysenteriae, and the treatment is effective if treated as dysentery or amoebic dysentery.

Treatment

1. *Treatment principles* fortifying the spleen and stomach, reserving the essence and stopping diarrhea.
2. *Commonly used maneuvers* rubbing, pressure kneading, and scrubbing.
3. *Commonly used acupoints and areas zhōngwǎn* (RN 12), *qìhǎi* (RN 6), *guānyuán* (RN 4), *tiānshū* (ST 25), *zúsān lǐ* (ST 36), *píshū* (BL 20), *wèishū* (BL 21), *dàchángshū* (BL 25), *bāliào* (BL 31 to 34), the lumbosacral region, and the abdomen.
4. *Operational methods*

   a. The patient is supine, with the practitioner to the right. Use the right hand to perform counter-clockwise rubbing all over the abdomen for two to three minutes.
   b. Next, use the index and middle fingers to apply finger kneading on both sides of *tiānshū*.
   c. Apply palm rubbing on *zhōngwǎn*, *qìhǎi,* and *guānyuán* for three to five minutes.
   d. Apply finger kneading on bilateral *zúsānlǐ* for one to two minutes.
   e. Have the patient change to a prone position with the practitioner standing at the left side. Use the index and middle fingers to perform kneading on bilateral back points. The points may include

píshū, wèishū, dàcháng shū, and *bāliào* (BL 31 to 34). Knead each point for one to two minutes.

f. Lastly, use the hypothenar to perform horizontal scrubbing on acupoints such as *bāliào, píshū,* and *mìngmén* (DU 4).

Self-preventional Methods

1. You should be in a supine position. With hands overlapped, use the entire palm to perform counter-clockwise kneading rubbing on the lower and upper abdomen, each area for three to five minutes, until there is feeling of heat generated by friction penetrating to the interior of the abdomen.
2. Remain in the same position as above. Apply finger kneading on bilateral *zhōngwǎn* and *tiānshū* respectively, one minute per point.
3. Change to a sitting position, and apply finger kneading on bilateral *zúsānlǐ* for about a minute.

Precautions

1. Help the patient to overcome the mental burden due to the illness.
2. Make sure you stick to a healthy and moderate diet, pay attention to personal hygiene, and avoid cold, greasy, or spicy food.

Everyday Exercises

1. What are the routine examinations for functional or chronic diarrhea?
2. How is tui na treatment performed for people suffering chronic diarrhea?

Day 3

CONSTIPATION

Constipation refers to a common malaise characterized by condensed and hardened feces, and prolonged and difficult defecation although there is a desire to defecate. Even though constipation can be caused by an organic intestinal disease, the majority of cases are related to the functional disorder of the nerve regulating the defecation reflex. Many other factors may also contribute to constipation, including insufficient motor power for defecation, changes in the routine of daily life, low fiber in the food, and decreased enterocinesia. In addition, people recovering from illness, post-partum women, or the elderly with insufficient qi, blood or body fluids, tend to have constipation. Over-dependence on laxatives or enema abuse can also contribute to the problem.

Clinical Manifestations

1. Reduced bowel movements, dry and hard stool with decreased volume, and difficult defecation.
2. Palpation can detect accumulated feces with mild tenderness in the left lower quadrant where the descending colon is located.
3. Defecation of hard feces can cause anal pain, fissure, and bloody stool, which in turn, would cause fear of the pain, so it makes bowel movement even more difficult.
4. If the patient suffers constipation for an extended period of time, accumulated fecal toxins in the body may lead to fatigue, weakness, headache, dizziness, abdominal pain, bloating, and loss of appetite. It may also result in problems such as hemorrhoids and anal fissure.

Diagnosis and Differentiation

Generally, the diagnosis of constipation can be made based on clinical manifestations. However, it still needs to be differentiated from the following diseases:

1. *Partial intestinal obstruction* Symptoms are abdominal pain, vomiting, abdominal distension, no bowel movements, or gas. X-ray examination shows a ladder-like fluid covering in the intestinal cavity.
2. *Anorectal diseases* Problems such as inflammation, hemorrhoids, and anal fissure may cause spasms of the anal sphincter and lead to constipation.

Treatment

Tui na has a fairly good treatment effect on functional constipation.

1. *Treatment principles* enhancing intestinal motility, promoting normal bowel movements.
2. *Commonly used maneuvers* rubbing, finger kneading, pressure kneading, and scrubbing.
3. *Commonly used acupoints and areas dàhéng* (SP 15), *qìhǎi* (RN 6), *guānyuán* (RN 4), *píshū* (BL 20), *wèishū* (BL 21), *dàcháng shū* (BL 25), *bāliào* (BL 31 to 34), *zhīgōu* (SJ 6), *zúsānlǐ* (ST 36), and the upper abdomen.
4. *Operational methods*

   Basic operations
   a. The patient is supine, with the practitioner sitting on the patient's right. Operate with agile and gentle finger kneading on the upper abdomen for one to two minutes, and gradually transition to the lower abdomen.
   b. Perform whole-palm or thenar kneading on lower abdomen acupoints *qìhǎi* and *guānyuán*, each point for two to three minutes.
   c. Apply pressure kneading with the thenar for three to five minutes along the surface anatomical path equivalent to that of the colon. Start working on the ascending colon on the lower right abdomen, then the transverse colon and lastly, the descending colon, for a total of three to five minutes (see Figure 113). Afterwards, focus on the left *dàhéng* and perform finger kneading for one to two minutes.

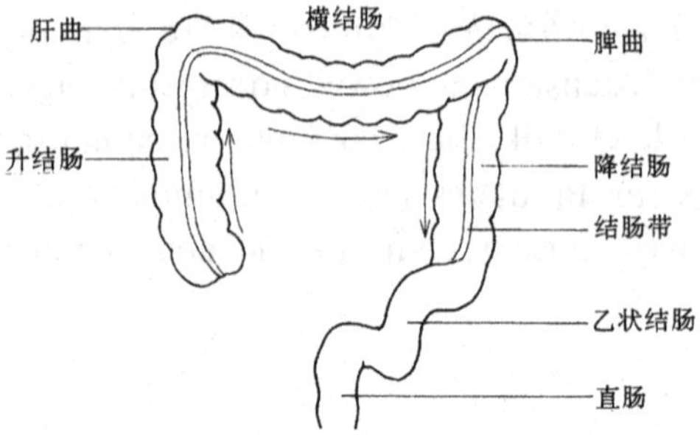

升结肠	-	ascending colon
肝曲	-	hepatic flexure
横结肠	-	transverse colon
脾曲	-	splenic flexure
降结肠	-	descending colon
结肠带	-	colic band
乙状结肠	-	sigmoid colon
直肠	-	rectum

Figure 113 Colon schematic

d. Perform thenar kneading top-down along the anatomical path of the descending colon on the left abdomen for two to three minutes. End the abdominal operation by using the palm to rub the abdomen.
e. Use finger kneading on both sides of *zhīgōu* and *zúsānlǐ*, one minute for each point.
f. The patient changes to a prone position. Perform double-finger kneading on back *shu* points, including *píshū*, *wèishū*, *dàchángshū* and *bāliào*. Operate on each point for one to two minutes.
g. Lastly, apply hypothenar scrubbing on the lumbosacral area in a top-down order along the path of *dumai* and both sides of *bāliào*.

- *Treatment based on pattern differentiation*

a. For decreased appetite, chest and abdominal fullness, and belching: more emphasis on kneading and rubbing of *zhōngwǎn*, foulage on hypochondriac area, and pressure kneading on *nèiguān*.

b. For patient with anal disease: finger kneading *cháng qiáng* (DU 1) for one to two minutes, and enhance finger kneading on *bā liào*.

Self-preventional Methods

1. *Rubbing the abdomen* Lie supine, and with hands overlapped, use the entire palm to rub the abdomen in a clockwise direction for eight to ten minutes.
2. *Kneading acupoints* Perform finger kneading on *zhī gōu* and *zú sān lǐ*, one minute for each acupoint.

Precautions

1. Drink sufficient boiled water, about 300 to 500 ml with a bit of salt in it every morning. Eat more vegetables, fruits, and other foods containing good amounts of fiber.
2. Develop a regular bowel routine. Go to the toilet regularly on a fixed schedule even if there is no desire to defecate.
3. Enhance the strength of the abdominal muscles by doing more physical exercises. Exercises to help strengthen the levator ani muscles (the muscles that make up the pelvic floor) is good for those with anal diseases.
4. Avoid laxative abuse.

Everyday Exercises

1. What is constipation? What are its main clinical manifestations?
2. How would you use tui na to treat constipation?

Day 4

CHRONIC CHOLECYSTITIS

Cholecystitis, which is inflammation of the gallbladder, is more common in adult obese women, and is caused by obstruction in the bile ducts, bacterial infection, cholestasis, or gallstone formation. Cholelithiasis, on the other hand, is the presence of gallstones in the gallbladder. Cholecystitis and cholelithiasis in clinical practice often reinforce and accompany each other.

Clinical Manifestations

The patient feels pain and discomfort on the right hypochondrium, ranging from a light pricking to a severe stabbing and cramping pain. The pain may radiate to the right scapular, and is induced by a rich meal or high-fat diet, and accompanied by indigestion, nausea, and vomiting. There is muscle tension, tenderness, and percussion pain on the upper right quadrant of the abdomen. According to the severity of the inflammation, varying degrees of muscle resistance can occur.

Upon the onset of chronic cholecystitis, there is an elevation of WBCs, and X-ray examination can reveal stones in the gallbladder Gallbladder imaging may reveal poor contracting function of the gallbladder. Ultrasound techniques may also reveal thickening and roughness of the gallbladder wall.

Diagnosis and Differentiation

The more obvious the pain, tenderness, muscle resistance, and inflammation on the upper right quadrant of the abdomen, the more serious is the problem. As mentioned, X-rays and ultrasound are helpful in diagnosing the disease. Clinically, it needs to be differentiated from the following conditions:

1. *Gastritis and ulcerous gastritis* The onset of gastritis pain is often postprandial, about half an hour after a meal, and usually not severe.

The onset of ulcerous gastritis pain follows a certain rhythm and usually lasts a longer time, often more than a week.

2. *Acute pancreatitis* The pain and tenderness are mostly located on the upper left quadrant of the abdomen, with increased serum amylase. Biliary tract disease often induces acute pancreatitis.
3. *Acute appendicitis* It may be mistaken for cholecystitis. Appendicitis is more common in younger people, while cholecystitis is more common in older people, unless the patient has a family history of cholecystitis.

Treatment

1. *Treatment principles* comforting the liver, benefiting the gallbladder, resolving stagnant qi, and relieving pain.
2. *Commonly used maneuvers* pressing, rubbing, kneading, disjoining pushing, scrubbing, and foulage.
3. *Commonly used acupoints and areas* the right *rìyuè* (GB 24) and *zhāngmén* (LR 13), *géshū* (BL 17), *gānshū* (BL 18), *dǎnshū* (BL 19), *yánglíngquán* (GB 34), *dǎnnáng* (EX-LE 6) and *qiūxū* (GB 40), the right hypochondrium, and the upper abdomen.

4. *Operational methods*
   *Basic operation*s

   a. The patient should be lying on his or her left side, with the practitioner sitting posterior to the patient. Apply agile and gentle rubbing maneuver on the right hypochondrium of the patient for three to five minutes; then, perform finger kneading on *rìyuè*, *zhāngmén,* and *qīmén*, one minute for each acupoint.
   b. Have the lie supine, with the practitioner sitting to the patient's right. Apply thenar or whole palm kneading on the upper abdomen and right hypochondrium, one minute for each area; then use disjoining pushing on the lower chest and upper abdomen. Do this 20 to 30 times for each area.
   c. Next, apply pressure kneading on *yánglíngquán*, *dǎnnáng,* and *qiūxū* for about one minute for each acupoint, until patient experiences a soreness *de*-qi sensation.

d. Have the patient in either prone or sitting position. Use your index finger, middle finger, or thumb to apply the finger kneading method on the back *shu* points, such as *géshū*, *gānshū,* and *dǎnshū*, about one minute per acupoint.
e. The last step is to perform scrubbing on *dǎnnáng* until the patient senses the heat from the friction. End the operation by using foulage on both hypochondria.

Treatment based on pattern differentiation

f. For patients with more severe cholecystitis pain: first, find the tender spots near *yánglíngquán* and *dǎnnáng*, and then apply relatively heavy yet gentle pressing or pressure kneading on the acupoints to resolve urgent pain.
g. For patients with gastrointestinal symptoms: focus more on kneading *zhōngwǎn* (RN 12), and pressure kneading *zúsānlǐ* (ST 36).

Self-preventional Methods

1. *Push-rubbing on the right hypochondrium* Use the entire palm to perform the pushing rubbing maneuver on the right hypochondrium from the inside out for three to five minutes. If one hand is tired, use the other hand to continue the maneuver.
2. *Finger kneading on the abdominal acupoints* Apply finger kneading on *zhōngwǎn*, right *zhāngmén* and right *qīmén*, about one minute for each acupoint.
3. *Finger kneading on acupoints of the extremities* Apply finger kneading on *yánglíngquán* and *dǎnnáng* for one minute each.

Precautions

1. Adopt a healthier diet, and avoid greasy food and other food that is not easy to digest.
2. If your condition worsens, consider surgery.

Everyday Exercises

1. What are the main clinical manifestations of chronic cholecystitis?
2. How should we use tui na therapy to treat chronic cholecystitis?

Day 5

SEQUELAE OF GASTRIC SURGERY

Sequelae is the term used for any abnormal condition resulting from a previous disease, treatment, or injury. Sequelae of gastric surgery refers to any anatomical, physiological, or metabolic disorders after stomach surgery. In the following sections we will discuss a few of such sequelae that can be treated with tui na.

Peristalsis Disorder of Remnant Stomach

Gastric peristalsis in the normal stomach is able to perform the functions of storing, stirring, mixing, digesting, and transporting the chyme to the duodenum. After stomach surgery, gastric tensility is often decreased, with a weakened emptying capability due to temporary gastric remnant movement disorders, resulting in food retention or stomach expansion.

Within one to two days after surgery, symptoms such as epigastric pain, nausea, and vomiting are often observed clinically, and can last for some ten days to several weeks. Gastrointestinal barium X-ray examination can reveal reduced gastric tensility, motility, retention, and expansion.

Dumping Syndrome

Dumping syndrome, also known as postprandial early onset syndrome, often occurs upon eating among post-surgical patients between the first and the third week, and especially after eating a large amount of carbohydrates. The symptoms are epigastric discomfort and nausea, sometimes accompanied by belching, vomiting, abdominal flatulence, and sometimes a feeling of urgency to pass motion. At the same time, there may be dizziness, vertigo, and even syncope, and the patient may feel extreme weak, with profuse sweating and pallor. In more serious situations, low blood pressure may occur so that the patient has to stop eating immediately.

Postgastrectomy Malnutrition

A gastrectomy (a partial or full surgical removal of the stomach) can cause gastrointestinal anatomical and physiological changes, as well as nutritional malabsorption, resulting in a series of clinical symptoms including diarrhea, weight loss, anemia, and vitamin deficiency. This condition is called post gastrectomy malnutrition.

Treatment

Tui na therapy can achieve results that Western drugs cannot in treating digestive ailments, especially those after gastrointestinal surgery.

The appropriate time for receiving tui na treatment is generally four weeks after the surgery.

1. *Treatment principles* fortifying the spleen and the stomach, promoting absorption, enhancing gastric function.
2. *Commonly used maneuvers* finger, double-finger, or palm kneading; scrubbing and spinal pinching.
3. *Commonly used acupoints and areas* *zhōngwǎn* (RN 12), left *liángén* (ST 21), *liángqiū* (ST 34), *zúsānlǐ* (ST 36), *xiàjùxū* (ST 39), *nèiguān* (PC 6), *wèishū* (BL 21), *píshū* (BL 20), *sānjiāoshū* (BL 22), upper abdomen, and the spine.
4. *Operational methods*
   Basic operations
   a. The patient is supine, with the practitioner sitting to the patient's right. Employ gentle kneading using the entire palm on the upper abdomen for about one minute with moderate force to make the patient get used to the operation.
   b. Apply finger kneading on *zhōngwǎn* and left *liángmén*, two to three minutes for each acupoint. Use moderate force to make the patient feel comfortable. Apply palm kneading for two to three minutes on the upper abdomen. Alternate between acupoints and the upper abdomen, for about 20 minutes.
   c. Continue the operation with the patient supine. Apply finger kneading on *nèiguān* bilaterally for one to two minutes, then *liángqiū*, *zúsānlǐ,* and *xiàjùxū*, each for one to two minutes.
   d. With the patient prone, stands to the patient's right. Apply double-finger kneading on *píshū*, *wèishū,* and *sānjiāoshū* until the patient gets the soreness *de*-qi sensation. Next, apply horizontal scrubbing

with the hypothenar until the patient feels the heat. Then, perform spinal pinching for three to five times starting from the sacroiliac area, going up to the lumbar, passing the thoracic segment, and reaching the cervicothoracic area. While pinching on *píshū* and *wèishū*, increase the intensity of spinal pinching or add lift pinching to enhance the stimulation on these acupoints.

Self-preventional Methods

1. Use one hand to apply clockwise kneading rubbing in the abdomen for about a minute.
2. With hands overlapped and the entire palm placed on the mid-upper abdomen, apply clockwise kneading rubbing for three to five minutes. Do the same for the upper left abdomen.
3. Use both thumbs for finger kneading on bilateral *liángqiū* and *zúsānlǐ*, for one to two minutes for each acupoint, until *de*-qi sensation is reached.

Precautions

1. After a gastrectomy, the patient should be served with high-calorie, easy-to-digest, and nutritious food.
2. It is good to eat multiple meals in a day in smaller proportions, supplemented with a little bit of vinegar, since vinegar can aid digestion and kill bacteria.
3. Chew carefully and swallow food slowly to reduce the workload of the stomach.
4. A large amount of carbohydrates is not appropriate for patients with dumping syndrome. Acquire the habit of taking soup during a meal and drinking water between meals.
5. Lie down and rest for a while after eating.
6. For patients with delayed postprandial syndrome, eat a little bit of candy during the onset to relieve the symptoms.
7. Avoid tobacco and alcohol. Balance work and rest. Establish a regular routine.

Everyday Exercises

1. How would you perform tui na on patients with sequelae of gastric surgery?
2. What are the precautions for a patient with gastric surgery sequelae?

Day 6

POLYNEURITIS

Polyneuritis, also known as peripheral neuropathy or never ending neuritis, is an inflammation of multiple nerves at once. Individuals with polyneuritis can experience paralysis, pain, loss of sensation, and tingling sensations in the affected nerves. The following are some possible causes of polyneuritis:

1. Systemic infections caused by bacteria or viruses: influenza, mumps, scarlet fever, dysentery, herpes zoster, infectious mononucleosis.
2. Nutritional deficiencies or metabolic disorders: athlete's foot disease, diabetes, and pellagra.
3. Heavy metal poisoning: arsenic, mercury, lead, copper, bismuth, manganese, antimony.
4. Organic compounds: carbon disulfide and organic phosphorus.
5. Drugs: sulfonamides, furan, and barbiturates.
6. Others: connective tissue diseases, cancer, genetic and other risk factors of unknown etiology.

Clinical Manifestations

1. Symmetric sensory, motor, and nutritional dysfunction on distal limbs.
2. Sensory disturbances: fingers and toes experience abnormal sensations such as tingling, itching, or burning, or a feeling as if one is wearing gloves or socks.
3. Dyskinesia: weakness, muscle atrophy, tenderness, diminished or disappeared tendon reflexes of the hands and feet.
4. Nutritional dysfunction: mostly profuse sweating or no perspiration, and coldness on hands and feet; thin and bright or dry and cracked skin; crisp nails and hyperkeratosis.

Diagnosis and Differentiation

1. Diagnosis is based on symptoms such as symmetric abnormality of the limbs; distal sensory, motor, and nutrition disorders; and impaired tendon reflexes.

2. Patients at an early stage may lack typical clinical manifestations. Seek professional care as soon as possible.
3. Clinically, it should be differentiated from the following diseases:

   a. *Periodic paralysis* There is no clear sensory disturbances of feeling like wearing gloves or socks; the duration is short-term with quick recovery.
   b. *Poliomyelitis (polio sequelae)* The muscle paralysis is asymmetric for the majority of cases, and there is no reduced skin sensation.

Treatment

1. *Treatment principles* strengthening the force of muscles, preventing muscle atrophy, and promoting early recovery of the nervous function.
2. *Commonly used maneuvers* rolling, grasping, finger kneading, and scrubbing.
3. *Commonly used acupoints and areas* shǒusānlǐ (LI 10), *wàiguān* (SJ 5), *hégǔ* (LI 4), *yújì* (LU 10), *láogōng* (PC 8), *zúsān lǐ* (ST 36), *nèiting* (ST 44), *sānyīnjiāo* (SP 6), *yǒngquán* (KI 1), muscle groups of the hands, feet, forearms, and calves.

4. *Operational methods*
   Operations on upper limbs

   a. The patient is supine, with the practitioner sitting at the side of the patient. First, use the rolling method on various extensors and flexors of the forearm, the palm, and the dorsum of the hand, back and forth for three to five minutes. Then, apply the grasping maneuver on the ulnar and radial muscles (see Figure 114) and the thenar and hypothenar muscles, back and forth for five to ten times.
   b. Perform finger kneading on *shǒusānlǐ*, *wàiguān*, *hégǔ*, *yújì* and *láogōng*, one minute per acupoint. Apply the same method on the interosseous muscles on the dorsum and lateral side of the hand (see Figure 115).
   c. Lastly, apply scrubbing on the extensor and flexors of the forearm.

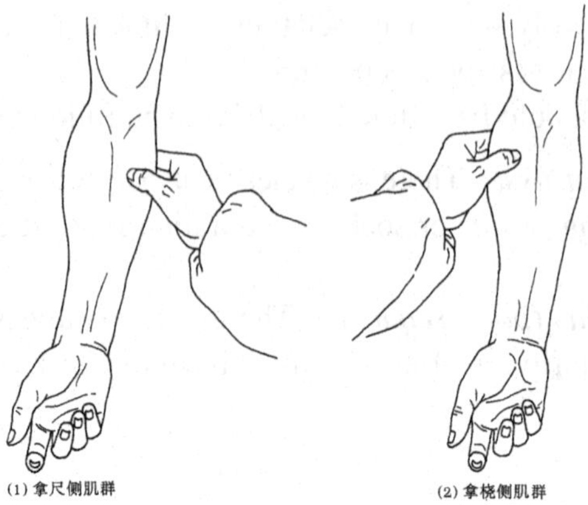

拿尺侧肌群	-	grasping the ulnar muscles
拿桡侧肌群	-	grasping the radial muscles

Figure 114 Grasping the muscle groups of the ulnar and radial sides

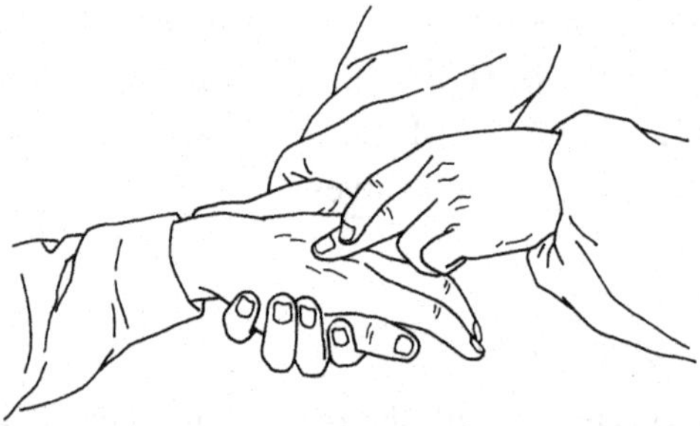

Figure 115 Finger kneading on the interosseous muscles on the dorsum of the hand

Operations on lower limbs

a. The patient is supine, with the practitioner sitting at the side of the patient. First, apply rolling or palm-heel kneading to the anterolateral leg, then down to the anterior tibialis muscle. Continue down to reach the dorsum of the foot, for a total of up to three to five minutes.
b. Apply finger kneading on *xuèhǎi* (SP 10), *zúsānlǐ*, *yánglíngquán* (GB 34), *sānyīnjiāo*, *jiěxī* (ST 41) and *nèiting*, one minute on each acupoint.

c. Apply finger kneading on the dorsal interosseous muscle for about two minutes; then apply scrubbing on the anterior tibialis muscle until there is a sensation of heat.
d. Have the patient in a prone position, and apply the rolling method with the focus on the triceps of the calf, going down to the Achilles tendon for three to five minutes.
e. Apply finger kneading on *chéngshān* (BL 57), *kūnlún* (BL 60), *shēnmài* (BL 62) and *yǒngquán*, each for one minute. Then, apply grasping starting from the triceps, and working all the way down to the Achilles tendon, two to three times. Lastly, perform scrubbing on the triceps and the pelma till the patient feels the heat.

Self-Preventional Methods

1. Be persistent with functional exercises of the extremities, including gripping strength, flexion, extension, and rotation.
2. Use the opposite hand to apply foulage or kneading alternately at the ends of the extremities, including the fingers, toes, wrists, ankles, forearms, and calves.

Precautions

1. Keep the extremities warm, and avoid burns.
2. Avoid tobacco and alcohol.
3. Send the patient to hospital immediately during the acute phase of infection, as there could be paralysis of the respiratory muscle in addition to quadriplegia.

Everyday Exercises

1. What are the characteristics of sensory disturbances and motor disorders on a patient with polyneuritis?
2. What are the treatment principles of tui na for a patient with polyneuritis? Give examples on how to operate on the upper limbs.

WEEK 6

Day 1

FACIAL NEURITIS

Also known as Bell's palsy, this condition refers to the peripheral facial paralysis caused by acute non-suppurative inflammation of the facial nerves in the stylomastoid foramen (i.e., facial nerve tube). It may be related to virus infection with various degrees of facial nerve edema, compression, and degeneration of the myelin or axon, leading to paralysis. It has acute onset and rapid development of complete facial paralysis, mostly on one side. It can affect people of any age, but predominantly young men.

In Chinese medical practice, it is believed that the disease often occurs in individuals with qi and blood deficiency. They contract the wind-cold pathogen that causes stagnant qi in meridians on the face, which further leads to immobilized blood failing to nourish the tendons. Therefore, it is often referred to as "wry mouth and eyes" or facial paralysis.

Clinical Manifestations

Patients often find out about wry mouth in the washroom in early morning after waking up. There is ipsilateral paralysis of the mimeticfacial muscles, with the following manifestations:

1. Disappeared forehead wrinkles, expanded eye cleft, and flattened nasolabial fold.
2. Crooked philtrum ditch, drooping mouth, and face dragged to the contralateral side.
3. Food easily resides in the gap between the ipsilateral cheek and teeth, often with saliva trickling down from the ipsilateral side of the mouth.

4. May be accompanied by diminished or disappeared gustatory sense in the front 2/3s of the tongue, and tears with ectropion of the lower eye lid.
5. Pain on the ipsilateral ear and mastoid.

Diagnosis and Differentiation

Key Diagnostic Criteria

1. There is acute onset, with sudden facial muscle paralysis.
2. The patient is not able to frown, close the eyes, show the teeth, blow air, or pout. Figure 116a shows left peripheral facial paralysis.
3. With the patient's eyes closed, the ipsilateral eye ball rolls on the top. Since the oculi rimae is not able to shut, the sclera exposes, which is a positive sign for Bell's palsy (see Figure 116b).

Differential Diagnosis

1. *Acute infectious polyneuritis* Facial paralysis is often bilateral, with limb paralysis and protein cell separation in cerebrospinal fluid.
2. *Mumps, parotid gland tumor, or acoustic neuromas* The onset of facial paralysis is slow, and can also damage other cranial nerves.
3. *Cerebral hemisphere lesions (e.g., cerebrovascular accident)* Facial paralysis is limited to motor disorders of contralateral facial muscles

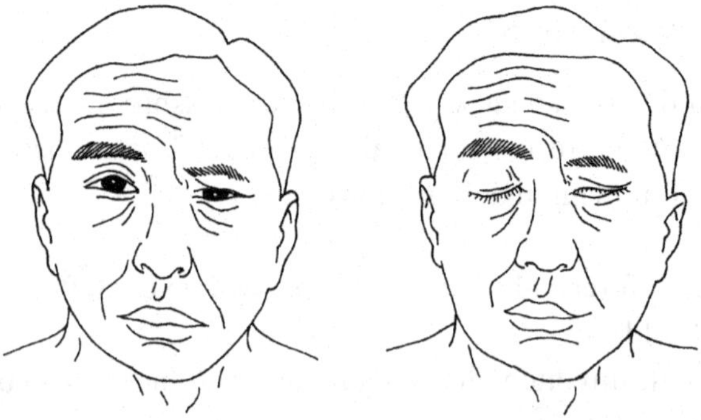

(a) (b)

Figure 116 Left peripheral facial paralysis (a) and Bell's sign (b)

below the lesion, while the facial muscles above the lesion remain normal, and it is often accompanied with paralysis of limbs. Such facial paralysis is known as central facial paralysis.

Treatment

1. *Treatment principles* dispelling wind, unblocking the collaterals, invigorating blood and scattering stasis.
2. *Commonly used maneuvers* finger and thenar kneading, grasping, rubbing, smearing, and pinching.
3. *Commonly used acupoints and areas yìntáng* (EX-HN 3), *sìbái* (ST 2), *yángbái* (GB 14), *jīngmíng* (BL 1), *tàiyáng* (EX-HN 5), *dìcāng* (ST 4), *jiáchē* (ST 6), *yíngxiāng* (LI 20), *shuǐgōu* (DU 26), *chéngjiāng* (RN 24), *fēngchí* (GB 20), *hégǔ* (LI 4), orbicularis oculi muscle, orbicularis oris muscle, facial area, and mastoid.
4. *Operational methods*

   a. The patient is supine, with the practitioner sitting at the patient's right side. First, apply finger kneading on facial acupoints including *tàiyáng*, *sìbái*, *yángbái*, *dìcāng*, *jiáchē*, and *yíngxiāng*.
   b. Then, apply thenar kneading on the ipsilateral site, and alternate between finger and thenar kneading for about ten minutes. Generally speaking, the forces applied on the ipsilateral side are relatively more intensive to make the patient experience the *de*-qi sensation.
   c. Next, apply smearing on the orbicularis oculi and orbicularis oris muscles (see Figure 117), and combine finger kneading on acupoints and thenar kneading on the face for two to three minutes.
   d. Apply facial pinching (see Figure 118), followed by finger rubbing on the ipsilateral mastoid (see Figure 119) for one minute and grasping on *fēngchí* for five to ten minutes.
   e. Finally, apply light and gentle thenar kneading for three to five minutes on the contralateral face, and end the operation with grasping *hégǔ*.

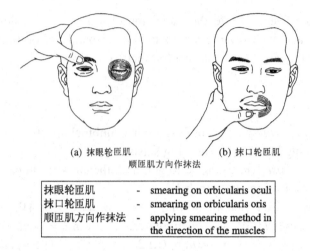

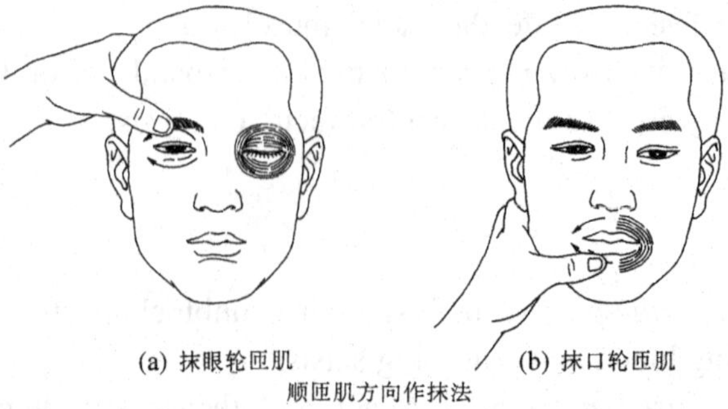

抹眼轮匝肌	-	smearing on orbicularis oculi
抹口轮匝肌	-	smearing on orbicularis oris
顺匝肌方向作抹法	-	applying smearing method in the direction of the muscles

Figure 117 Smearing on orbicularis oculi and orbicularis oris muscles

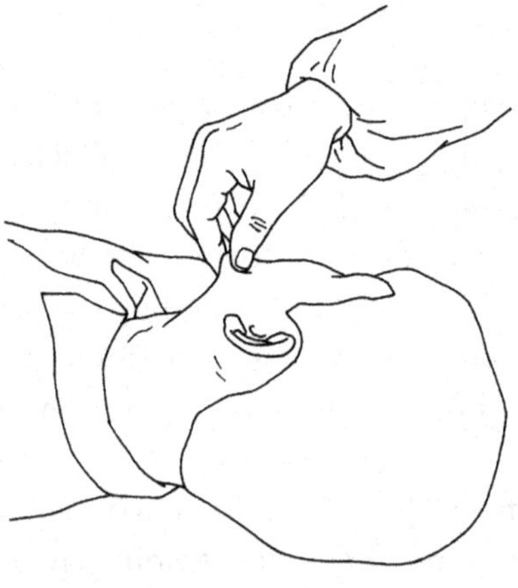

Figure 118 Facial pinching

Self-Preventional Methods

1. Apply kneading and pinching daily on the paralyzed facial muscles.
2. Apply kneading on *fēngchí*, *hégŭ,* and *jiáchē*, and smearing on orbicularis oculi and orbicularis oris muscles.
3. A hair dryer can be used as a tool for thermal therapy on the paralyzed facial muscle and the mastoid. However, take precautions to prevent burns.

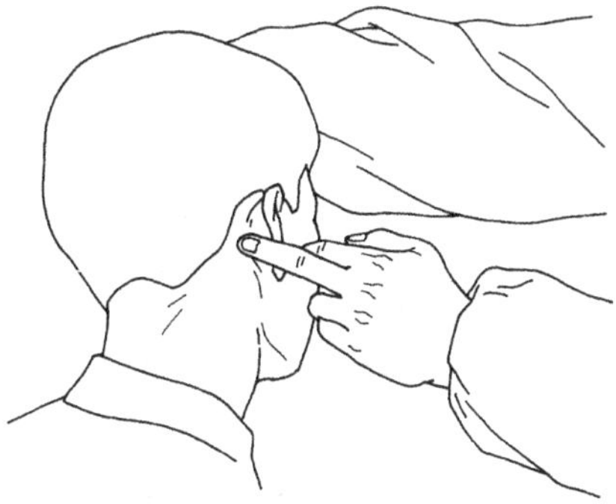

Figure 119 Finger rubbing the mastoid

Precautions

1. The practitioner should have his or her nails cut prior to performing tui na on the face. A novice tui na practitioner should use a therapeutic towel to prevent the skin from being broken.
2. Use eyeshades, eye ointment, or eye drops to protect the exposed cornea and prevent conjunctivitis.
3. Keep the face warm, especially when going out in winter.
4. Seek professional treatment to have the functions of the facial nerves restored as soon as possible.

Everyday Exercises

1. What are the major differences between peripheral facial paralysis and central facial paralysis?
2. How would you perform tui na for a patient with peripheral facial paralysis?

Day 2

DYSMENORRHEA

Dysmenorrhea is a common condition experienced in young women. It refers to the pain in the lower abdominal or lumbosacral pain before, during, or after her menstrual period. Sometimes the pain is severe enough to even cause shock.

If dysmenorrhea occurs upon menarche (a woman's first menstrual period), it is known as primary dysmenorrhea, and is usually caused by uterine hypoplasia or malposition, and cervical stenosis. If the first onset of dysmenorrhea occurs a while after menarche, it is known as secondary dysmenorrhea, and is mostly caused by endometriosis and chronic pelvic inflammation.

In Chinese medical practice, it is believed that the condition is usually a result of qi-blood stagnation, sluggishness of damp-cold, or damp-heat accumulation. When there is blockage of qi movement in the lower abdominal area, there would be stasis in the meridians and vessels, causing lower abdominal pain.

Clinical Manifestations

Lower abdominal pain often occurs a few days before, or on the first day of, menses, and some patients may experience associated lumbosacral pain, distended breast pain, and sluggish flow. Symptoms may gradually alleviate and disappear after the first or second day. Dysmenorrhea is often accompanied by other systemic symptoms, such as irritation, nausea, vomiting, dizziness, and cold limbs. Pain and other symptoms disappear naturally after menstruation.

In severe cases, the patient may suffer pallor and profuse sweating, and pain so debilitating that she is unable to engage in work or study.

Diagnosis and Differentiation

Lower abdominal pain is an important diagnostic evidence of this condition. Of course, abdominal pain is also indicative of many other conditions. Therefore, in addition to obtaining a detailed medical history of the patient, it is necessary to perform general and gynecological examinations to identify the problem.

Treatment

Tui na treatment needs to be applied two weeks prior to menstruation, once every other day for the two weeks. The next treatment course should start two weeks prior to the next cycle.

1. *Treatment principles* moving qi, invigorating blood, warming the meridians, dissipating cold, dispelling blood stasis, and relieving pain. Generally, tui na should be done for three consecutive months as a treatment course for the best results.
2. *Commonly used maneuvers* rubbing, finger kneading, grasping and scrubbing.
3. *Commonly used acupoints and areas* *guānyuán* (RN 4), *xuèhǎi* (SP 10), *yīnlíngquán* (SP 9), *sānyīnjiāo* (SP 6), *bāliào* (BL 31 to 34), *tiáojīng* (an extra point located lateral to *yǒngquán*, i.e. KI 1, between the fourth and fifth metatarsal bone), lower abdomen and the lumbosacral region.
4. *Operational methods*

   Basic operations

   a. The patient is supine, with the practitioner sitting at her right. First, perform finger rubbing gently on the lower abdomen with *guānyuán* as the center in a clockwise direction. Then, apply finger kneading on *guānyuán*, preferably invoking the soreness *de*-qi sensation. Alternate between rubbing and finger kneading maneuvers on the lower abdomen for about ten minutes.
   b. Apply finger kneading on menstrual regulating points such as *xuèhǎi*, *yīnlíngquán,* and *sānyīnjiāo*, for two minutes each. Focus more on *xuèhǎi* and *sānyīnjiāo* by alternating between heavier and lighter stimulation for an extended length of time, as they are the main acupoints.
   c. Have the patient lie prone, with the practitioner sitting to her right. Perform finger kneading on *bāliào* to end the operation.

Treatment based on pattern differentiation

The patient should be supine, with the practitioner sitting at her right.

a. *For patients with qi stagnation and blood stasis* In addition to the basic operation, add kneading rubbing on the hypochondriac area and finger kneading on *gānshū* (BL 18) and *géshū* (BL 17).
b. *For stagnant damp-cold* Apply additional kneading on the lower abdomen, and add scrubbing on *bāliào* until the patient feels the heat generated from the friction.

Self-Preventional Methods

1. Lying supine, place overlapped palms over the lower abdomen to apply clockwise pressure kneading for three to five minutes.
2. Apply finger kneading on *xuèhăi* and *sānyīnjiāo*, each for one to two minutes.
3. Be persistent with the self-preventative method, and do it once or twice daily.

Precautions

1. Exercise more in between menstrual periods.
2. Pay attention to personal hygiene during the menstrual period.
3. Keep warm during the menstrual period. Avoid exposure to cool air during summer while asleep. Avoid exposure to the rain and strenuous activities during the menstrual period.
4. Eat warm food, and avoid overeating of cold and raw food, including cold fruits, or very spicy food.
5. Rest well when dysmenorrhea attacks.
6. Before and during the menstrual period, maintain a happy mood, avoid disputes or negative mental stimuli, and relax. Do not be afraid of the condition.
7. If the patient has received tuina treatment for an extended period of time without significant results, she should have a gynecological examination.

Everyday Exercises

1. What is dysmenorrhea, and what are the two types of dysmenorrhea?
2. When in the menstrual cycle do you treat dysmenorrhea using tui na? How would you treat it?

Day 3

ACUTE MASTITIS

Acute mastitis is a condition characterized by breast swelling, pain, and blockage of milk flow among lactating women. It is commonly known as "breast boils" in Chinese. It is often due to several reasons, such as the breasts being squeezed more than usual, insufficient cleaning, or broken nipples during breast-feeding. Bacteria, mainly *Staphylococcus aureus*, gets into the ruptured nipples and spread along the breast ducts, leading to inflammation and edema of the breast ducts, which blocks the milk from being excreted. When milk accumulates, it in turn creates a favorable environment for the bacteria to grow.

Clinical Manifestations

1. Red and swollen breasts, pain or burning sensation, blocked milk flow on ipsilateral breast.
2. Palpation can detect obvious agglomeration and tenderness. The size of the agglomeration has a positive correlation with the severity of the mastitis. The bigger the size, the greater the range of breast duct blockage. Likewise, a smaller mass indicates a smaller range of blocked ducts.
3. In addition to local symptoms, the condition is often accompanied by severe systemic symptoms including fever, chills, headache, aching joints, and poor appetite.
4. Ipsilateral axillary lymph node enlargement and tenderness can be detected.

If the condition does not get treated, and there is persistent fever, it can often lead to formation of abscesses, which then requires surgical drainage.

Diagnosis

Key Diagnostic Criteria

1. Women during lactation suffers breast redness, swelling, pain, and sluggish milk flow.

2. There is local agglomeration and tenderness.
3. There is ipsilateral axillary lymph node swelling and tenderness.
4. Fever; blood tests show increased WBCs and neutrophils.

Treatment

The characteristics of mastitis are blocked breast ducts and milk accumulation, for which tui na is an effective external treatment.

1. *Treatment principles* reducing swelling, resolving masses, and unblocking milk ducts.
2. *Commonly used maneuvers* rubbing, finger kneading, disjoining pushing.
3. *Commonly used acupoints and areas* *dànzhōng* (RN 17), *zhāngmén* (LR 13), *qīmén* (LR 14), *géshū* (BL 17), *gānshū* (BL 18), *qǔchí* (LI 11), *sānyīnjiāo* (SP 6), and the ipsilateral breast.
4. *Operational methods*
   a. The patient sits with the practitioner sitting at the patient's rear left. First, apply double-finger kneading on bilateral *géshū* and *gānshū*, each for one to two minutes. Next, standing at the back of the patient, use both hands to perform finger rubbing for one to two minutes on the hypochondria where *zhāngmén* and *qīmén* are located (see Figure 120).
   b. The patient lies supine, with the practitioner sitting to her right. Use finger rubbing on *dànzhōng* for one to two minutes; then apply disjoining pushing on the same points for ten to 20 times.
   c. The patient remains supine. Use the entire palm to apply push-rubbing to the ipsilateral breast. Take the right breast as an example: start from the bottom close to the midline, transition to the upper lateral side, and reach the top near the midline, making it a clockwise operation that lasts for two to three minutes (see Fig. 121). Next, perform finger kneading with the agglomeration as the centre, and operate toward the outer loop around the mass for three to five minutes. Apply these two maneuvers alternately. Since the patient will already be experiencing breast swelling and pain, the

manipulations must be gentle. This step is the key tui na procedure in treating acute mastitis.

The above procedures can be supplemented with finger kneading on acupoints including *qŭchí* and *sānyīnjiāo*, about one minute each. For patients with fever, increase the intensity while operating on *qŭchí*.

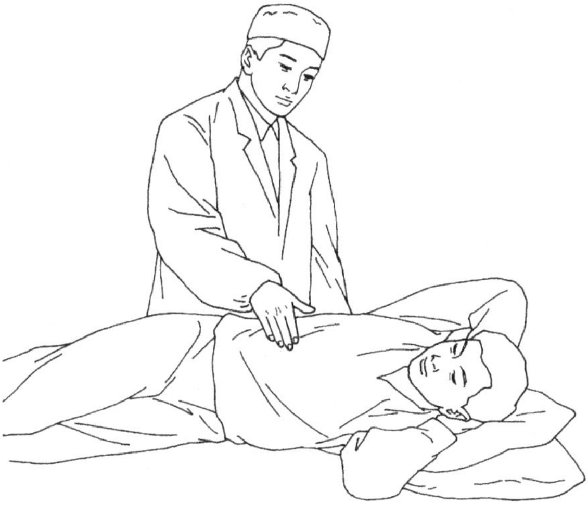

Figure 120 Rubbing the hypochondrium

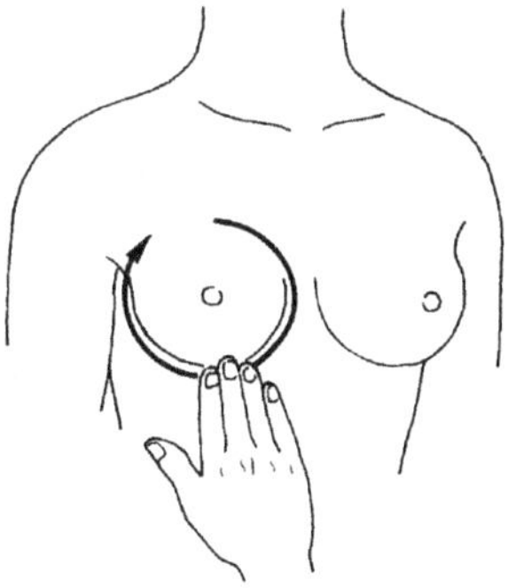

Figure 121 Push-rubbing the breast

Self-Preventional Methods

1. Apply finger kneading on *dànzhōng* and *sānyīnjiāo*, approximately one minute for each acupoint.
2. Use the entire palm to apply push-rubbing around the breast for two to three minutes.
3. Perform grasp-pinching on the upper lateral area of the breast.
4. For individuals with higher tolerance to pain, apply pressure kneading on the breast lumps for two to three minutes. Alternatively, the patient may ask the spouse to perform the procedure. (See Figure 122.)

Precautions

1. Develop the habit of regular and timely breast feeding, and pay attention to the oral hygiene of the baby as well as hygiene of the breasts and nipples.
2. Use a hot towel, heat patch, or hot-water bottle on the affected area to relieve the pain and dissipate the masses.
3. Use a breast pump to pump out accumulated milk on a regular basis in order to reduce the accumulation of milk and promote breast duct patency.
4. For a severely ill patient with obvious systemic symptoms, seek professional care. In extreme circumstances, surgical treatment may be necessary.

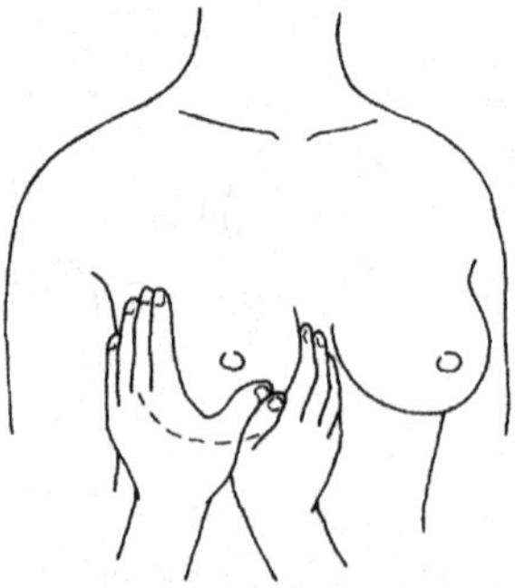

Figure 122 Pressure kneading on the breast lumps

Everyday Exercises

1. What is acute mastitis? What precautions can one take to prevent this condition from developing?
2. What are the tui na treatment principles for acute mastitis? How would you perform tui na for this condition?

Day 4

SHOULDER PERIARTHRITIS

This condition generally refers to the chronic changes with aseptic inflammation of the soft tissues of shoulder, including the joint capsule, synovial capsule, muscles, tendons, tendon sheaths and ligaments, or degenerative changes that cause shoulder pain and restricted range of motion on shoulder joints. In Chinese medical practice, it is called "leaking shoulder wind," while the Japanese refer to it as "fifties shoulder" or "frozen shoulder." It is commonly seen among people in their 50's, and more in women than in men. However, during the past ten years, there have been a tendency for the onset of the disease to occur at a younger age.

The exact cause of shoulder periarthritis is not entirely clear. Yet it may be related to factors such as degenerative changes of the soft tissue on the shoulder, trauma, chronic strain, decreased shoulder activity, cold stimulation and endocrine disorder. In Chinese medical practice, it is believed that the condition is due to long-term strain and insufficient qi and blood, combined with exposure to exterior wind-cold-damp pathogen, causing the failure of the blood to nourish tendons, further leading to the contracture of disused tendons.

Clinical Manifestations

1. Mostly unilateral, and a very small number of patients would have synchronous bilateral onset of the condition.
2. At the early stages, the patient experiences a dull kind of pain in the shoulder. Then, it develops into continuous pain, which can range from a stabbing pain to a severe pain, often radiating to the arms.
3. The pain is more severe in the night. The patient often wakes up due to a cramped sleeping position triggering the pain, and is unable to go back to sleep.
4. During the day, the pain is often intensified because of tiredness and exposure to cold air.

5. The mobility of the shoulder joint — flexion, extension, adduction, abduction, internal rotation, external rotation, and circumduction — is restricted, and the condition gradually worsens. Patients often lose normal life skills, such as combing the hair, dressing, and tightening up a belt due to the shoulder pain and limited mobility, causing great frustration.
6. At the late stages, due to adhesions of the soft tissue, the shoulder joint becomes stiff with loss of motor function, resulting in muscle atrophy, especially of the deltoid muscle.
7. Physical signs a shrugged shoulder (see Figure 123) and obvious tenderness around the acromion, coracoid, and long head of the biceps.

Diagnosis and Differentiation

Key Diagnostic Criteria

1. Upper shoulder pain and restricted shoulder joint function that gradually worsens without other causes.
2. If the shoulder X-ray radiography excludes bone and joint diseases, the diagnosis of shoulder periarthritis can be confirmed.

Differential Diagnosis

If the patient is elderly, has a frail physique, has been suffering a progressive weight loss, and experiences severe back pain that worsens in the

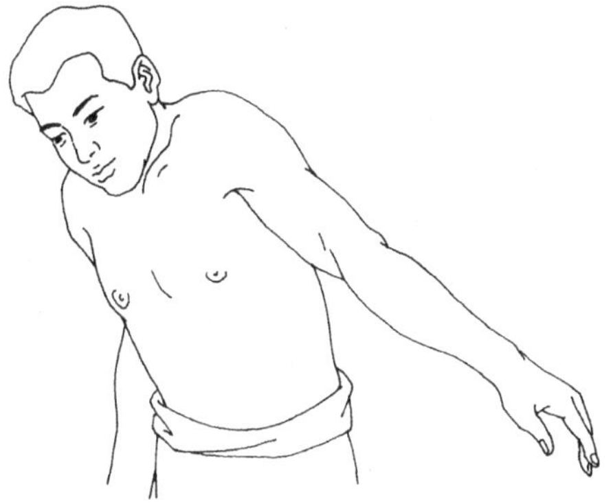

Figure 123 Shrugged shoulder phenomenon of frozen shoulder

night, there is a high chance that a tumor is the cause. Further examination and tests would be required.

Treatment

1. *Treatment principle* soothing the meridians, unblocking the collaterals, loosening up adhesions, and benefiting the joint.
2. *Commonly used maneuvers* rolling, rubbing, palm rubbing, shaking, and joint motion method.
3. *Commonly used acupoints and areas jiānyú* (LI 15); *jiānqián* (also known as *jiānnèilíng*, EX-UE) and *jiānzhēn* (SI 9); *jiānsānxuè*, which is the name given to three combined acupoints, literally meaning "triplet shoulder points"; *tiānzōng* (SI 11), *jiānjǐng* (GB 21), *qǔchí* (LI 11), *āshìxué,* and the shoulder.
4. *Operational methods*
    a. Here we use the right shoulder as an example. The patient is supine, with the practitioner standing to the right of the patient in order to work on the right shoulder. Apply rolling or palm-heal pressure kneading on the anterior edge of the upper arm and transition to *jiānqián* for three to five times. The operation should be coordinated with passive shoulder abduction and external rotation. Next, apply the rolling maneuver and transition to the deltoid on the lateral side of the shoulder with one hand supporting the elbow of the patient to perform passive shoulder adduction.
    b. The patient sits with the practitioner standing posterior to the ipsilateral side. Use one hand to perform the rolling maneuver on the lateral aspect of the shoulder and with the other hand holding the distal limb, do passive shoulder extension, internal rotation, and elbow flexion (see Figure 124).
    c. Next, apply finger kneading on the *jiānsānxuè*, *tiānzōng,* and *āshìxué*, followed by scrubbing the shoulder, grasping *qǔchí*, rotating the shoulder joint, and shaking the upper limb. End the operation by applying the grasping maneuver on *jiānjǐng*.

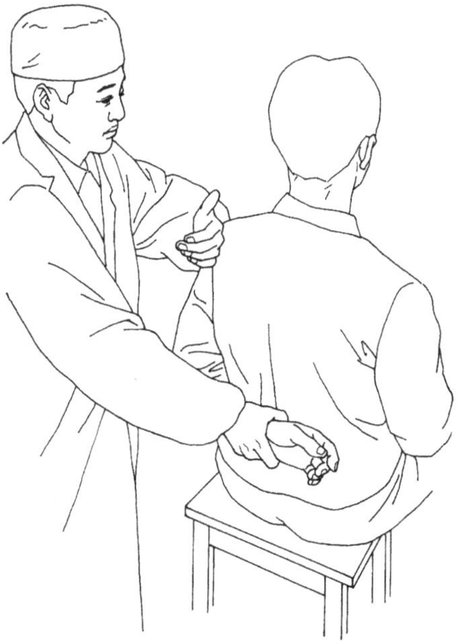

Figure 124 Passive backward shoulder extension

Self-Preventional Methods

1. *Patting the shoulder and pounding the waist* Stand with feet apart, the distance equivalent to the shoulder width, and with upper limbs naturally hanging down. Making the torso the centre, rotate left and right to drive the movement of patting the shoulder and pounding the waist. While rotating to the left, use the left hand and pound the waist with the dorsal side of the loose fist, and the right palm to pat the shoulder joint (see Figure 125). Repeat the maneuver on the right side. Work alternate sides for four sets of eight beats each.
2. *Pulling the wrist from behind* Stand with the ipsilateral arm extended to the back, and internally rotate and touch the spine. The healthy arm also extends to the back to pull the ipsilateral wrist. Try to further extend as far as possible to reach the contralateral spine, going up from the lumbar region to the thoracic area and pull.
3. *Others* The patient can also mimic wall climbing (see Figure 126), dragging the pulley (see Figure 127), or engage in other activities that involve lifting up the arms and moving the shoulder joints in all directions.

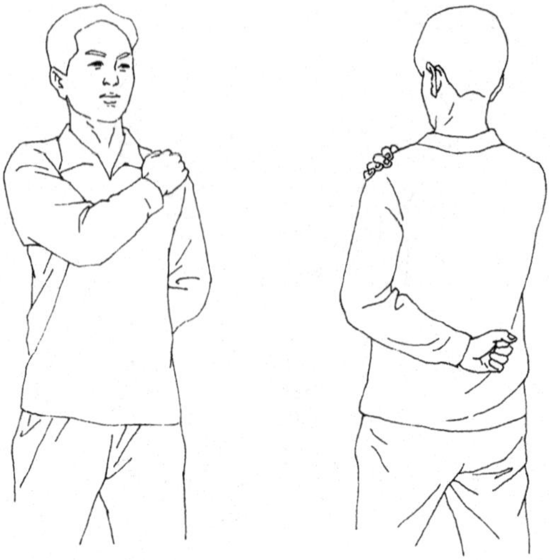

(1) 正面　　　　(2) 背面

正面 - anterior view	
背面 - posterior view	

Figure 125 Patting the shoulder and pounding the waist

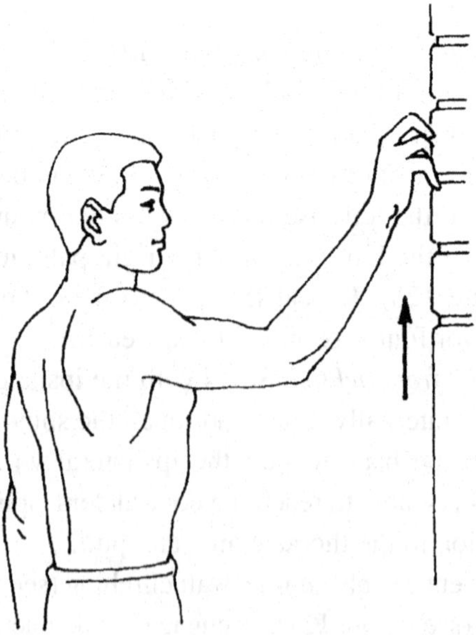

Figure 126 Mimic wall climbing

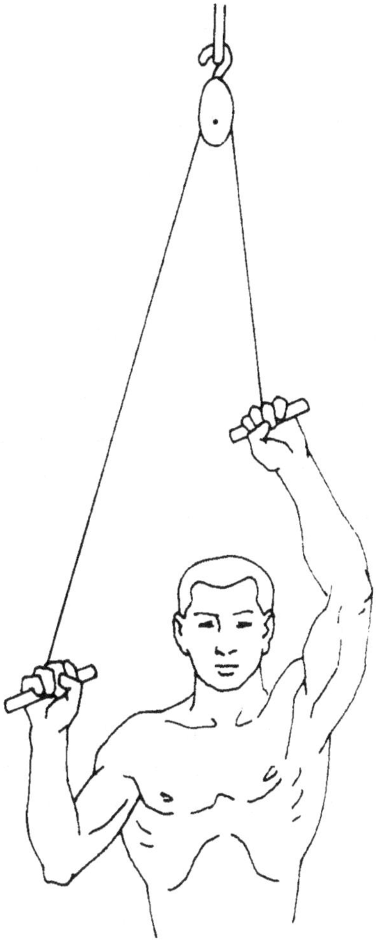

Figure 127 Dragging the pulley

Precautions

1. Keep the shoulder warm. Avoid cold showers in summer. Add shoulder pads in winter.
2. Be persistent with joint function exercises.

Everyday Exercises

1. What is shoulder periarthritis?
2. How is tui na treatment done for shoulder periarthritis?

Day 5

HUMERAL EPICONDYLITIS

Humeral epicondylitis, also known as tennis elbow, is a condition characterized by localized pain at the lateral epicondyle of the elbow, affecting wrist function. The occurrence of this condition is related to work that requires repetitive forceful pronation and supination of the forearm extensor, and wrist activities for an extended period of time. It can result in conditions like partial tendon injury, periostitis of the lateral condyle, anular ligament degeneration of the radial head, tendon bursitis of the forearm extensor, subcutaneous vascular strangulation of the nerve bundle, and the radial nerve neuritis of the articular branch. A similar condition can be found for the medial epicondyle, but its occurrence is lower.

Clinical Manifestations

1. Localized pain on the lateral aspect of the elbow which radiates to the forearm, and often affects the ability to grip items or twist a towel.
2. Localized tenderness on the lateral condyle of the humerus, the brachioradial is joints, or the annular ligament.
3. The pain worsens upon flexion and forearm rotation against resistance.
4. The patient would have decreased gripping power without obvious swolling on the elbow, and the range of motions is unrestricted.
5. X-ray examination shows that the elbow joint is normal.

Diagnosis

1. The disease often occurs among people with labor-intensive jobs involving the forearm, and is more common in middle-aged men.
2. The localized pain on the lateral side of the elbow corresponds to the referencing tenderness of the particular examination.
3. Resistance test of the forearm makes the pain worse.
4. X-ray examination is necessary to rule out bone and joint diseases.

Treatment

1. *Treatment principles* rectifying the tendons, unblocking the meridians, resolving spasms, and relieving pain.
2. *Commonly used maneuvers* rolling, pressure kneading, plucking, scrubbing, and passive joint movement.
3. *Commonly used acupoints and areas qǔchí* (LI 11), *shǒusānlǐ* (LI 10), *āshìxué*, and the lateral aspect of the elbow and the forearm.
4. *Operational methods*

   a. Here we use the right elbow as an example. The patient sits with the ipsilateral arm flexed to the front and placed on the treatment table. The elbow needs to be slightly bent, with a pillow underneath and the practitioner standing to the right.

      i. Apply the rolling maneuver on the radial side of forearm muscles in conjunction with passive forward and backward rotation;
      ii. Now, focus on the humeral epicondyle while using the rolling method with the passive flexion and extension of the elbow (see Figure 128).
      iii. Repeat the operation in (ii) and (iii) alternately for about ten minutes.

   b. Then, use one hand to support the ipsilateral elbow and the other hand to grab the ipsilateral wrist to perform passive elbow flexion and extension.
   c. Next, apply pressure kneading on the *āshìxué*, *qǔchí,* and *shǒusānlǐ*, about one minute per acupoint.
   d. Apply plucking, grasping, and scrubbing on the radial side of the wrist extensor, and scrubbing to the epicondyle of the humerus.
   e. For patients who have suffered severe pain for a long time, add fomentation to the epicondyle of the humerus.

Self-Preventional Methods

1. Use the heel of the contralateral palm to apply pressure kneading on the radial side of the wrist extensor for two to three minutes.

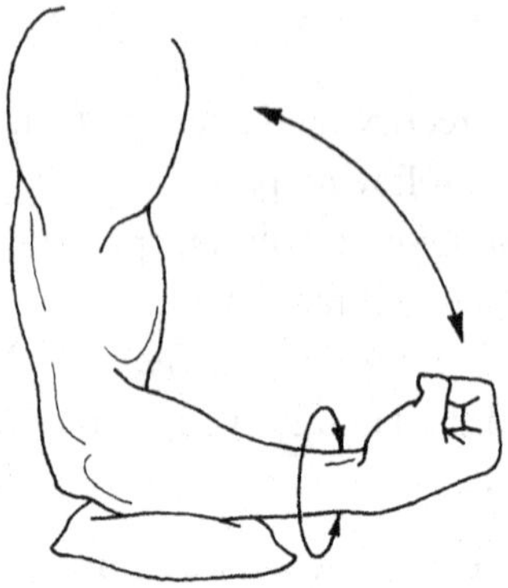

Figure 128 Maneuvers for tennis elbow and passive movements

2. Apply finger kneading on *āshìxué* and *qŭchí*, each for one minute.
3. Apply scrubbing on the lateral epicondyle of the humerus and the radial side of the wrist extensor until the heat from the friction can be felt.

Precautions

1. Reduce the intensity of work, and properly balance work and rest.
2. To avoid further injury, tui na treatment should not be too strong.
3. Be persistent with the treatment.
4. Keep the affected area warm.

Associated Topic — Radial Head Subluxation

Radial head subluxation is a common injury of the upper extremities in infants and young children. It is also known as nursemaid's elbow. The radial head in a young child is not yet completely developed, the diameters of the head and the neck of the radial bone are almost equal, and the annular ligament is generally weak. A sudden pull of a child's forearm, or an action like wearing or taking off clothes may cause the entrapment of the annular ligament between the radial head and the capitellum humerus, leading to partial dislocation of the radial head.

Key Diagnostic Criteria

1. Sudden crying of a child after the arm has been pulled, with the elbow semiflexed, forearm mildly pronated, and the hand unable to lift or grab.
2. There is mild to moderate tenderness on the radial head. Passive elbow flexion and forearm rotation can make the pain more obvious and lead to crying of the child. No obvious swelling on the elbow can be found.
3. X-ray examination does not detect any abnormality. If there is a history of falling, be aware of clavicular or humeral supracondylar fracture.

Tui Na Reduction Maneuver

With a parent holding the child, the practitioner sits opposite the child. Hold the ipsilateral elbow with one hand, while with the other hand apply the traction method to the wrist and rotate the forearm. A crisp snapping sound can be heard during the supination. The symptoms disappear afterwards, and the elbow and forearm can move freely. The elbow can flex and child can lift the arm or grab objects, indication a successful reduction of the radial head.

Generally, there is no need for a plaster cast. At the same time, the parents should be informed not to overstretch the arm of the child, so as to prevent habitual dislocation. After the child turns eight or nine, the condition is self-limited and subluxation rarely happens again.

Everyday Exercises

1. What is lateral epicondylitis of the humerus, and what are the self-preventative procedures?
2. How do we prevent radial head subluxation?

Day 6

STENOSING TENOSYNOVITIS

The tendon sheath (see Figure 129) is a protective synovial sheath around the tendon, which supports ligaments, avoids friction between the bone and the tendon, prevent oppression from other tissues, and ensures full range of mobility of the tendon. Excessive long-term friction between the tendon and the tendon sheath causes inflammatory changes including edema, thickening, and exudation of the synovium. Repeated trauma or protracted inflammation will result in proliferation, adhesion, and thickening of fibrous connective tissue, thickening of the sheath wall, and adhesions between the tendon and sheath wall. As a result, the thickened sheath compresses the tendon, making it swollen and enlarged, so that when the tendon moves through the narrowed fibrous tube, it makes a snapping sound (see Figure 130). This condition is called stenosing tenosynovitis, and often occurs in manual operators. It affects more women than men.

The etiology and pathology of all types of tenosynovitis are the same; the only difference lies in the areas affected. Our discussion will be based on where the incidence occurs.

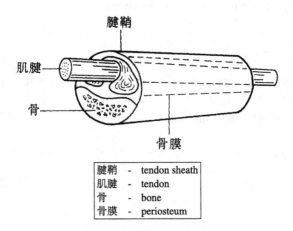

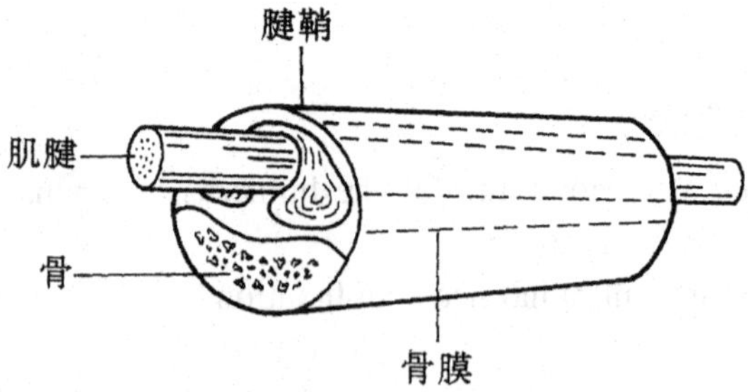

腱鞘	-	tendon sheath
肌腱	-	tendon
骨	-	bone
骨膜	-	periosteum

Figure 129 Tendon sheath

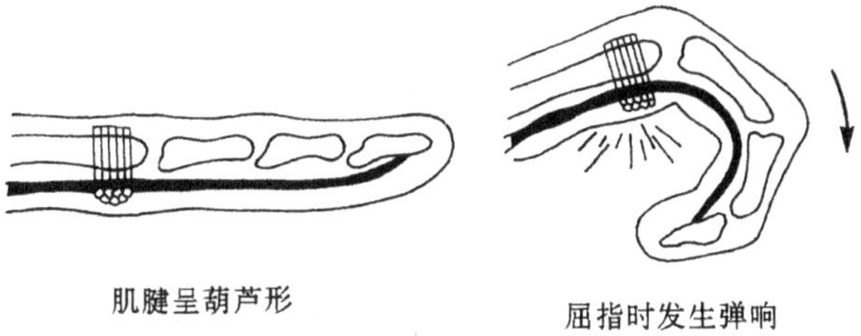

肌腱呈葫芦形	-	bulging tendon
屈指时发生弹响	-	snap sound while flexed

Figure 130 Finger tenosynovitis

Clinical Manifestations

1. *Stenosing tenosynovitis of the radial styloid process* Localized pain at the radial styloid process with slow onset and gradually aggravation. The thumb is weakened with restricted mobility. When the wrist moves toward the ulnar side, the pain worsens. Mild swelling and tenderness can be found on the radial styloid. A specific sign of the disease is a positive result on ulnar deviation fist test.
2. *Flexor tendon tenosynovitis (also known as snapping finger or trigger finger)* The patient finds limited mobility of the ipsilateral finger only in the morning or after laborious work, with localized pain on the palm or soreness of the metacarpophalangeal joint. Along with the narrowing of the tendon sheath, the compression results in gourd-shaped swelling and enlarged tendon, and it is difficult for the swollen portion to pass through the narrowed area of the sheath when the tendon slides. Therefore, the finger is stuck, appearing to be locked in a straight or flexed state. If it is forced to pass through, a triggering or snapping sound would take place.
3. *Peripheral inflammation of the radial wrist extensor tendon* Pain on the dorsum of the wrist, with a bulge at the lower 1/3 radial side of the forearm extensor. There is tenderness on the radial side of the wrist extensor muscle, and a cord-shaped swelling can be detected, with crepitus found at the lower 1/3 radial side of the forearm extensor.

Diagnosis

See clinical manifestations.

Treatment

1. *Treatment principles* soothing the tendon, unblocking the collaterals, benefiting the joints.
2. *Commonly used maneuvers* rolling, pressure kneading, twiddling, smearing, and scrubbing. In addition, fomentation and passive movement of the joints can be used.
3. *Commonly used acupoints and areas*

   a. *Stenosing tenosynovitis of the radial styloid process qǔchí* (LI 11), *shǒusānlǐ* (LI 10), *lièquē* (LU 7), *hégǔ* (LI 4), and the radial styloid process.
   b. *Flexor tendon tenosynovitis nèiguān* (PC 6), *wàiguān* (SJ 5), and *āshìxué*.
   c. *Peripheral inflammation of the radial wrist extensor tendon shǒusānlǐ* (LI 10), *wàiguān* (SJ 5), *nèiguān* (PC 6), and the radial surface of the forearm extensor.
4. *Operational methods*

Stenosing tenosynovitis of the radial styloid process The patient sits with the ipsilateral arm placed on the treatment table and a pillow under the wrist; the practitioner stands at the side of the patient.

a. First, apply the rolling maneuver on the area of the radial styloid process, starting with gentle force and gradually increasing the intensity. At the same time, coordinate with passive movements of making a fist and moving to the ulnar side for ten to 15 times.
b. Perform finger kneading on *lièquē*, *hégǔ*, *qǔchí* and *shǒusānlǐ*, about one minute per acupoint.
c. Apply plucking on the tender spots of the affected tendon perpendicularly for ten to 15 times.
d. Lastly, apply smearing on the radial styloid process.

Flexor tendon tenosynovitis The patient assumes the same position as above.

a. Apply the rolling method on the medial side of the forearm, especially where the lesion is located on the palm. Add moderate passive movement of wrist flexion, finger flexion, and finger extension for five to ten minutes.
b. Apply finger kneading and plucking alternately to the enlarged tender spots of the palmar aspect of the flexor tendon of the metacarpophalangeal joint, coordinating with passive movements of the metacarpophalangeal flexion and extension.
c. Apply smearing and twiddling on the flexor tendon and rotating the metacarpophalangeal joint.

Peripheral inflammation of the radial wrist extensor tendon The patient assumes the same position as above.

a. Apply rolling on the forearm extensor tendon from the elbow to the wrist in conjunction with passive forearm pronation and supination, and wrist flexion and extension for about ten minutes.
b. Finger kneading on *nèiguān*, *wàiguān*, *shǒusānlǐ* and *āshìxué* with firm but not intense stimulation.
c. Finally, end the operation with plucking and scrubbing.

Self-Preventional Methods

1. *Stenosing tenosynovitis of the radial styloid process* Apply finger kneading on *lièquē* for two to three minutes, coordinating with fist-making, and moves toward the ulnar side. Then, use the palm to scrub the radial styloid process until the heat generated from the friction is felt.
2. *Flexor tendon tenosynovitis* Apply finger kneading on tender points of the flexor tendon for two to three minutes. Then, perform smearing along the path from the proximal limb to the distal end in conjunction with passive movement of the metacarpophalangeal flexion.
3. *Peripheral inflammation of the radial wrist extensor tendon* Use the thenar to apply kneading on tender spots of the radial wrist extensor tendon for three to five minutes, with the forearm actively pronating

and supinating for ten to 20 times. Apply the scrubbing maneuver on the radial side of the wrist extensor muscle.

Precautions

1. Keep the affected area warm, and balance work with rest.
2. Cooperate with the treatment; the disease can be cured through conservative treatment. For refractory condition with unsuccessful tui na treatment, consider local nerve block or surgical treatment.

Everyday Exercises

1. What is tenosynovitis?
2. How would you apply tui na treatment for tenosynovitis of the radial flexor tendon?

WEEK 7

Day 1

GANGLION CYST

Ganglion cysts are swellings formed on or around the joints and tendons in the hand or foot. Most ganglion cysts are attached to the joint capsule, or to the joint cavity in the tendon sheath. The wall of the cyst is made up of fibrous tissue and the cyst is filled with clear gelatinous mucus. One or more cysts can develop. It is more common in young and middle-aged people, and in women than in men.

The etiology of the condition is unknown. Generally speaking, it is related to trauma or chronic strain. Some believe ganglion cysts are the result of myxoid degeneration of the joint capsule or specific tissues of the tendon sheath, while others believe they are due to the herniated protrusion of the joint capsule or tendon sheath membrane.

Clinical Manifestations

Ganglion cysts often occur on the dorsal side of the wrist, on the radial palmar surface of the wrist, or on the dorsal aspect of the foot near the dorsal artery. The onset is slow; initially the cysts are occasionally seen as small lumps above the skin, and they present little or mild pain. When they occur on the wrist area, the fingers may feel some weakness.

The cyst appears as a hemispherical fixed mass that originates underneath the skin and appears higher than the skin. It has a smooth surface and does not adhere to the skin, being attached to the deeper tissue. Cysts are capsule-like; some are hard while others feel soft to the touch. When a cyst occurs in the membrane of the tendon sheath, it has an irregular spherical shape. If it occurs on the distal flexor tendon sheath, it is as hard as cartilage and the size of a grain. Pain would occur with pressure or holding an object.

Diagnosis

See clinical manifestations.

Treatment

Due to the fact that the conservative treatment of ganglion cysts on different locations is the same, we will discuss the treatment for the ones on the wrist.

1. *Extrusion* The patient sits with the technician standing facing the patient. First, rub the site where the cyst is located, pushing it up and down, and left to right to loosen it up. Next, hold the patient's wrist with both hands to perform traction, at an angle between the wrist and your hands to increase the space between the wrist joints on its dorsal side. Then, place overlapped thumbs on the cyst with the angle switched from the palmar side to the dorsal aspect, and squeeze the cyst to make it rupture (see Figure 131). This maneuver is called double-handed extrusion. It takes time and practice to master such a technique; therefore, if it is unsuccessful the first time round, try it multiple times.

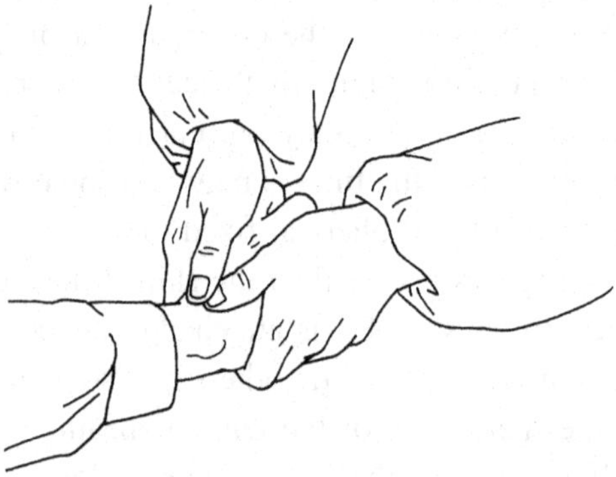

Figure 131 Double-handed extrusion

Another extrusion method is to use a single hand. Use one hand to apply traction on the ipsilateral wrist, and with the thumb of the other hand, press hard on the cyst (see Figure 132).

After applying the extrusion method to the cyst, dress the area with a small cotton pad and a bandage, and leave it on for two to three days.

2. *Piercing extrusion* Check with the proper authorities if this is within your scope of practice. Prior to the operation, the area receiving the operation must be disinfected, and the injection and piecing equipment sterilized. First, disinfect the skin area that is to be treated. Inject 2–3 ml of 1% lidocaine into the subcutaneous cyst, and use

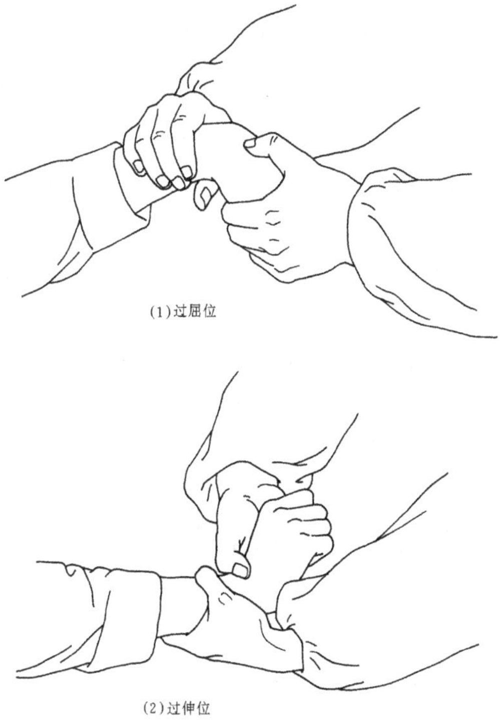

过屈位	-	hyper-flexed position
过伸位	-	hyper-extended position

Figure 132 Single-handed extrusion

a manufactured sterilized three-edged needle to pierce the cyst from different directions. Then, use the thumb to squeeze the cyst and extrude the content. Dress the area and keep the bandage on for two to three days.

If the above methods are unsuccessful or if the cyst recurs repeatedly, consider surgery to remove the cyst.

Carpal Tunnel Syndrome

The palmar side of the wrist is made up of a tough transverse carpal ligament and carpal bones, such as the hamate, capitate, trapezium, and trapezoid, to form a bone-fibrous canal called the carpal tunnel (see Figure 133). The flexor tendons and median nerve pass through the tunnel. Carpal tunnel syndrome is caused by pressure in the carpal tunnel compressing the median nerve.

There are many factors responsible for increased pressure in the carpal tunnel. Some of these are:

1. *Trauma* An example would be wrist fractures, including distal radius and scaphoid fractures, and dislocation such as semilun are dislocation.

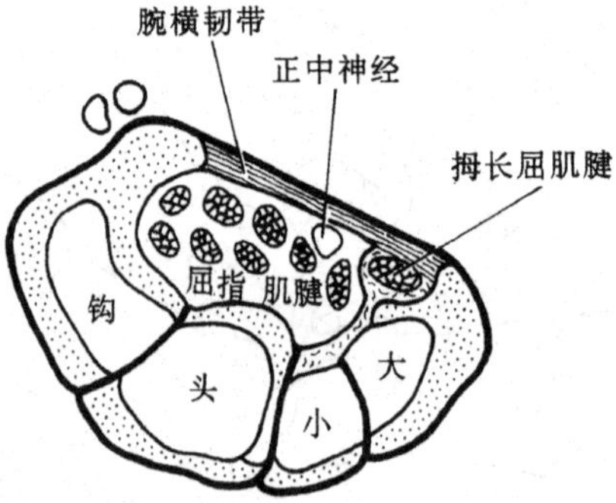

腕横韧带	-	transverse carpal ligament
正中神经	-	median nerve
拇长屈肌腱	-	flexor pollicis longus muscle tendon

Figure 133 The carpal tunnel

2. *Palmar or dorsal hyper flexion and strain* This would cause hypertrophy of the transverse carpal ligament.
3. *Endocrine changes* These are hormonal changes that occur in pregnant or postmenopausal women, or in other conditions such as mucinous edema, acromegaly, hypothyroidism, and diabetes.
4. *Increased tube volume* If the flexor muscle pulp is positioned too low or the lumbrical muscle positioned too high while entering the carpal tunnel,
5. *Space-occupying lesions* There may be tendon sheath cysts, lipoma, or other types of tumor inside the carpal tunnel.
6. *Rheumatism* This may cause synovitis of the tendon sheath within the carpal tunnel.

Clinical Manifestations

1. The main symptoms are numbness, tingling, or burning pain in the thumb and fingers, especially the index and middle fingers, and the radial half of the ring finger. The numbness or pain often radiates to the hand, elbow, and shoulder.
2. The pain often occurs at night or in the early morning; the thumb feels weak and handles things clumsily.
3. The skin of the hand controlled by the median nerve has diminished or absent sense of feeling. The abduction ability of the thumb is weakened, with gradual atrophy of the thenar muscle.
4. When the middle of the wrist flexor is tapped by a reflex hammer, it can cause radiating pain in the area that the median nerve serves.
5. If the patient pushes the dorsal aspect of the wrists against each other to make it a complete flexion, and hold this position for a minute, there will be radiating numbness on the ipsilateral thumb, index finger, and middle finger.

Lateral wrist radiography can be used to ruled out other bone and joint lesions.

Diagnosis

See clinical manifestations.

Treatment

1. *Treatment principles* soothing the tendons and unblocking the collaterals.
2. *Commonly used maneuvers* rolling, pressing, finger kneading, rotating, smearing, and scrubbing.
3. *Commonly used acupoints and areas nèiguān* (PC 6), *dàlíng* (PC 7), *yújì* (LU 10), the palmar aspect of the forearm, wrist, and palm.

4. *Operational methods*:

   a. The patient sits up or lies supine, and the practitioners its or stands by the patient's side. First, apply rolling on the palmar aspect of the ipsilateral forearm, wrist, and palm, up and down from the forearm to the palm, with more focus on the palmar side of the wrist and lateral side of the palm. Coordinate with passive movements of the wrist flexion, and a little bit of ulnar and radial deviation of the wrist. This procedure should last for about ten minutes.
   b. Apply finger kneading on *nèiguān*, *dàling*, and *yújì*, for one minute each. Focus more on *dàlíng* with a certain pressure, and combine with slight passive wrist flexion and extension. Then, continue with the same method on *yújì, coordinating with grasping on hégŭ* (LI 4) and the the nar, and the tendon-rectifying method. This procedure should last for three to five minutes.
   c. Rotate the wrist in all directions, such as up and down, clockwise and counter-clockwise. Then, apply smearing on fingers with the focus on the thumb, index finger, and middle finger.
   d. Finally, apply scrubbing on the palmar side of the forearm, the carpal area, and the thenar eminence.

Self-Preventional Methods

1. Use the contralateral finger to perform kneading on *nèiguān*, *dàlíng*, *yújì,* and *hégŭ.*
2. Use the heel of the palm or the nar to apply kneading on the palmar side of the forearm, the carpal area, and the lateral aspect of the palm for a total of five to ten minutes.

Everyday Exercises

1. How would you treat a wrist ganglion cyst using tui na?
2. What is the carpal tunnel? What is carpal tunnel syndrome and how would you treat it with tui na?

Day 2

ISCHEMIC CONTRACTURE OF THE FOREARM MUSCLES

Ischemic muscle contracture is caused by insufficient blood supply to the muscles, resulting in degeneration and subsequent formation of scar and contracture, affecting the limb's normal physiological functions. It is one of the serious complications that may occur after traumatic injury. It is good practice to be prepared for occurrence of it during traumatic events in order to prevent it. Once it occurs, treat it as early as possible and try to maximize the preservation of the basic functions of the limbs.

Besides insufficient blood supply to the muscles, often seen in supracondylar or forearm fractures, Other contributing factors may include poor reduction, or not being reduced, too tight a dressing or external fixation, substandard bundling, forearm soft tissue injury, vascular injury, or the limb being compressed for too long after the occurrence of a coma. All of the above can cause insufficient blood supply to the limbs or torso.

Muscle ischemia causes the muscle cells to swell, followed by central necrosis. Later, the muscle cells are gradually replaced by scar tissue, resulting in the muscle losing elasticity and remaining contracted. The muscular contracture can further result in the secondary compression of the nearby nerves, causing nerve injury. If the condition occurs in childhood without proper treatment, it can have a negative impact on bone development, and lead to the ipsilateral limb being shorter and thinner than the other one. It may also cause deformities such as permanently flexed wrist and fingers or a pronated forearm.

Clinical Manifestations

The condition can be confirmed when the following symptoms present:

1. Sudden severe pain of the injured limb after being externally fixed.
2. Weakened or even disappeared radial arterial pulse with fingers in a flexion state, and aggravated pain while being passively straightened.

3. Swelling, coldness, and cyanosis on distal limbs with diminished or absent senses.

Diagnosis

See clinical manifestation.

Treatment

This is a very difficult problem encountered in the process of trauma. Tui na therapy in the early stages of the condition can improve the blood circulation of the affected limb. Certainly, tui na is not the panacea. If the trauma is of the oppression of bone ending, reduction process and internal fixation are appropriate. If there is vasospasm, thrombus formation, or vascular rupture, take appropriate measures in order to restore the blood supply of the forearm.

1. *Treatment principles* After ruling out problems of other systems such as the bones and blood vessels, and immediate removal of any external restraints or dressings, apply appropriate tui na technique as soon as possible to improve blood circulation of the ipsilateral limb.
2. *Commonly used maneuvers* finger kneading, grasping, rotating, smearing, twiddling, and passive joint movement.
3. *Commonly used acupoints and areas* *qŭchí* (LI 11), *dàlíng* (PC 7), *yújì* (LU 10), *láogōng* (PC 8),and the palmar side of the forearm.
4. Operational methods
   The condition may occur at any stage after a bone fracture. It is not appropriate to perform either tui na or passive joint movements at the fractured end of the bone, especially during the early stages, since this is the period for the granulation tissue to repair fractured fragments by connecting them together. Fibrous callus takes two to three weeks to form. Therefore, tui na maneuvers can only be done on the distal part of the limb.

   a. The patient should either sit up or lie supine, with the practitioner sitting or standing by the patient's side. Apply twiddling and smearing on the fingers, and increase the intensity of the maneuver at the finger tips to increase blood circulation.

b. Apply finger kneading on *dàlíng*, *yújì* and *láogōng*. The manipulation must not be too forceful.

For patients in mid to late stages(8–12 weeks) after the occurrence of the fracture, and if X-rays show a fuzzy line of the fracture and a visible callus, distal and local treatment can be performed as follows:

a. Apply gentle rolling or palm-heel kneading on the palmar side of the fore arm multiple times, from the proximal to the distal side, back and forth for about ten minutes.
b. Apply finger kneading on the forearm flexors with moderate and gentle, yet in-depth force to reach the deeper muscles, starting from the proximal ends of the radial or ulnar flexors to the distal ends. Put more focus on *qŭchí*, *shŏusānlĭ* (LI 10), *nèiguān* (PC 6), and *dàlíng*. This procedure should total up to about ten minutes. Sometimes it can be performed with the first step alternately.
c. Moderately flex and extend the elbow and wrist, and rotate the forearm. Start with a smaller range and gradually increase it. The passive movement should not force the joints to reach their maximum range of motion.
d. Apply finger kneading on *yújì* and *láogōng*, each point for about one minute.
e. Apply twiddling on finger joints, smearing all fingers, and enhance the stimulation of the fingertips.
f. Apply grasping on the forearm flexors and *hégŭ* (LI 4); rotating the wrist and the meta carpophalangeal joints with a small amplitude.

If tui na maneuvers cannot improve blood circulation in one to two weeks, seek hospital care or surgery as soon as possible.

Self-Preventional Methods

1. Perform wrist flexion and fist-making exercises with a targeted quantity on a regular schedule every day. Complete two to four sets of eight beats each time, and gradually increase the number of sets.

2. Use the contralateral fingers to perform kneading maneuver on the flexors of the affected arm.

Everyday Exercises

1. What is chemic contracture of the forearm muscles and what are the major risk factors?
2. How can we confirm the diagnosis of ischemic contracture of the forearm muscles?

Day 3

DISTAL RADIOULNAR JOINT INJURY

Distal radioulnar joint injury is also known as distal radioulnar joint separation or wrist triangular fibro cartilage injury. Distal radioulnar joint injury occurs when there is an increased gap between joints, causing tears of the wrist triangular fibro cartilage and damage of the surrounding ligaments. (See Figure 134.)

The rotational movement of the forearm is completed with the coordination of the proximal radioulnar joint, distal radioulnar joint, and in terosseous membrane of the forearm. Under normal circumstances, the ulna in the distal radioulnar joint does not move. Instead, the ulnar notch of the radius circles around the ulnar head, using it as the axis and rotating in a 150° arc to complete pronation and supination. The wrist cartilage plate is an isosceles triangular shaped fibro cartilage, with its tip attached to the base of the ulnar styloid process. At the same time, the bottom of the triangle is attached to the edge of the distal ulnar notch of the radius, with its front and back connecting to the synovium of the articulation. Thus, the distal radioulnar joint and wrist radial articulation are separated into two joint cavities, and its physiological function is to limit hyper-rotation of the forearm.

During the rotation of the forearm, when the carpometacarpal area encounters resistance, or the forearm continues the rotation with the palm immobilized, the distal radioulnar joint is against the shearing force from

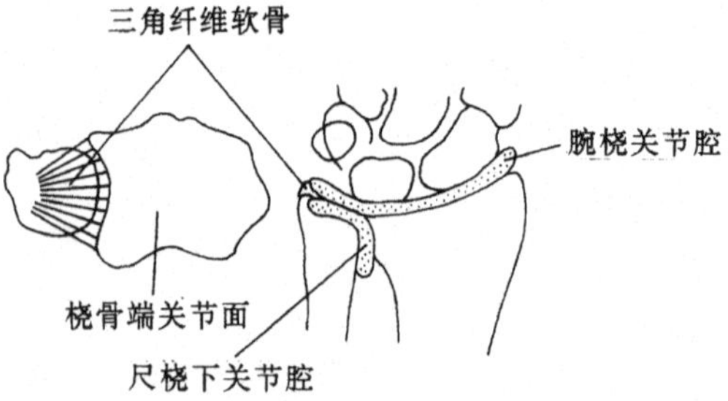

Figure 134 Wrist cartilage plate

the rotation or separating injury force, causing the damage to the radioulnar joint and the wrist triangular fibro cartilage.

Clinical Manifestations

At the early stage, the ulnar aspect of the dorsal side of the wrist may have different degrees of swelling with wrist pain, which is aggravated when the wrist is rotated in activities such as twisting a towel and opening a bottle. A small number of patients would experience a snapping sound. Wrist gripping strength decreases, making it difficult to lift heavy items.

There is tenderness on the dorsal aspect of the distal radioulnar articulation, with the location equivalent to the midpoint on the dorsum of the wrist, a little closer to the ulnar side. The distal radioulnar joint is flaccid with a loose ulnar head and easy to be pushed. Dorsal wrist pain intensifies when the forearm rotates. If the wrist is forced to flex, pronate, and tilt toward the ulna, with external force to squeeze and rotate it, the pain in the distal radioulnar joint worsens, a positive result for the cartilage plate compression test.

Wrist X-ray examination can confirm whether there is separation of the distal radioulnar joint and dislocation of the ulnar head. During the iodine contrast of the wrist joint, if the contrast agent enters into the distal radioulnar joint space, the rupture of the triangular fibro cartilage plate can be confirmed.

Diagnosis and Differentiation

Key Diagnostic Criteria

1. Significant trauma history, such as falling and spraining the wrist in dorsiflexion, or excessive force used during the pronation of the forearm.
2. Wrist pain, weakness, diminished gripping strength.
3. Tenderness and joint laxity on distal radioulnar joint.
4. Positive for cartilage plate compression test.
5. Wrist X-ray shows separation of the distal radioulnar joint.

Differential Diagnosis

1. *Scaphoid fracture* There is a history of trauma or falling, and pain is located on the radial side of the wrist. Swelling and tenderness are obvious at the snuff box. X-rays can confirm the diagnosis.
2. *Aseptic necrosis of the carpal lunate bone* There is a history of trauma or chronic strain, and obvious tenderness on the midpoint of the dorsum of the wrist, equivalent to the location of the lunate. Vertical compressing along the third metacarpal bone causes pain; laxity of the distal radioulnar joint is not sensed. X-rays can be helpful in the diagnosis.

Treatment

1. *Treatment principles* using reduction manipulation during the acute stage of the injury; soothing the tendons and invigorating the collaterals to reduce chronic damage.
2. *Commonly used maneuvers* traction, support lifting and reduction, finger kneading, and scrubbing.
3. *Commonly used acupoints and areas* *wàiguān* (SJ 5), *yángchí* (SJ 4), *yánggŭ* (SI 5), *yănglăo* (SI 6), *shénmén* (HT 7), the distal forearm, and the cubit.
4. *Operational methods*

    a. *Diorthosis maneuver in acute stage* Patient should sit with the upper arm abducted, the practitioner standing at the ipsilateral side. Hold the ipsilateral limb at the the nar and hypothenar areas using both hands and apply continuous pulling traction. Note that the force of the traction does not need to be great; it is the enduring force that matters. This is the basic reduction technique for all fractures and dislocations. After a few minutes of traction, use a thumb to suppress the prominent distal ulna and make it "flattened from being protuded."Continue with the method of traction, support lifting, and reduction. Upon the completion of the diorthosis, wrap the wrist with elastic bandage for six to eight weeks or dress it with medicinal cream to dissolve stasis and relieve pain. Then, fasten the ipsilateral arm with a sling and wrap it around the neck to make the arm fixed in front of the chest.

b. *Treatment in chronic phase* Apply finger kneading on *wàiguān*, *yángchí*, *yánggŭ*, *yănglăo,* and *shénmén*, for one to two minutes each. While treating the distal forearm, focus more on the dorsal aspect, combining it with moderate passive movements including pronation, wrist flexion, and extension. However, avoid forearm supination and wrist tilting to the ulnar side. In addition, apply scrubbing at the dorsal and ulnar aspects of the distal forearm until the patient feels the heat from the friction. Upon completing the tui na maneuver, protect the wrist with a bracer, and fasten the wrist with a sling and wrap it around the neck.

Self-Preventional Methods

1. Apply the finger kneading method daily with the focus on *wàiguān* and the tender spots.
2. Apply scrubbing on the dorsal and ulnar aspects of the distal forearm.
3. Continue to use the sling to protect the wrist.

Precautions

1. It is preferable to have X-rays of both forearms for comparison.
2. Protect the wrist immediately to avoid further injury from laborious work after the diagnosis is confirmed.
3. If conservative treatment fails, surgery may be considered.

Everyday Exercises

1. What is the relationship between the distal radioulnar joint and the triangular fibro cartilage?
2. What is the reduction method in acute phase of distal radioulnar joint injury?

Day 4

PERIPHERAL NERVE INJURY

Peripheral nerves consist of motor, sensory, and autonomic fibers, and belong to the lower motor neurons. The injury to lower motor neurons can lead to conditions including obvious muscle atrophy, flaccid paralysis, diminished or disappeared tendon reflexes, pain, sensory disturbances, vasomotor barriers, and nutritional disorders. Tui na can help to improve muscle function, prevent deformity, and benefit rehabilitation of the nerve tissue. Common peripheral nerve injuries are described below.

Median Nerve Injury

The median nerve originates from the brachial plexus, and is related to C5–C8 and T1. It innervates muscles such as the forearm pronatorteres, flexor carpi radialis, palmaris long us, finger flexors, opponens pollicis, and the thenar muscle.

Clinical Manifestations

The extent of paralysis in the muscles depends on where the injury occurs on the median nerve. For example, thenar muscle atrophy causes the following condition: flattened fingers leading to "ape hand" deformity (see Figure 135); obstruction of the palmar opposition function of the thumb; and sensory disorder of the radial half at the palmar aspect, and the dorsal finger tips of the index and middle fingers, especially the distal end of the thumb, index and middle fingers.

Diagnosis

See clinical manifestation.

Treatment

Refer to tui na treatment for carpal tunnel syndrome.

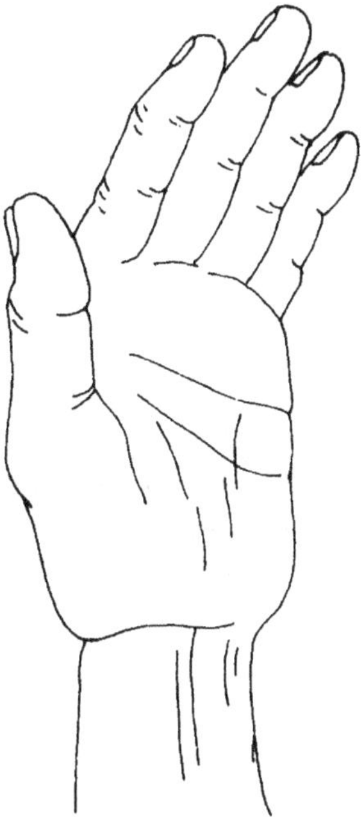

Figure 135 "Ape Hand" due to median nerve paralysis

Ulnar Nerve Injury

The ulnar nerve originates from the C8 and T1 roots. It innervates the forearm flexor carpi ulnar is, hypothenar muscles, and intrinsic muscles of the hand.

Clinical Manifestations

Injury of the ulnar nerve results in the "claw hand"(see Figure 136). The patient has difficulty gripping things between the fingers, and there is atrophy of the hypothenar muscle. If the disease lasts over a long time, atrophy of the interosseous muscles, especially in the dorsal side of the hand, may be very significant. Sensory disturbances of the skin involves the ulnar side of the palm, the little finger, the ulnar half of the ring finger, the dorsal aspect of the 4th and 5th finger, and a half of the 3rd finger. Furthermore, the ulnar edge of the hand may appear to be cold, dry, pale, or flushed, and sometimes there may be skin blisters and nail changes.

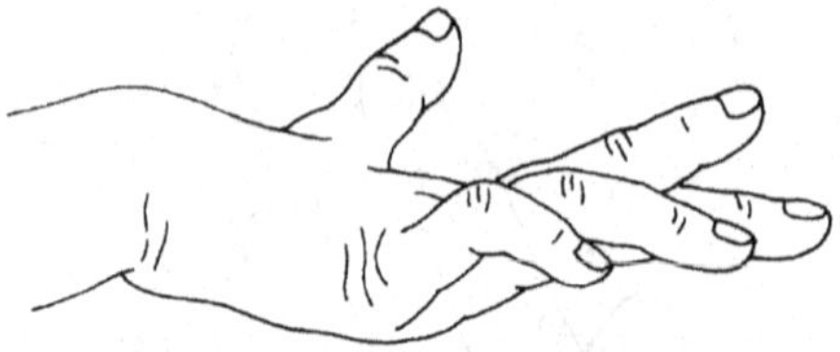

Figure 136 "Claw Hand" due to paralysis of the ulnar nerve

Often, the median nerve and ulnar nerve can be injured at the same time. When this happens, the wrist is slightly straightened, the hand tilting to the ulna, and thumb abducted with muscle atrophy of both the thenar and hypothenar. Other signs are flattened palm, paralysis of all the flexors, inability of wrist flexion and hand flexion, and sensory disturbances in areas where the median nerve and ulnar nerve is innervated.

Diagnosis

Refer to clinical manifestations.

Treatment

1. *Commonly used maneuvers* rolling, grasping, finger kneading, twiddling, scrubbing, smearing, and rotating.
2. *Commonly used acupoints and areas shàohăi* (HT 3), *xiăohăi* (SI 8), *yánggŭ* (SI 5), *hòuxī* (SI 3), *shàofŭ* (HT 8), ulnar side of the forearm, ulnar aspect of the palm, and between the metacarpal bones.

3. *Operational methods*

   a. The patient is supine or sitting, with the practitioner sitting or standing according to the patient's position. Apply the rolling maneuver from the proximal ulnar side of the forearm down to the distal ulnar aspect of the palm, back and forth several times. Increase the intensity on muscles for deeper penetration. This procedure should last for about ten minutes.
   b. Apply grasping on the ulnar side of the forearm muscles, then grasping on the hypothenar muscles with increased stimulation for two to three minutes.

c. Apply finger kneading on *shàohǎi*, *xiǎohǎi*, *yánggǔ*, *hòuxī*, *shàofǔ*, and the gaps between the metacarpophalangeal bones for three to five minutes. This is a very important step.
d. Rotate the wrist and all of the metacarpophalangeal joints. Then, apply the twiddling technique to the 3rd, 4th, and 5th fingers with more intensive stimulation on the fingertips. Next, apply the smearing maneuver to these fingers.
e. End the operation with scrubbing on the forearm flexor until the patient feels the warmth owing to the friction.

For those with median nerve injuries, apply manipulations on acupoints and muscles of the palmar side of the forearm, thenar, thumb, index, and middle fingers.

Radial Nerve Injury

The radial nerve originates from the roots of C5–C8, and is often related to T1. It innervates the radial side of the wrist extensor, extensor digitorum, and the skin from the dorsal forearm to the radial side of the wrist.

Clinical Manifestations

The most typical symptom of a radial nerve injury is wrist drop (see Figure 137). Examination can reveal dysfunction of the wrist extensor and the extensor digitorum, and loss of reflexes of the triceps tendon and radial perio steal membrane. There are obvious sensory disorders on the

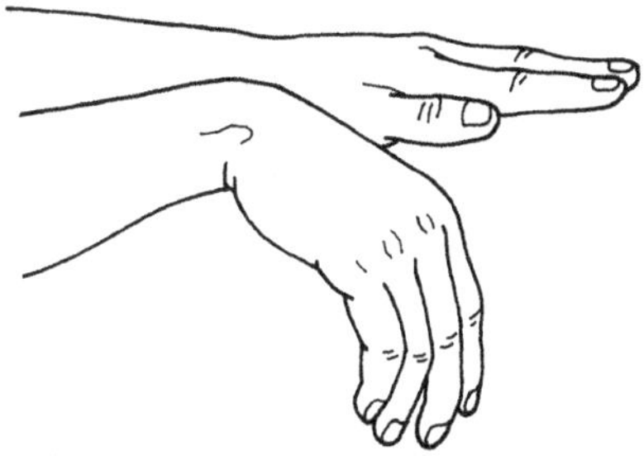

Figure 137 Wrist drop caused by radial nerve palsy (right hand)

dorsal side of the skin between the first and second metacarpal bones with the feeling of coldness and cyanosis. If the condition lasts, semi-flexing stiff contracture may occur between the wrist and fingers, accompanied by forearm, metacarpal, and carpal osteoporosis.

Diagnosis

Refer to clinical manifestation.

Treatment

1. *Commonly used maneuvers* rolling, grasping, finger kneading, twiddling, smearing, rotating, and scrubbing.
2. *Commonly used acupoints and areas* *qŭchí* (LI 11), *shŏusānlĭ* (LI 10), *yángxī* (LI 5), *hégŭ* (LI 4), *wàiguān* (SJ 5), *yángchí* (SJ 4), and the dorsal aspect of the forearm.
3. *Operational methods*

The patient lies supine or sits, with the practitioner in sitting or standing position.

a. Apply rolling on the dorsal forearm from the proximal to the distal end, back and forth several times, with the focus on the forearm extensors, for about ten minutes.
b. Alternate among the maneuvers of grasping on the forearm extensors, finger kneading on *qŭchí*, *shŏusānlĭ*, *yángxī*, *wàiguān* and *yángchí*, and grasping on *hégŭ* for about five minutes.
c. Apply twiddling and smearing the thumb, index, middle, ring, and little finger, as well as all the metacarpophalangeal and interphalangeal joints, and rotating the wrist and metacarpophalangeal joints to prevent them from semi-flexion stiff contracture.
d. Lastly, perform the smearing maneuver on the dorsal radial side of the forearm until the patient feels the heat.

Injury of the Common Peroneal Nerve

The common peroneal nerve originates from the sciatic nerve at the lower 1/3 of the thigh. When it passes by the fibular head on the lateral side of the popliteal fossa, it further branches out to the superficial peroneal nerve, deep peroneal nerve, and cutaneous nerve.

Clinical Manifestations

A typical symptom of an injured common peroneal nerve is foot drop. On the anterolateral side of the calf, muscle atrophy is obvious with functional impairment such as dorsiflexion of the foot and extension of the toes. There is also cutaneous sensory disorder on the anterolateral aspect of the calf and dorsal sensory disorder of the foot.

Diagnosis

Refer to clinical manifestations.

Treatment

1. *Commonly used maneuvers* rolling, finger kneading, grasping, plucking, twiddling, smearing, rotating, and scrubbing.
2. *Commonly used acupoints and areas xuèhǎi* (SP 10), *yánglíngquán* (GB 34), *zúsānlǐ* (ST 36), *jiěxī* (ST 41), *wěizhōng* (BL 40), *chéngshān* (BL 57), and the anterolateral aspect of the calf.

3. *Operational methods*

   a. The patient is supine, with the practitioner sitting at the patient's ipsilateral side. First, apply the rolling maneuver on the anterolateral aspect of the ipsilateral calf with emphasis on the tibialis anterior muscles, from the proximal side to the distal end until reaching the dorsum of the foot. Work back and forth several times for about ten minutes.
   b. Apply finger kneading on *xuèhǎi*, *zúsānlǐ*, *yánglíngquán*, and *jiěxī*, about one minute for each point. Then apply grasping on *wěizhōng* and *chéngshān*, and plucking the tibialis anterior muscle in an up-and-down movement several times. Finger kneading, grasping, and plucking may also be used alternately to increase the amount of stimulation.

c. Apply twiddling and smearing on all toes; then apply rotating on the ankle and toes. End the operation by scrubbing on the anterior tibial.

Everyday Exercises

1. What are the major signs and symptoms when there is an injury on the median, ulnar, radial, or common peroneal nerves?
2. Explain the general principles of tui na in treating common peripheral nerve injury.

Day 5

LÀOZHĚN (ACUTE STIFF NECK)

In Chinese, *làozhěn* literally means "fallen from the pillow" or "lost pillow." It is characterized by sudden neck stiffness. In the majority of patients, it is caused by improper sleeping position, or the pillow is either too high or too low, causing the head to slip from the pillow and the neck to lean to one side. However, in the case of some patients, it is due to wind-cold pathogen invading the meridians and blocking the qi and blood. Therefore, another Chinese name for the same condition is *làozhěnfēng*, meaning "pillow-fallen wind." The neck muscles involved in this condition, mainly the trapezius, sternocleidomastoid, and levator scapulae, would have spasms with sudden increased muscular tension, resulting in neck pain. The mild form of the condition lasts only for a day or two and is self-limiting, while the severe form may last for several days or weeks, affecting normal life and work. Clinically, the disease is fairly common. Tuina therapy is extremely effective for this condition.

Clinical Manifestations

The majority of patients would feel stiffness and pain on the neck with limited mobility after getting out of the bed in the morning. Sometimes, the discomfort makes the patient tilt his or her neck to one side, with the movements of the neck restricted in a certain direction. The area affected by the condition has significant muscle contracture associated with tenderness. In some patients, cord-shaped knots are palpable underneath the tenderness. For middle-aged individuals repeatedly affected by *laozhen*, or for those who have experienced the condition multiple times in a period of six months, there is a high possibility of cervical spondylosis.

Diagnosis and Differentiation

Key Diagnostic Criteria

1. Sudden neck pain in the early morning with limited mobility, forced activity making the pain worse.

2. No significant trauma, fever, or other predisposing factors, no radiating pain on upper extremities.
3. Localized tenderness on the muscles of the neck with noticeable muscle spasms; an X-ray examination can rule out lesions of the neck bones.

Differential Diagnosis

This disease should be differentiated from cervical spondylosis. Refer to the section on cervical spondylosis in Week 8.

Treatment

1. *Treatment principles* soothing the tendons, invigorating blood, warming the meridians, and benefiting the cervical spine.
2. *Commonly used maneuvers* rolling, grasping, plucking, passive movement of the neck, and supple menting with a fomentation patch.
3. *Commonly used acupoints and areas fēngchí* (GB 20), *jiānjǐng* (GB 21), *āshìxué*, *lièquē* (LU 7), *hòuxī* (SI 3), and muscles of the affected area.
4. *Operational methods*
   a. The patient sits with the practitioner standing at the rear oripsilateral side. For relatively severe neck pain, apply finger kneading first on *lièquē* and *hòuxī*. *Lièquē* is one of the four command points of the body, with the famous a dage "for problems on the head and neck, seek for *lièquē*." Kneading on the two points, which relieves the neck pain, pertains to the principle of "prescribe distal acupoints." At the same time, ask the patient to slowly move the head in all directions for one to two minutes.
   b. Perform gentle rolling around the tenderness, and gradually transition toward where the pain is most severe until it is somewhat alleviated. Then, while one hand continues to apply the rolling method, with your other hand, hold on to the patient's forehead, jaw, or head, and slowly perform passive neck flexion, extension, left and right lateral bending, and rotation for about five minutes.

c. Next, apply finger kneading on *fēngchí*, *jiānjǐng* and *āshìxué*. The *āshìxué* acupoint needs especially to be treated by alternating gentle and intensive forces. This procedure should also be supplemented by the passive movement of the neck, totaling up to about five minutes. Alternate the rolling and kneading maneuvers to create the synergy of varying stimulation.
d. When the neck pain is alleviated with improved mobility, apply the plucking maneuver on muscles suffering spasms, using mild force and gradually increasing it, and at the same time increasing the amplitude of the maneuvers. Based on the patient's tolerance to pain, plucking may be applied on muscles with spasms for three to five times, followed by thenar kneading method on the same area to ease the pain caused by the maneuver.
e. End the operation by grasping on *fēngchí* and *jiānjǐng*, and place a fomentation patch on the affected area.

Associated Topic – Fomentation

Fomentation is one of the external treatment methods in Chinese medicine with a history of more than 2,000 years. The *wei* method described in *Inner Classic*, literally meaning "hot press", is actually the fomentation method. There are dry hot presses and moist hot presses used in the treatment. *Kanlisha*, a medicinal sand granule, is one of the traditional dry hot press agents. In tuina practice, moist hot press is usually applied after the tuina procedures to enhance the curative effect and reduce local adverse reactions owing to excessive stimulation of tui na maneuvers.

Method of Fomentation

Depending on the condition, choose different Chinese medicinal herbs, put them into a muslin bag, tie it, and place it into a pot. Add the proper amount of water into the pot and boil it for about ten minutes. While it is still hot, soak a towel into the decoction, wring the towel to remove excess fluid, fold it into a square, and apply it on the desired area. When the towel cools down, repeat the procedure with a second towel. Do it twice to three times for each treatment, and once or twice in a day.

In order to enhance the penetration of the heat into the deeper tissues, gently pat on the towel where it is placed. Or, use the scrubbing maneuver to make the area warm, then apply medicinal fomentation to improve the therapeutic effect.

Precautions

1. The temperature of the towel used in fomentation should be 70°C ± 5°C (158°F ± 41°F). Too high a temperature would damage the skin, and too low would not achieve the result.
2. The fomentation treatment time is in direct proportion to the temperature of the fomentation media. If the temperature is higher, the fomentation treatment time would be shorter, about three to five minutes. By contrast, a lower temperature requires a longer treatment time, about five to ten minutes.
3. Watch closely while performing fomentation; for first-time patients especially, observation of the skin is necessary.
4. Tui na maneuver should be avoided on areas that have just received fomentation.
5. Keep the room warm to prevent the patient from contracting wind-cold.

Commonly Used Reference Formula in Fomentation

sāngzhī (Ramulusmori, 桑枝) 10 g, *hǎifēngténg* (*Caulis piperiskadsurae,* 海风藤) 20 g, *luòshíténg* (*Caulis trachelospermi,* 络石藤) 15 g, *jīxuèténg* (*Caulis spatholobi,* 鸡血藤) 20 g, *rěndōngténg* (*Caulis loniceraejaponicae,* 忍冬藤) 15 g, *zhāngmù* (*Cinnamomumcamphora,* 樟木) 25 g, *hónghuā* (*Floscarthami,* 红花) 10 g, *xīxiāncǎo* (*Herbasiegesbeckiae,* 豨莶草) 30 g

Everyday Exercises

1. What is *laozhen*? What are the key diagnostic criteria?
2. Please master the method and cautions of fomentation.

Day 6

TEMPOROMANDIBULAR JOINT DYSFUNCTION

The temporomandibular joint (TMJ), consisting of the condyle of the mandible and the temporomandibular joint fossa of the temporal bone, is a joint with intra-articular cartilage disc, and is the only joint with mobility in the head and face. The TMJ connects the mandible to the skull.

TMJ dysfunction (or TMJ dysfunction syndrome) is mostly caused by acute or chronic injuries caused by external forces or often by chewing hard objects, resulting in damage to the articular disc and aseptic inflammation. Sometimes, it is due to over-excitation and lack of coordination during inhibition of the joint muscles, so that the joint is out of balance. It may also be due to poor dental occlusion, causing muscle cramps and pain around the TMJ. Lastly, congenital malformation of the joint can also be a cause of TMJ dysfunction.

Clinical Manifestations

The major symptoms of TMJ dysfunction are local chronic pain, tightness, and limitation of opening the mouth. For example, the patient may face difficulties while brushing the teeth with the mouth open, or while laughing. Sometimes, the mouth is suddenly out of control and remains open with a localized sharp pulling pain and a snapping sound. When a patient closes the mouth or unintentionally encounters a hard object while chewing food, pain and snapping may also occur. The severity varies, and recurrence is common. Initially, only one side is affected, but gradually the other side can get affected too, if the condition goes untreated. A small number of patients may experience symptoms such as hearing impairment, dizziness, and headache due to nerve entrapment.

Diagnosis and Differentiation

Key diagnostic criteria

1. Chronic localized pain at the TMJ.
2. Trismus, snapping sound with tenderness at the TMJ.
3. Organic changes of the TMJ have been ruled out.

Differential Diagnosis

1. *Fracture* Symptoms include an immediate onset of the condition, a significant history of trauma, local swelling, pain, loss of functions of opening and closing the mouth. X-rays of the TMJ can confirm the diagnosis.
2. *Rheumatoid arthritis* This condition often occurs in young women, and is characterized by a symmetrical attack on the small joints, typical rheumatoid hands and foot deformities, increased erythrocyte sedimentation rate (ESR), and positive rheumatoid factor test. X-rays can be helpful in the diagnosis.

Treatment

1. *Treatment principles* soothing tendons, benefiting the joints.
2. *Commonly used maneuvers* finger or thenar kneading, scrubbing, and fomentation.
3. *Commonly used acupoints and areas jiăosūn* (SJ 20), *ěrmén* (SJ 21), *xiàguān* (ST 7) and *jiáchē* (ST 6).
4. *Operational methods*

   a. The patient is supine or lying on the side, with the head tilted to one side, so that the affected side is facing up. The practitioners its to the patient's right. In order to prevent damage to the skin, a treatment towel can be placed on the affected area. First, apply thenar kneading around the TMJ to loosen up the temporal is muscle and soft tissue of the cheek. Do this for three to five minutes.
   b. Next, apply finger kneading on *jiăosūn*, *ěrmén*, *xiàguan,* and *jiáchē*. While operating on *ěrmén* and *xiàguān*, ask the patient to open and close his or her mouth. The manipulation needs to be slow with small amplitude so that the force of kneading can be passed into the deeper tissues of the diseased area. This part of the procedure should last for about ten minutes.
   c. Finally, apply scrubbing or fomentation on the affected area, and end the treatment with grasping on *hégŭ* (LI 4).

Self-Preventional Methods

1. Apply finger kneading on the TMJ area for three to five minutes in conjunction with mouth opening and closing.
2. Apply finger kneading on *hégŭ* for about one to two minutes.

Precautions

1. Avoid hard food.
2. Keep the TMJ area warm, preferably by wearing a face covering in the winter when going outside.
3. Alternate between the left and right side while chewing food to avoid over-use of one side and under-use of the other.

Associated Topic — TMJ Dislocation

TMJ dislocation is more common in the elderly and people of frail constitution. Depending on when it happened and the number of recurrences, it can be divided into new, old, and habitual dislocation. Another classification method is unilateral and bilateral dislocation, based on which side is involved. With regard to the position of the man dibularcondyle in relation to the TMJ glenoid fossa, the vast majority of cases are anterior dislocations, while posterior dislocations are rare.

Clinical Manifestations

Upon dislocation of the TMJ, the mouth is half opened and not able to close naturally. The patient may have symptoms including slurred speech, swallowing difficulties, and salivation. In unilateral dislocation, the lower jaw would tilt to the contralateral side, with a palpable pit in front of the ipsilateral tragus. In bilateral dislocation, the lower jaw is prolapsed and protruded with a palpable depression in front of both sides of the tragus.

Treatment

A new TMJ dislocation is relatively easier to treat; reduction (i.e., realignment of a body part in its normal position) is done inside the oral cavity.

Have the patient sit in a low chair with head, neck, and back resting against the wall. The practitioner should stand in front of the patient.

a. Use sterilized gauze to wrap both your thumbs, and insert them into the patient's mouth at the back-end of both sides of the molars between the upper and lower dentitions. Use the other fingers of both hands to grip both sides of the jaw (see Figures 138 and 138b).
b. Prior to the reduction operation, ask the patient to relax. Use both thumbs to push down the jaw and push it back firmly. At the same time, the other fingers need to coordinate to lift up the jaw. When a click is heard, it is the indication of a successfully reduction (see Figures 138c and 138d). Quickly remove the thumbs from the mouth to prevent them from being bitten owing to the reflective closure of the mouth.
c. For unilateral dislocation, use the thumb to firmly press and push the affected side, with the other thumb assisting it without exerting much force. The reduction method for a habitual dislocation is the same as for anew dislocation.
d. After the operation, use a four-tailed bandage to wrap around the mandibular, make a tie on the top of the head, and keep the bandage on fora day or two. The patient should avoid excessive movements of the mouth or biting on hard food for one to two weeks to prevent further and habitual dislocation. For individuals with habitual dislocation, ask them to sip a spoonful of vinegar and keep it in the mouth for half an hour. Then, use the bandage to stabilize the jaw.

Everyday Exercises

1. What are the main symptoms of temporom and ibular joint (TMJ) dysfunction?
2. How would you use tui na to treat TMJ dysfunction?

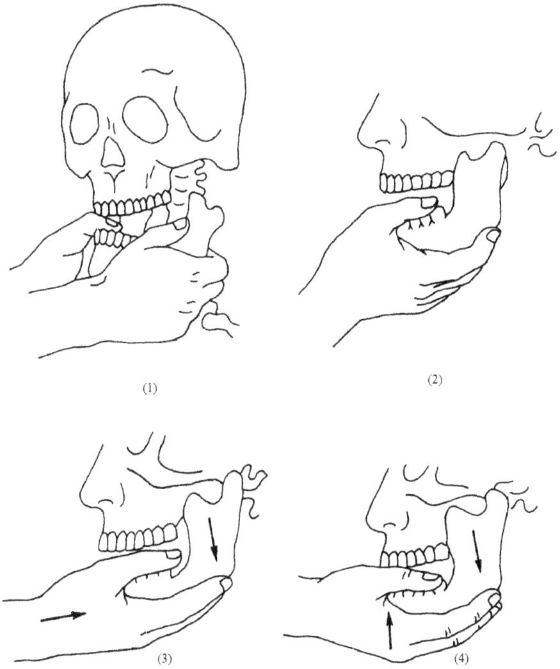

Figure 138 Reduction of TMJ dislocation

WEEK 8

Day 1

CERVICAL SPONDYLOSIS

Cervical spondylosis, also known as cervical spine syndrome, is a common disease in middle-aged people and the elderly. With age, the cervical intervertebral discs (see Figure 139) gradually degenerate, resulting in decreased elasticity; there is bulging of the discs, narrowed space between discs, vertebral edge hyperostosis, intervertebral instability, yellow ligament hypertrophy and degeneration, or hyperplasia of Luschka joints and secondary changes of small joints. The structural changes will inevitably lead to deformation of the cervical spinal canal or foraminal stenosis, resulting in direct stimulation and oppression and affect its blood supply. The structural or functional damage to the spinal nerve root, spinal cord, vertebral artery, and sympathetic nerve causes the series of clinical symptoms seen in cervical spondylosis.

Clinical Manifestations

1. *Cervical vertebra disorder* The patient suffers only slight neck pain, though he or she is unable to read and write for long periods of time; there is a normal range of motion of the neck in general, as well as an absence of radiating pain on the upper extremities.
2. *Cervical spondylotic radiculopathy* In addition to neck pain, symptoms include a significant radiating pain on the upper extremities with paroxysmal aggravation; a limited mobility of the neck or rigidity; weakness of the ipsilateral limbs with reduced gripping strength, and numbness of the fingers.

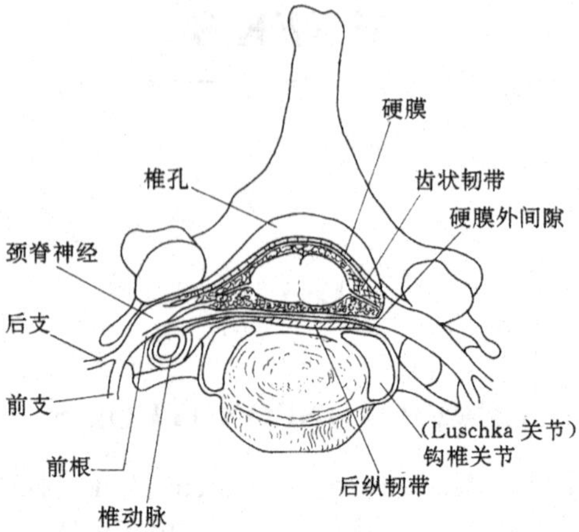

椎孔	-	vertebral foramen
颈脊神经	-	cervical spinal nerve
后支	-	posterior branch
前支	-	anterior branch
前根	-	anterior root
椎动脉	-	vertebral artery
硬膜	-	dura mater
齿状韧带	-	denticulate ligament
硬膜外间隙	-	epidural space
钩椎关节	-	Luschka joint
后纵韧带	-	posterior longitudinal ligament

Figure 139 Transverse view of a cervical vertebra

3. *Cervical spondylotic myelopathy* There is neck pain accompanied by limb numbness, stiffness, and decreased strength; the hand is unable to hold things or move freely; the patient has an awkward gait or may be unable to stand or walk, and in the most severe cases, there is paralysis. Some patients may experience zonesthesia over the chest and abdomen, creating an unusual discomfort. There may be fecal and urinary incontinence or dysuria.
4. *Cervical spondylotic vertebral arteriopathy* (CSA) General symptoms include neck pain, dizziness, and headache. Visual symptoms include diplopia, visual hallucinations, and decreased vision. There may also be cataplexy. These symptoms are often associated with head and neck rotation.

5. *Sympathetic cervical spondylosis* Symptoms include neck pain accompanied by migraine, dizziness, distension of the head, blurred vision, tinnitus, and deafness, arrhythmia, tachycardia, or bradycardia and precordial pain, cold limbs, decreased surface temperature, finger numbness and swelling, and hyperalgesia.

Diagnosis and Differentiation

1. *Cervicalvertebra disorder*
   Diagnosis Neck pain does not radiate to the upper extremities; passive movements of the neck are normal; cervical X-ray shows decreased or disappeared cervical physiological curvature and no other bone changes.
2. *Cervical spondylotic radiculopathy*
   Diagnosis Pain on the neck and arms; numbness of the fingers, pain and decreased strength in accordance with distribution of the nerve roots; skin hypesthesia; diminished or absent reflexes of the biceps and triceps tendons; limited neck mobility; paraspinal tenderness with radiating pain of the ipsilateral limb; positive results in head tapping test and brachial plexus traction test. Neck X-ray shows disappearance of the physiological curvature, narrowed disc space, vertebral hyperostosis, intervertebral foramen deformation, and Luschka joint hyperplasia.

Differential Diagnosis

a. *Rheumatology* There is no radiating pain, and the numbare as are not in accordance with the spinal nerve root segment distribution. Anti-rheumatic drugs alleviate the symptoms.
b. *Thoracic outlet syndrome* Although there is root pain on the upper extremities, it has its own unique signs, i.e., results turn out positive for intermittent fluctuation test, chest expansion test, and upper extremity over-outreach test. X-ray examination suggests redundancy of cervical ribs and transverse process.

3. *Cervical spondylotic myelopathy*
   Diagnosis Increased muscle tension and decreased muscle force of the limbs, tendon hyperreflexia, and occurrence of pathological reflexes.

Sensory disorder and dyskinesia occur below the level of the lesion; in advanced stages, spastic paralysis occurs. X-rays can show typical cervical spondylosis changes, and myelography can reveal the compression on the cervical spinal cord. Finally, CT and MRI scans can confirm the diagnosis.

Differential Diagnosis

a. *Cervical spinal cord tumors* Major characteristics of this disease are quadriplegic paralysis of the motor system, decreased or absent sensory ability below the level of cervical or the upper extremity of nerve tract type, and sphincter disturbances. X-rays show destruction of the vertebral arch and vertebral body, and inverted cup-shaped obstructions. An MRI scan can confirm the diagnosis.
b. *Syringomyelia* Slow onset, usually in adults younger than 30 years. At the early stage, segmental paresthesia and dissociative sensory disturbances occur; there is diminished or disappeared temperature sensation, with the danger of the patient getting burned unconsciously. Upper limb weakness and muscle atrophy from the distal to the proximal limb may affect the sacrospinal muscles. X-rays show the deformities of the skull and neck, with spinal angiography showing symmetrical enlargement of the spinal cord. MRI scans can confirm the diagnosis.

4. *Cervical spondylotic vertebral arteriopathy*
   Diagnosis Dizziness and nausea associated with head and neck rotation. Cervical X-rays show hyperplasia of the Luschka joint. Blood flow diagram of the vertebral basilar artery and vertebral angiography can help in the diagnosis.

Differential Diagnosis

a. *Meniere's syndrome* (*Meniere disease*) Symptoms include episodes of vertigo, tinnitus, deafness, nausea, vomiting, and nystagmus.
b. *Internal auditory artery spasms* The internal auditory artery originates from the basilar artery. Along with spasms on the ipsilateral side of the artery, acute progressive tinnitus and deafness will soon lead to hearing loss and sudden onset of severe vertigo. Several hours later, the hearing gradually improves and the vertigo is also alleviated.

5. *Sympatheticcervical spondylosis*
   Diagnosis There are clinical manifestations of sympathetic dysfunction and nerve root irritation. X-rays show signs of cervical spondylosis.

Differential Diagnosis

a. *Nerve (sensory) disease or autonomic nervous dysfunction* There are no significant signs or symptoms of nerve root or spinal cord involvement; X-rays do not show signs of cervical spondylosis.
b. *Angina pectoris* The patient has a history of coronary heart disease. An angina attack often occurs after physical activities, emotional turbulence, a big meal, or exposure to cold. It does not last long, usually lasting from a few seconds to an hour, and is all eviated after rest or an intake of nitroglycerin tablets.

Treatment

1. *Treatment principles* regulating qi and blood, soothing tendons, unblocking collaterals, resolving spasms, and relieving pain.
2. *Commonly used maneuvers* rolling, pressure and finger kneading, grasping, plucking, shaking, and passive movements.
3. *Commonly used acupoints and areas fēngchí* (GB 20), *fēngfŭ* (DU 16), *jiānjĭng* (GB 21), *tiānzōng* (SI 11), *āshìxué*, *qŭchí* (LI 11), *lièquē* (LU 7), *hégŭ* (LI 4), neck, shoulder, and four limbs.
4. *Operational methods*
   Basic operations
   a. The patient sits with the practitioner standing at his or back. Apply gentle rolling on the upper and middle parts of the contralateral trapezius, and gradually transition to the ipsilateral trapezius and work on its upper and middle portions. This is the adaptive stage of the treatment and it should last for one to two minutes.
   b. Apply finger kneading on *fēngchí jiānjĭng,* and *āshìxué* for about a minute each, and coordinate with appropriate passive movements, including neck flexion and extension, and left and right lateral flexion and rotation.

c. Apply the rolling maneuver with the focus on the trapezius and supraspinatus, coordinating with passive movements of the neck in all six directions for about five minutes.
d. Lastly, apply pressing and plucking on painful spots, i.e., *āshìxué*. Then, apply grasping on *jiānjǐng*, pressure kneading on *lièquē* and *qǔchí*, and scrubbing the shoulders and back to end the treatment.

The procedure above is indicated for cervical vertebra disorders and is a fundamental operation in treating other types of cervical spondylosis.

Treatment Based on Pattern Differentiation

- *Cervical spondylotic radiculopathy* Upon completing the fundamental operation above, apply fixed point pressing and rotating maneuver on the neck. This maneuver uses a thumb pulp to press on a cervical paraspinal tender point. Flex the other elbow and use the cubital fossa to hold the mandible of the patient; gently lift it up, and slowly rotate the cervical vertebra once or twice. The napply neck support-lifting and stretching maneuver– use both hands to hold the mandible of the patient, slowly lifting up the cervical vertebra for a good stretch three to five times. Apply tuina maneuvers on the ipsilateral upper limb where the spinal nerves distribute.
- *Cervical spondylotic myelopathy* Upon completing the fundamental operation above, have the patient assume a prone position. Apply rolling on the back along the bladder meridian, and intense pressing along *du mai* for five to eight minutes. Then, apply rolling along the bladder meridian, starting from the hip, passing the posterior side of the thigh, calf, and all the way to the Achilles tendon, supplemented with intense pressing of *huántiào* (GB 30), finger kneading on *wěizhōng* (BL 40), grasping on *chéngshān* (BL 57), and the Achilles tendon for three to five minutes. Get the patient to change to the supine position. Apply the rolling maneuver on the anterolateral aspect of the leg, from the thigh to the dorsum of the foot for three to five minutes, supplemented by passive movement of the lower extremity and pressure kneading on *zúsānlǐ* (ST 36), *yánglíngquán* (GB 34), and *jiěxī* (ST 41). Lastly, get the patient to sit, and apply tuina maneuvers on both the upper limbs with the focus on the hands for three to five minutes.

- *Cervical spondylotic vertebral arteriopathy* Upon completing the fundamental operation above, first, apply enhanced finger kneading on both sides of the neck for three to five minutes. Then, add various head tuina manipulations: disjoining pushing of the forehead, smearing, pressing, five-finger grasping, and scattering sweeping for three to five minutes.
- *Sympathetic cervical spondylosis* Upon completing the fundamental operation above, add head tuina, same as the second part of treating CSA, and pressure kneading on *bǎihuì* (DU 20). Then, add finger kneading on *dànzhōng* (RN 17), *nèiguān* (PC 6), and *sānyīnjiāo* (SP 6) for approximately three to five minutes.

Self-Preventional Methods

1. *Finger kneading on paraspinal cervical muscles* With the four fingers close together, use the finger pulps to apply kneading along the paraspinal cervical muscles top-down, back and forth for about three to five minutes, with hands alternating.
2. *Double-handed intense pressing on fēngchí* Use both thumbs to apply intense pressing on the bilateral *fēngchí* simultaneously, supplemented by pressure kneading for about a minute.
3. *Finger kneading on qǔchí and lièquē* Use both thumbs to perform the maneuver on the bilateral acupoints, each for about a minute.
4. *Neck movements* Slowly perform flexion, extension, left and right rotation, left and right lateral bending, and clockwise and counterclockwise movements.

Precautions

1. Avoid high pillows.
2. Change body positions every now and then, for those who need to work at the desk for a long time.
3. Avoid brute, violent force and substandard passive movements while using tuina to treat the patient.
4. If tuina is not very effective for a patient with cervical spondylotic myelopathy, or the disease has a chronic progressive trend, surgery should be considered.

Everyday Exercises

1. What is cervical spondylosis? What are the clinical types for this condition?
2. Describe the fundamental operation of tuina in treating cervical spondylosis.

Day 2

SUDDEN HYPOCHONDRIAC BURST INJURY

Pain caused by underestimating a heavy object and overstraining oneself by attempting to carry it, or using an abnormal posture to carry, lift, and move a heavy object, is called sudden hypochondriac burst injury. In Chinese medical practice, it is commonly known as *cha qi*, literally "stitched qi", belonging to the scope of the chest wall injuries. It is believed that the root cause is abnormal qi movement with a sudden onset triggered by injury factors.

Clinical Manifestations

1. Unilateral chest and back pain.
2. The patient is unable to speak loudly, take a deep breath, or cough without feeling pain.
3. Aggravation of pain while moving, such as when the patient changes his or her lying position;
4. The pain is of a broad range, vague, shifts around, and without a fixed point.
5. When the pain is aggravated, there is local muscle tension and tenderness.

Diagnosis and Differentiation

Diagnosis

The patient has a significant history of incidences that might have triggered the injury. There is hypochondriac pain without fixed tenderness; absence of fixed pain point against the chest wall, shallow breathing; Chest X-rays show no abnormalities.

Differential Diagnosis

1. *Soft tissue contusion injury of the chest wall* This is the result of direct impact against the chest wall and fixed sore spots, often accompanied

by swelling and bruises. Local tenderness is evident. X-rays show no bone lesions.

2. *Costal chondritis* There is no significant history of trauma; there is chronic onset; a hard bulge is found at the costal cartilage with obvious tenderness; local skin temperature may increase, but the skin is not flushed. X-rays show no bone changes.
3. *Rib fracture* There is a significant history of trauma. There is local pain, bruising, deformity, and obvious tenderness or bone fricative after the injury. An X-ray examination can confirm the diagnosis of rib fractures.

Treatment

1. *Treatment principles* regulating qi and blood, comforting the chest, and relieving pain.
2. *Commonly used maneuvers* finger rubbing, finger kneading, disjoining pushing.
3. *Commonly used acupoints and areas* *dànzhōng* (RN 17), *zhōngfǔ* (LU 1), *zhāngmén* (LR 13), *qīmén* (LR 14), *fèishū* (BL 13), and the hypochondriac area.
4. *Operational methods*
   The patient is supine with the practitioner standing at the right side of the patient. First, apply finger rubbing on the ipsilateral *zhōngfǔ* followed by *dánzhōng*, *zhāngmén,* and *qīmén* for one to three minutes to smooth out the local qi and blood flow. Second, in the same position, apply finger kneading and disjoining pushing (see Figure140) on the hypochondriac area where the pain is relatively severe for three to five minutes. The two steps can be performed alternately. Next, get the patient to shift to a sitting position. Apply finger kneading on *fèishū* and *nèiguān* (PC 6), followed by foulage of the affected hypochondrium to end the treatment.

Self-Preventional Methods

1. Palm kneading on the hypochondrium: use the contralateral palm to knead the ipsilateral hypochondrium for two to three minutes.

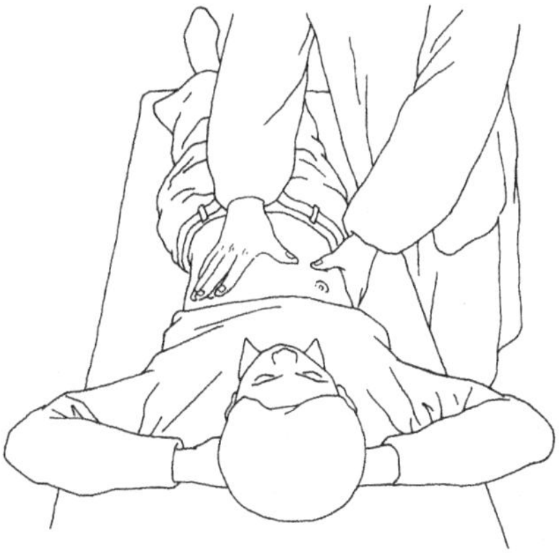

Figure 140 Disjoining pushing the tenderness on the chest

2. Finger kneading on *dànzhōng* and *nèiguān*: use the index finger or the thumb to apply kneading on *tánzhōng* and *nèiguān*, for a minute on each acupoint.

Precautions

1. Avoid laborious work after recovery.
2. Relax, and if the pain is severe, oral analgesics and sedatives may be needed under a physician's order.

Associated Topic — Thoracic Facet Joint Disorders

Thoracic facet joint disorder refers to the upper back pain caused by the injuries of thoracic facet joints, costal-vertebral joints, and the joints of the costal transverse process.

Clinical Manifestations

There is immediate occurrence of upper back pain, right after a crisp sound is heard. There is discomfort in supine or prone position, or when turning over while lying down. Deep breathing and coughing can make the symptoms worse.

Diagnosis

Onsetis sudden. There is a history of traumaendured due to traction and careless turning of the body. There is paraspinal thoracic tenderness with increased tension of the surrounding back muscles.

Treatment

1. *Treatment principles* spinal reduction maneuvers.
2. *Commonly used maneuvers* rolling, intense pressing, and finger kneading.
3. *Commonly used acupoints and areas huàtuójiájǐ* (also known as *jiájǐ*, EX-B 2) and sacrospinal muscles.
4. *Operational methods*

   Reduction with intensepressing

   Caution: this maneuver is forbidden in patients with heart diseases.

   a. Have the patient lie prone with a soft cushion in front of the chest, and the practitioner standing to the right. First, apply rolling on the ipsilateral back by starting from distant locations and gradually moving to the diseased site, up and down, back and forth alongs acrospinal muscles for three to five minutes.
   b. Remain in the same position. Perform finger kneading on the corresponding *jiájǐ* points where the tenderness is located to relax the sacrospinal muscles.
   c. Lastly, place one thumb on the tender spot, the entire palm of the other hand pressing the previous thumb. Ask the patient to take a deep breath. When the patient is at the end of the inhalation, follow the trend of the breath with a sudden pressing At this point, a snapping sound can often be heard indicating the reduction. If the reduction is successful, symptoms of the disorder will no longer exist.

   Vertebral stretching with chest out (Fig. 141)

   Have the patient sit on a bench, with the practitioner standing posterior to the patient.

   a. Follow steps (a) and (b) above to loosen up tensed muscles.
   b. Ask the patient to hold his or her occipital area by clasping the hands tightly together. Then, supporting and holding on to both elbows of the patient, flex one knee to prop it against the diseased

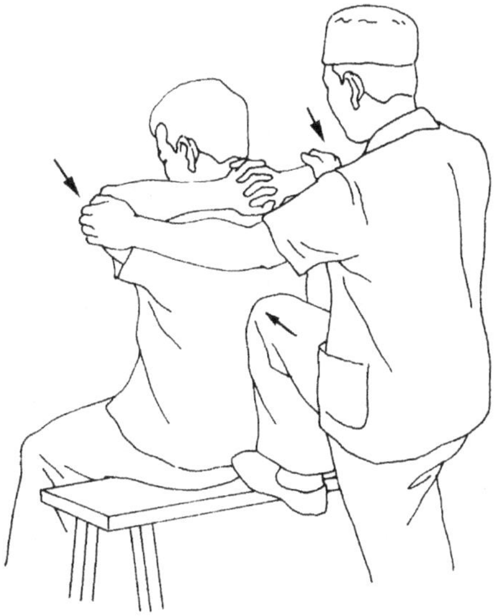

Figure 141 Vertebral stretching with chest out

spinous process, and place the foot on the bench to get ready for the next step.

c. Now, here comes the most important part of the operation. Ask the patient to take a deep breath, and right at the moment of the inhalation, use your hands to pull back the patient's elbows, while using your knee to push the patient's back forward (see Figure 141). The combination completes the action of vertebral stretching with chest out. A crisp snapping sound is a sign of successful reduction, though it is not mandatory to produce this sound.

Everyday Exercises

Memorize the main differential diagnosis of a sudden hypochondriac burst.

Day 3

ACUTE LUMBAR SOFT TISSUE INJURY

This condition is more common in young adults, especially manual workers, and people who lack physical exercise or those who rarely participate in laborious work. Most of the time, it occurs when the person moves or lifts a heavy object with incorrect posture, or is involved in excessive flexion, extension, and torsion beyond the normal physiological range of motion or individual's limit, causing soft tissue injuries of the waist that may include muscles, ligaments, or synovial membrane.

Since this condition may damage different tissues, the manipulations are different. It is therefore extremely important to categorize the condition correctly. In addition, the condition must be handled well during the acute phase to avoid future problems.

Acute Lumbar Injury

Acute lumbar injury often affects one side of the sacrospinal muscles.

Clinical Manifestations

1. Immediate back pain and limited lumbar movement with difficulties in walking; in severe cases, the patient cannot stand or walk at all.
2. Forced waist position, unilateral spasms of lumbar muscles with obvious tenderness, movement of the waist in all directions is limited, and sometimes the pain is so severe that the patient is not able to withstand the physical examination.

Diagnosis

1. Significant history of trauma.
2. Pain on one side of the lumbar muscles.
3. Ipsilaterallumbar muscle spasms, increased muscle tension with tenderness.
4. Waist X-rays rule out bone lesions.

Treatment

1. *Treatment principles* invigorating blood, dissolving stasis, resolving spasms, and relieving pain.
2. *Commonly used maneuvers* rolling, pressure kneading, grasping, scrubbing, fomentation, and passive movements.
3. *Commonly used acupoints and areas āshìxué, huántiào* (GB 30), jūliào (GB 29), wěizhōng (BL 40), and sacrospinal muscle.
4. *Operational methods*
   a. The patient is prone, with the practitioner standing at the ipsilateral side. First, work on the distal acupoints. Perform finger kneading on *wěizhōng* for about a minute.
   b. Next, apply rolling on ipsilateral sacrospinal muscles for three to five minutes. It must start from non-painful areas to the most painful area, and the force of the manipulation must be mild to start with and gradually become intense, so that the patient can endure the treatment.
   c. Apply finger kneading and plucking alternately on *āshìxué* for two to three minutes. Then apply scrubbing on the same spot until the warmth is felt.
   d. In addition, coordinate oblique pulling maneuver with passive knee and hip flexion. If the condition allows, apply fomentation to the patient as the last procedure of the operation.

Injury of the Supraspinous or Interspinous Ligament

Injury of the supraspinous or interspinous ligaments is the result of strong traction while the body is in excessive anterior flexion. Tuina accelerates the circulation of local blood and lymph of the ligament tissue lacking blood supply, therefore contributing to the repair of damaged tissue.

Clinical Manifestations

1. Tearing pain in the posterior central lower back that is exacerbated with anterior flexion; limited mobility of the waist.
2. The tender point is located superficially above the spinous process in the posterior midline or between the two spinousprocesses.

Diagnosis

1. History of injury due to excessive anterior flexion of the waist.
2. Superficial supraspinous or intraspinous tenderness.
3. Local nerve block provides instant relief for the pain.

Treatment

1. *Treatment principles* invigorating blood, dissolving stasis, harmonizing *ying* qi, and relieving pain.
2. *Commonly used maneuvers* finger kneading, scrubbing, and fomentation method. Avoid any passive movements.
3. *Commonly used acupoints and areas āshìxué, bāliào* (BL 31 to 34) and *wěizhōng* (BL 40).
4. *Operational methods*
   a. The patient is in the prone position, with the practitioner standing to one side. Select the distal *wěizhōng* to perform finger kneading for a minute or two.
   b. Apply finger kneading on *bāliào* with the focus on *shàngliáo* (BL 31) and *cìliáo* (BL 32) for two to three minutes.
   c. Gradually transition to the painful area, and apply finger or thenar kneading on the injured area of the supraspinous or intraspinous ligaments for five to ten minutes.
   d. Be aware that tissue repair can only be boosted with gentle maneuvers and adequate rest. Any movement of the waist would aggravate the damage to the injured ligament tissue. (See Figure 142.)

Synovial Membrane Incarceration of Intervertebral Joints

This condition often occurs in the lumbosacral intervertebral joints, accounting for 50% to 60% of acute soft tissue injuries of the lower back. (See Figure 143.)

Clinical Manifestations

1. Lower lumbar pain with limited mobility, especially posterior extension.

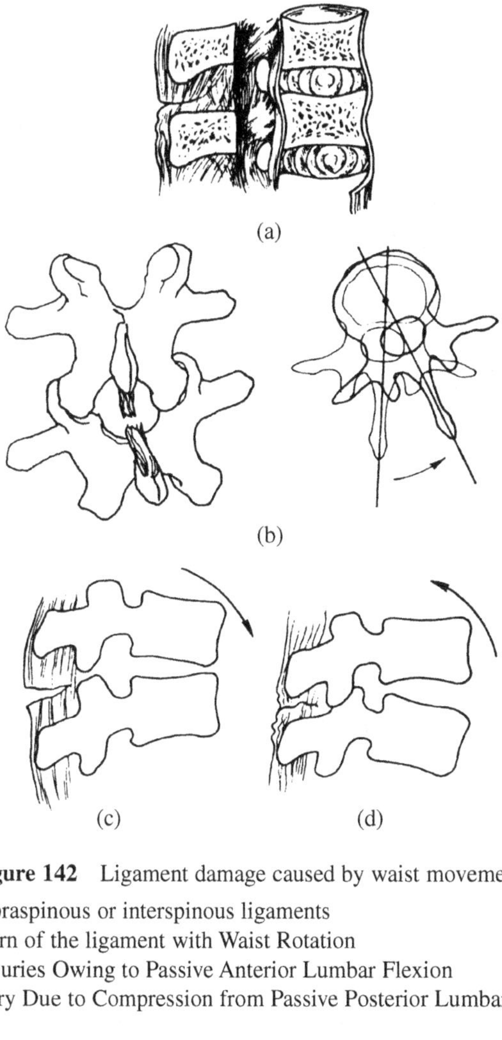

Figure 142 Ligament damage caused by waist movements

a. Injuries of Supraspinous or interspinous ligaments
b. Aggravated Torn of the ligament with Waist Rotation
c. Aggravated Injuries Owing to Passive Anterior Lumbar Flexion
d. Ligament Injury Due to Compression from Passive Posterior Lumbar Extension

2. Disappearance of the physiological curvature of the waist, and local muscle spasms.
3. The tender spots are often confined at an intervertebral joint near the spinous process without radiating pain to the lower limbs.

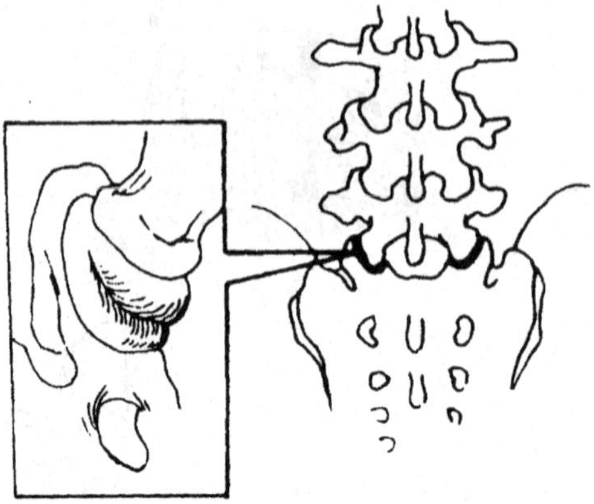

Figure 143 Diagram of Synovial membrane incarceration of intervertebral joints

Diagnosis

1. History of sudden low back pain while straightening or rotating the waist, with lumbar muscle spasms and disorders of posterior extension of the waist.
2. Lumbosacral joint tenderness.
3. Lumbar X-rays are normal.

Treatment

1. *Treatment principles* reduction of dislocated joints, alleviating the urgency, and relieving pain.
2. *Commonly used maneuvers* rolling, pressure kneading, intense pressing and oblique pulling.
3. *Commonly used acupoints and areas guānyuánshū* (BL 26), *xiǎochángshū* (BL 27), *kūnlún* (BL 60), the waist and hips.
4. *Operational methods*:
   a. The patient is in the prone position, with the practitioner standing at the affected side. Apply rolling or palm-heel pressure kneading on the lumbosacral area, glutea, and the posterior side of the thigh with the main focus on the lumbosacral region to relax the spasms of the lumbar muscles. This manipulation should last eight to ten minutes.
   b. Apply intense pressing on *guānyuánshū*, *xiǎochángshū,* and *kūnlún*, for five to ten times each to alleviate pain.

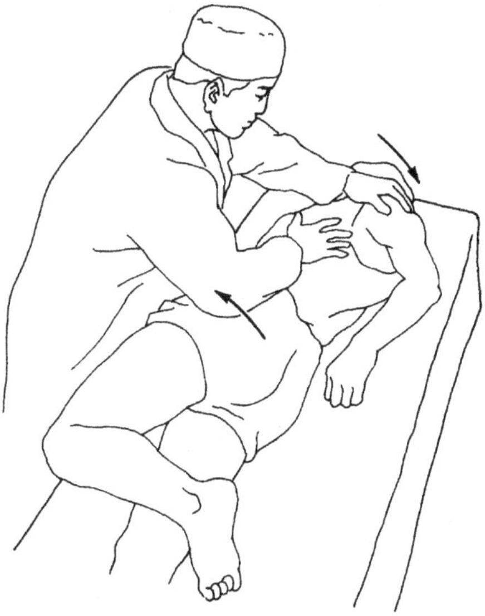

Figure 144 Oblique pulling maneuver

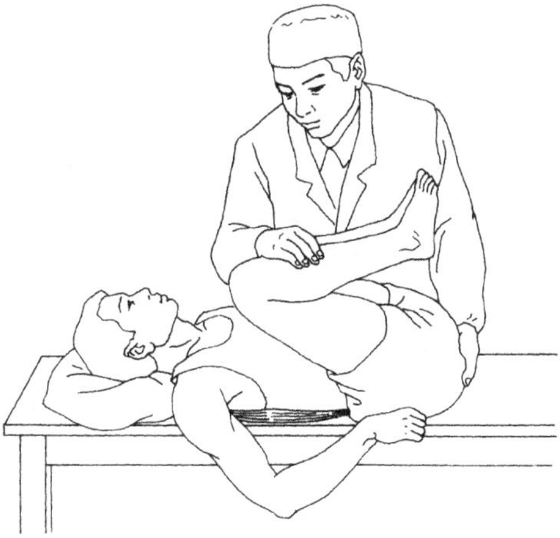

Figure 145 Passive movement of bilateral knee and hip flexion

c. Ask the patient to lie on his or her side, and perform the oblique pulling maneuver (see Figure 144). Or have the patient supine with the practitioner standing at the affected side, and apply passive flexion of the knee and hips (see Figure 145). Both techniques enable diaplasis of incarcerated synovial membrane. However, the manipulation should not be violent. A snapping sound should not be forced while performing oblique pulling.

Precautions

1. The treatment should be based on pattern differentiation. Avoid careless manipulation.
2. The manipulation needs to be applied according to the natural tendency of the body. Use gentle yet skillful techniques to solve the problem. Avoid rude and substandard passive movements.
3. The recovery of injured ligament tissue is very slow, approximately four to six weeks. Do not force success. Avoid any passive movements. It is appropriate to coordinate treatment and rest simultaneously. It is better for the patient to sleep on a hard bed.
4. Even if the patient is able to get instant relief with tuina maneuvers, the patient suffering acute lower back injury should avoid waist movements for three to five days to facilitate the repair of damaged tissue and prevent further problems.

Everyday Exercises

1. What specific conditions does acute lumbar soft tissue injury include? What are the main symptoms for each of them?
2. Why should patients with supraspinous or interspinous ligamentinjury avoid any passive movements?
3. Try to memorize the precautions associated with acute lumbar soft tissue injuries.

Day 4

THE THIRD LUMBAR TRANSVERSE PROCESS SYNDROME

The third lumbar transverse process syndrome is also known as lumbar muscle strain. L3 (see Figure 146) is the center of the lumbar spine, and the prominence of the forward physiological curvature of the lumbar vertebrae. It serves as the pivot of the waist for flexion, extension, lateral flex, and rotation. The transverse processes of L3 on both sides are the longest and bear the most lever force, with lumbar muscles, ligaments and other tissues attached. Waist movements in any direction expose the L3 transverse processes to repeated pulling and friction, thus allowing chances for injuries to occur.

The condition is mostly due to delayed or improper treatment after acute lumbar muscle injury, leading to sequela symptoms. The condition can be the result of poor posture or overloading of the psoae over time, causing muscular fatigue. It can also be due to variations in the anatomical structure of the lower back. In Chinese medical practice, it is believed to be due to pathogenic wind, cold and dampness lingering in the waist.

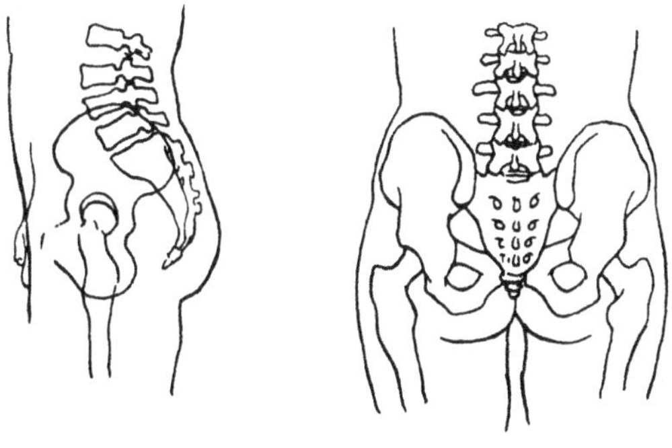

(a) (b)

Figure 146 Diagram of lateral aspect of the L3 vertebra

a. Lateral Aspect: L3 in the Forefront of the Lumbar Protrusion Arc with the Upper and Lower Edges Leveled
b. Antero posterior View: L3 Transverse Process Is the Longest

Clinical Manifestations

1. Main symptoms: chronic and intermittent soreness, pain, weakness of the waist.
2. Difficulty in maintaining the same body position and aggravated symptoms in the waist after laborious work.
3. Absence of obvious signs in the chronic stage. Hypertonia of the psoae upon acute attack with restricted motor function, tenderness on the top of the L3 transverse process with palpable subcutaneous knots.
4. Tendon reflexes of the lower limb are symmetrical; skin sensation, muscle strength, straight leg raise test are normal.

Diagnosis and Differentiation

Key Diagnostic Criteria

1. The diagnosis of the disease is mainly based on the history and clinical manifestations mentioned above, especially the tenderness on L3 transverse process. If other organic changes are excluded, the diagnosis can be confirmed.
2. Waist X-rays do not provide significant diagnostic evidence. However, it can be used for the purpose of differential diagnosis.

Differential Diagnosis

1. *Lumbar disc herniation* In addition to lower back pain, it is associated with ipsilateral sciatica showing paroxysmal exacerbation, limitation in the straight leg raise test, paraspinal tenderness, and radiating pain along the affected limb.
2. *Lumbar tumor* The occurrence of lumbar tumors is highly likely in middle-aged and older patients with progressive lower back pain that worsens in the night, pain that is not relieved after symptomatic treatment. The tumor may be in the spinal cord or caudaequina. There may be fecal and urinary incontinence, saddle area (i.e., perineum) numbness and tingling, and paralysis of both lower extremities.

3. *Lumbospinal tuberculosis* Symptoms include lower back pain with fever, anemia, weight loss, and increased ESR. Pick-up test shows positive. X-rays show bone destruction and greater psoas abscess.
4. *Perinephritis* Symptoms include low back pain accompanied with fever, increased WBC count, percussion pain in the kidney area.
5. *Gynecological diseases* The female patient experiences lower back pain with periodic changes.

Treatment

1. *Treatment principles* relieving lumbar muscle spasms, loosening up adhesions, and improving muscle strength.
2. *Commonly used maneuvers* rolling, pressure kneading, plucking, grasping, scrubbing, and fomentation.
3. *Commonly used acupoints and areas* *āshìxué*, *shènshū* (BL 23), *jūliào* (GB 29), *huántiào* (GB 30), *wěizhōng* (BL 40), and lower back.
4. *Operational methods*
   a. The patient is prone with the practitioner standing at the affected side. Apply rolling or palm-heel kneading to the ipsilateral soft tissue distal from the affected area and work the way up to the waist, back and forth for five to eight minutes.
   b. Then focus on the surrounding area of the pain, and apply finger kneading on *āshìxué* for a minute or two.
   c. Take *āshìxué* as the center and perform disjoining pushing to rectify the surrounding tendons.
   d. Apply the rolling method to the waist, or palm-heel kneading along both sides of the bladder meridian down from the gluteal area to the posterior thigh, up and down and back and forth for three to five times.
   e. Apply intense pressing on *shènshū, jūliào, huántiào,* and *wěizhōng* for five to ten times. If the waist movement is limited, passive movement of the waist can be selected according to the specific circumstances.
   f. Maintain the same body position. First, the practitioner needs to locate it (see Figure 147). With both thumbs overlapped, apply

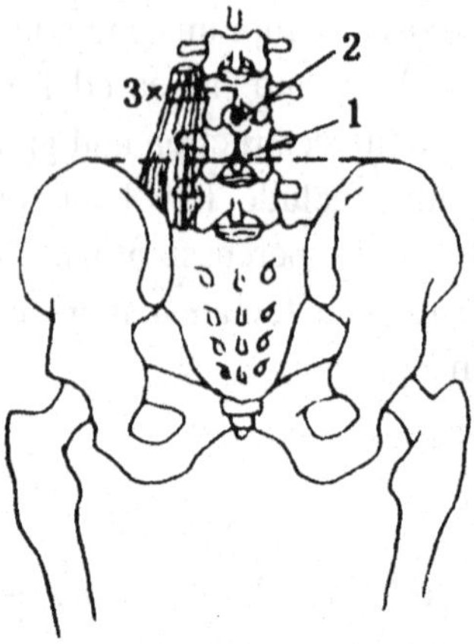

Figure 147 Allocating L3 transverse process

1. L4 Spinous Process: Leveled with the Line Connecting the Iliac Crests
2. L3 Spinous Process: Right above L4 Spinous Process
3. Apex of the L3 Transverse Process: the Bony Protrusion Lateral from Lumbar Spinal Muscle, Outside of the Upper Edge of the L3 Spinous Process

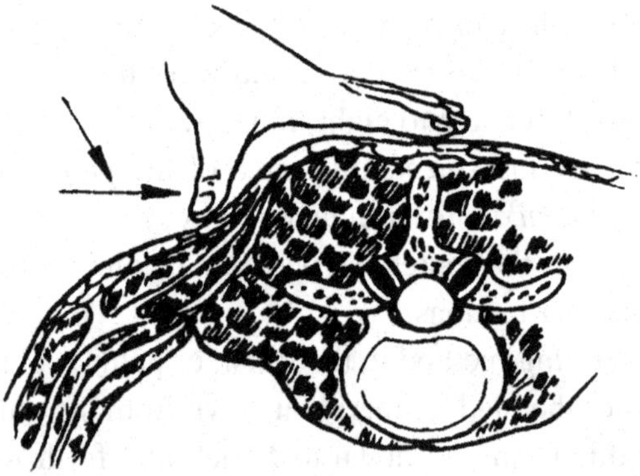

Figure 148 Plucking on L3 transverse process

plucking in a down and inward direction on L3 transverse process (see Figure 148) for ten to 15 times, followed by finger kneading for one to two minutes. Lastly, end the operation with localized scrubbing or fomentation.

Self-Preventional Methods

1. *Tuina on the tender spots* In sitting or prone position, both hands making loose fists, use the inter phalangeal joints of the thumbs or the metacarpophalangeal joints of index fingers as the focal point, and apply left-and-right plucking or up-and-down pushing on the tender point of L3 transverse process. Do it for four to eight sets of eight beats each.
2. *Exercises of the back and lumbar muscles* Figure 149 shows strengthening exercises for the back and lumbar muscles. The exercises are (a) five-point supporting, (b) three-point supporting, (c) bridge arch, (d) chest and spine stretching, (e) stretching spine with leg lifted, and (f) flying swallow sipping water. As we go from (a) to (f), the exercises gradually increase in difficulty and in the physical strength needed to carry them out. The training should be in accordance with the physical condition of the patient. Start with the easier exercises, then slowly progress to the more difficult ones, gradually increasing the time you spend on them. It is important to be persistent and exercise daily. Make sure you do not exhaust yourself. It is not necessary to complete all six exercises every day. Lastly, exercises (a) and (b) are not appropriate for patients with cervical spondylosis.

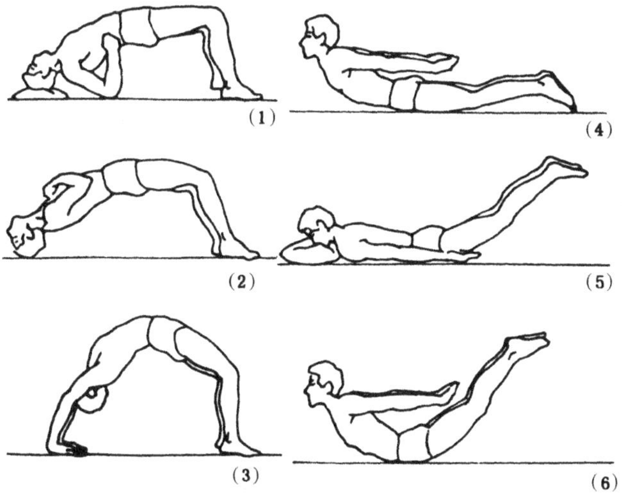

Figure 149 Exercising the back muscles

Precautions

1. Seek timely treatment for acute waist injury.
2. Pay attention to, and adjust, unhealthy postures.
3. Use a wide waist belt to support and protect the waist, and sleep on aahard bed.
4. Stay warm, and avoid exhaustion.

Everyday Exercises

1. How would you locate the L3 transverse process?
2. How would you exercise the lumbar muscles?

Day 5

DEGENERATIVE LUMBAR SPONDYLITIS

The condition has various names, such as traumatic spondylitis, hypertrophic spondylitis, senile spondylitis, and spinal vertebra arthritis.

Bone spurs, also known as osteophytes, are sometimes formed in the process of lumbar degeneration. Osteophytes form naturally on the back of the spine as a person ages. Osteophytes can occur at any edge of the vertebrae, but they are more common at the anterior edge, and less common at the posterior edge. It is mainly because the former has more chances to be squeezed. Figure 150 shows how osteophyes are formed. The longitudinal ligament of a normal disc is firmly attached to the vertebrae(see Figure150a). However, when there are degenerative changes to the disc, the intervertebral space narrows, leading to a flaccid longitudinal ligament, so that the disc material enters the space between the periosteum and the posterior longitudinal ligament (see Figure 150b). Over time, fibration and calcification of the herniated disc material would occur, which finally leads to the formation of osteophytes (see Figure150c). X-rays can detect osteophytes. Generally, the presence of osteophytes

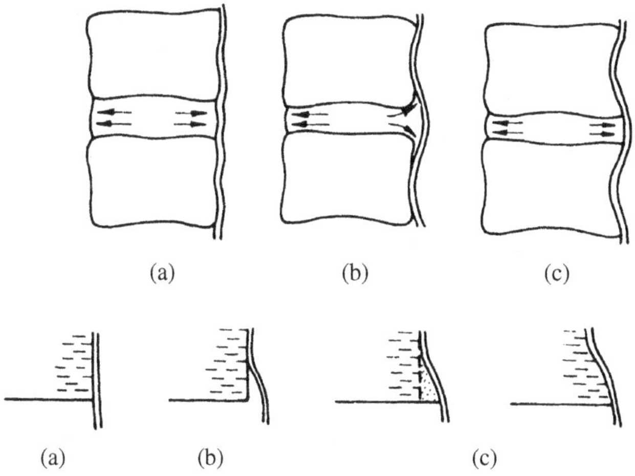

Figure 150 Mechanism of osteophyte formation

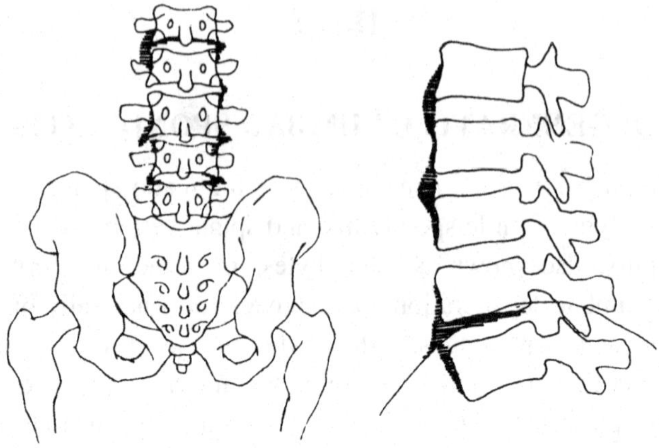

(a) (b)

Figure 151 Bone bridge

means there is degenerative change of the lumbar vertebrae; however, an X-ray examination should not be the only diagnostic evidence of degenerative lumbar spondylosis.

Investigations have shown that patients with osteophytes do not necessarily have low back pain, and vice versa. If there is lower back pain, one needs to seek professional help and identify the cause immediately, so that early symptomatic treatment can be given. Another academic view is that bone spurs can enhance the stability of the spine. In particular, when bone bridges are formed between the vertebrae, the contact area increases, with the activities of the waist severely restricted. On the other hand, the waist is often not painful anymore. The formation of bone bridges (see Figure 151) is more commonly found in the elderly. Statistics show that the incidence of degenerative changes on the lumbar vertebrae increases with age; low back pain peaks at the age of 45 years, then declines in the following years.

Clinical Manifestations

1. Patients are often middle-aged people with chronic low back pain, generally not accompanied with systemic symptoms. Early symptoms are not obvious; there is only soreness, fatigue, and distended pain, resulting in slightly restricted waist activities.

2. Factors that aggravate lumbar pain are trauma, exhaustion, cold, bad posture, and body position. More obvious pain occurs in the morning or when standing up after sitting for a long time, but the symptoms can be significantly reduced or even disappear after doing physical activities.
3. Some individuals may experience zonesthesia, while others find that the low back pain often radiates to the hips and thigh.
4. In mild cases, there is no positive sign. Tenderness, sacrospinal muscle spasms, and increased muscle tension can only be detected while palpating the affected area. The lumbar spine flattens with limited waist mobility.
5. X-ray examinations show a visible sharpened vertebral edge, osteophyte formation, relatively narrowed disc space, and disappeared physiological lumbar curvature.

Diagnosis and Differentiation

Diagnosis

The condition can be diagnosed based on medical history, age of the patient, clinical manifestations, and results of lumbar X-rays.

Differential Diagnosis

Ankylosing spondylitis This condition occurs in young adults aged 20 to 30 years with progressive development, often accompanied by systemic symptoms such as fever, weight loss, and a history of morning stiffness. The sacroiliac joint is often the first to be affected. X-rays can detect calcification or ossification of the posterior longitudinal ligament; generally at its late stage, a condition of so-called "bamboo spine" occurs, leading to a round-looking deformity of the entire spine.

Treatment

1. *Treatment principles* strengthening the waist, supplementing the kidney, unblocking the collaterals, relieving pain.
2. *Commonly used maneuvers* rolling, palm-heel pressure kneading, scrubbing, and fomentation.

3. *Commonly used acupoints and areas āshìxué, shènshū* (BL 23), *dàchángshū* (BL 25), *huántiào* (GB 30), *yánglíngquán* (GB 34), *kūnlún* (BL 60), and the lumbar segments of the spine.
4. Operational methods
   a. The patient is prone, with the practitioner standing at one side. First, apply rolling or palm-heel pressure kneading on both sides of the lumbosacrospinal muscles, up and down and back and forth repeatedly for five to eight minutes.
   b. For patients with waist muscle spasms, add intense pressing. Then, apply finger kneading on tenderness spots, shènsh*ū*, dàchángsh*ū*, and b*ā*liào (BL 31 to 34). The two manipulations can be repeated alternately twice or three times.
   c. Next, apply scrubbing on du mai and bilateral bladder meridian along the lumbar section until the heat from the friction is felt. This maneuver can strengthen the waist and relieve pain.
   d. Then, apply finger kneading on yánglíngquán and k*ū*nlún to strengthen the bones and relieve lumbago. For patients with more serious low back pain, end the therapy with fomentation.

Self-Preventional Methods

Same as that for the third lumbar transverse process syndrome on page

Precautions

1. Exercise the lumbar and back muscles.
2. Avoid work requiring long-term weight-carrying and bending using the waist.
3. Sleep on a hard bed. Keep the vulnerable area warm, and use a waist protector if necessary.

Everyday Exercises

1. What is an osteophyte?
2. What is the correct way to treat osteophytes of the lumbar spine?

Day 6

KIDNEY DEFICIENT LUMBAGO

In Chinese medical practice, it is believed that "the waist is the house of the kidney." The kidneys regulate bone health and generate bone marrow. Kidney essence deficiency causes the loss of nourishment of the lumbar spine, leading to soreness, weakness, and continuous pain that is aggravated with laborious work, and is alleviated with good rest. Pressing and kneading make the affected area comfortable, and violent forces make it suffer. As a disease in the category of chronic lumbago, the pain is the result of several causes. The first one is innate deficiency in conjunction with over-exhaustion or weakness owing to long-term illness. Other reasons include feebleness due to aging and intemperate sex, leading to depletion of kidney essence and the kidneys' inability to nourish the lumbar spine. As a result, lumbago (which is pain or discomfort in the lower back) occurs.

In modern Western medicine, this type of lumbago is mostly related to declining adrenal cortex hormone levels, particularly sex hormones, and insufficiency of protein. The patient could also be suffering from osteoporosis, a metabolic bone disease. Osteoporosis occurs due to a reduction in the number of osteoblasts, which are cells that are responsible for bone formation, resulting in the bone matrix becoming deficient. Osteoporosis of the spine may often present biconcave deformity (see Figure 152) that could easily lead to compression fractures even with a minor injury, although the histologic analysis and chemical composition of the bones are normal.

Clinical Manifestations

1. Vague and lingering low back pain, soreness, distension, and fatigue; soreness and weakness of the knees and feet.
2. In patients suffering from yang deficiency: pallor, cold hands and feet, shortness of breath, fatigue, lower abdomen spasms, pale tongue, deep and thready pulse.

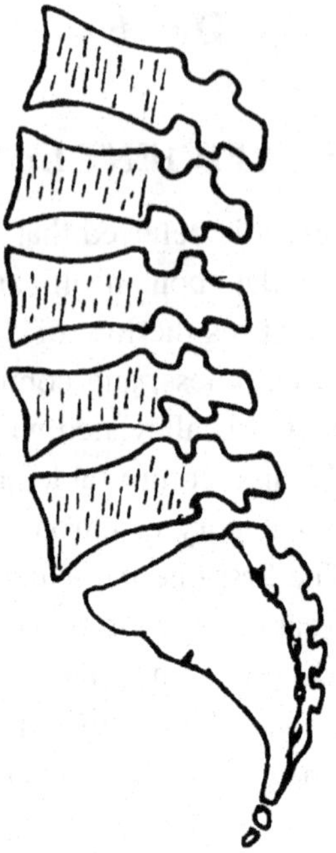

Figure 152 Biconcave deformity of the spine

3. In patients suffering from yin deficiency: facial flushing, vexing heat in palms and soles, dry mouth and throat, red tongue with very little coating, thin and rapid pulse.
4. No obvious and fixed points of tenderness in the waist, no significant motor dysfunction. If the patient has suffered the condition for a long time, there may a tendency of kyphosis and decreased height.
5. X-rays show signs of osteoporosis without other bone lesions. In severe cases, there may be changes similar to compression fractures and biconcave deformity.

Diagnosis

1. Persistent dull pain without clear and fixed tenderness in the elderly; lumbar motor function is normal.
2. Lumbago due to kidney essence deficiency should be considered in elderly feeble individuals whose chief complaint is one of soreness and

weakness of the waist and lower limbs. However, physical examinations and laboratory tests of serum calcium, phosphorus, and alkaline phosphatase all show normal results. In addition, the disease pattern needs to be differentiated based on the data collected through the four TCM diagnostic methods.

3. Waist X-ray examination shows a general decline in bone density, reduction of trabecular bone, biconcave or wedging malformation of lumbar vertebrae, and other signs of osteoporosis.

Treatment

1. *Treatment principles* supplementing the kidney, strengthening the waist, and relieving the lumbar pain.
2. *Commonly used maneuvers* finger or thenar kneading, scrubbing, and spinal pinching.
3. *Commonly used acupoints and areas* *géshū* (BL 17), *píshū* (BL 20), *wèishū* (BL 21), *shènshū* (BL 23), *qìhǎishū* (BL 24), *yāoyángguān* (DU 3), *zúsānlǐ* (ST 36), and the lower back.
4. *Operational methods*
   a. The patient is prone with the practitioner to his or her left. First, apply bilateral-finger kneading on back *shu* points with the index finger on the left point, and the middle finger on the same point on the right. The maneuver should follow a top-to-bottom order, back and forth for about ten minutes.
   b. Next, focus on the *píshū*, *wèishū*, *shènshū*, and *yāoyángguān* with the finger kneading or thenar kneading method, about a minute or two for each acupoint. Then apply the same maneuver on *wěizhōng* and *zúsānlǐ*, each for a minute. *Shènshū*, *yāoyángguan,* and *wěizhōng* enhance yang, supplement the kidney, and resolve lumbago while *píshū*, *wèishū,* and *zúsānlǐ* strengthen the stomach and replenish the foundation of postnatal constitution. The combination has the function of supplementing the spleen and benefiting the kidney, making it the key treatment method for this disease.
   c. Apply spinal pinching on the back along *du mai* and both sides of the bladder meridian, starting from the sacrococcygealarea, and working your way up to the cervicothoracic section. Then, apply intense manipulations to stimulate *píshū*, *wèishū,* and *shènshū.*

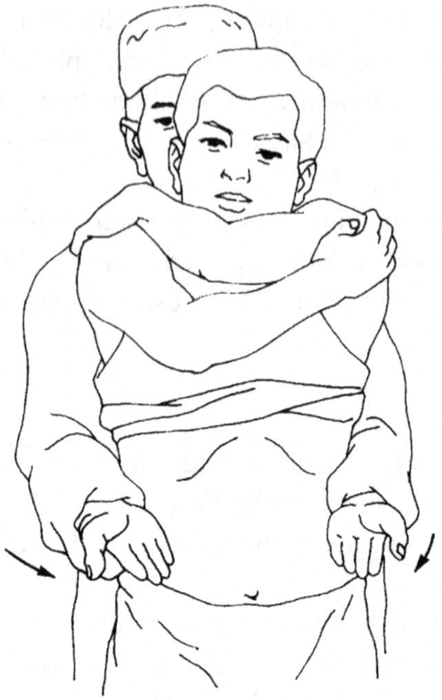

Figure 153 Scrubbing *Dai Mai*

d. With the patient sitting, apply scrubbing to the back of the patient on *du mai*, the bladder meridian, and *daimai* to warm the kidney and strengthen the waist (see Figure 153).

The entire operation should be gentle. Avoid brute force.

Lumbago can also be treated using an integrative approach. Therefore, Chinese and Western medicine may be used together if that is within the scope of the tuina practitioner.

1. *Treatment with Chinese medicine*

   a. For those with more of yang deficiency: *YòuGuīWán* (Right-Restoring Pill, 右归丸) may be chosen to warm the kidney yang.
   b. For those with more of yin deficiency: *ZuǒGuīWán* (Left-Restoring Pill, 左归丸) may be chosen to nourish the insufficient kidney yin.

c. For those with no apparent yin or yang pattern: *Qīng É Wán* (Rejuvenated Lady's Pill, 青娥丸) may be used to tonify the kidney and resolve lumbago.

The appropriate dosage of the above should be twice daily, 6 grams each time.

2. *Western medical treatment* The patient may seek western medical treatment from a physician when it is necessary.
3. *Supplements* The treatment may be supplemented with calcium and vitamins under professional guidance.

Precautions

1. Participate in appropriate exercise and physical work to stimulate osteoblast activities for the benefit of bone formation, so that it prevents further aggravation of muscular atrophy and osteoporosis from disuse of the waist tissue.
2. Make sure the food you eat is rich in protein, calcium, and vitamins, especially vitamins C and D, in order to recover the loss of protein and calcium in the bone due to osteoporosis.
3. Tuina maneuvers need to be gentle. Never apply excessive force and unnecessary passive movements of the waist and legs to prevent fractures.
4. Avoid being exhausted from work and physical activities.
5. Avoid cold and damp places.

Everyday Exercises

1. How would you differentiate lumbago of kidney yin deficiency from that of kidney yang deficiency?
2. How would you use tuina therapy to treat kidney deficient lumbago? What are the precautions in dealing with the condition?

WEEK 9

Day 1

LUMBAR DISC HERNIATION

Lumbar disc herniation is due to the degeneration, damage, and fibrous anular disruption of the intervertebral disc. The condition allows the nucleus pulposus to bulge out posterior-laterally from the rupture of the annulus, compressing the spinal nerve or caudaequina, resulting in lower back pain and sciatica (see Figure 154). The condition occurs in young adults aged 20 to 45 years old, more in men than women. Clinically, it is mostly common on discs between L4 and L5 or L5 and S1.

Inter vertebral disc degeneration is a major factor leading to this condition. Another internal pathogenic factor, from the anatomical aspect, is the narrowed posterior longitudinal ligament and weakened postero-lateral edge of the fibrous ring. Patients often have a history of trauma, or are engaged in long-term manual labor, where weight-bearing activities put a strain on the inter vertebral disc. All of these chronic injuries can cause increased intradiscal pressure, resulting in a bulging out of the disc and consequent clinical symptoms, sometimes triggered by the exposure of the waist to exterior pathogenic cold. These pathogenic external factors only take effect when the disc itself has suffered degeneration.

Clinical Manifestations

1. The main symptoms of lumbar disc herniation are lower back pain and sciatica with paroxysmal aggravation under increased abdominal pressure caused by coughing, sneezing, and bowel movement.
2. Generally, the pain is relatively mild in the early morning, worsens owing to constant weight-bearing and inter vertebral pressure on the disc in the early afternoon, and eases with bed rest.

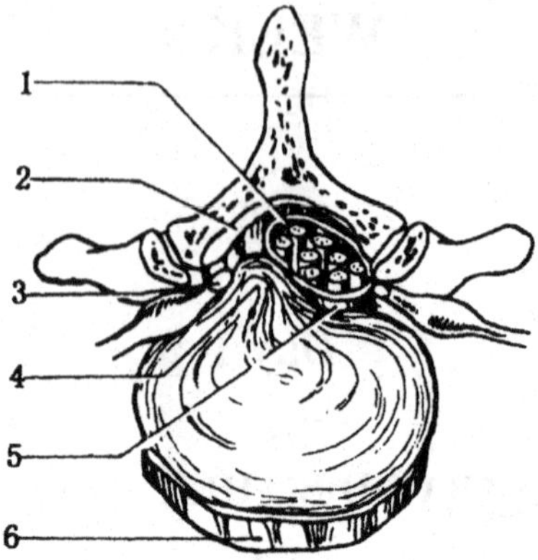

1. 马尾	-	Cauda Equina
2. 黄韧带肥厚	-	Hypertrophy of the Yellow ligament
3. 脊神经根	-	Spinal Nerve Root
4. 突出的髓核	-	Herniated Nucleus Pulposus
5. 后纵韧带	-	Posterior Longitudinal Ligament
6. 前纵韧带	-	Anterior Longitudinal Ligament

Figure 154 Lumbar disc herniation

3. The patient suffers from limited waist mobility, walking difficulties, and muscle atrophy of the lower ipsilateral limb.
4. The patient experiences saddle area numbness and tingling, and urination and defecation disorders if the protrusion compresses the caudaequina.
5. The patient has a limping gait, a disappeared physiological lumbar curvature, change of the lateral curve, waist movement disorders, sacrospinal muscle spasms, and paraspinal tenderness with pain radiating to the ipsilateral limb.
6. Straight leg raise test shows the affected limb to be significantly lower than the contralateral one.
7. The patient has diminished or disappeared reflexes of the knee and ankle, decreased extensor or flexor power, and cutaneous hypesthesia of the lower limb.
8. For patients with urine and fecal incontinence, and saddle area numbness and tingling, the sensation of perineal skin and the anal

reflex must be examined. If there is skin hypesthesia on the saddle area with disappeared levatorani reflex, it may be an indication of caudaequina tumor or central lumbar disc herniation. These conditions are not suitable for tui na therapy but need to be corrected with surgery.

9. Waist X-rays can exclude other organic lumbar lesions, and provide an evidence for the diagnosis of lumbar disc herniation.
10. Common positive signs of lumbar disc herniation under waist X-rays: flattened and laterally protruded lumbar vertebrae, narrowed or asymmetric inter vertebral spaces, vertebral hyperostosis of the upper and lower edge, prolapsed small bone fragment floating freely inside the spinal canal posterior to the inter vertebral disc, and instability of the lumbar spine.

Diagnosis and Differentiation

Key Diagnostic Criteria

1. A history of trauma or chronic injury of the waist.
2. The low back pain is often accompanied by sciatica with paroxysmal aggravation.
3. Relatively moderate waist and leg pain in the morning that increases in the afternoon, and decreases with rest. Pain on the ipsilateral limb worsens with increased abdominal pressure.
4. Flattened lumbar spine, lateral protrusion, limited lumbar movement, and sacro-spinal muscle spasms.
5. Paraspinal process tenderness, percussion, and radiating pain of the affected limb.
6. Straight leg raise $< 60°$, and positive enhanced straight leg raise test.
7. Weakened or disappeared lower limb tendon reflexes, skin hypesthesia and muscle weakness; and muscle atrophy of the ipsilateral limb in patients suffering from the condition for a long time.
8. Lumbo spinal X-rays: visible narrowing of the lumbar inter vertebral space and bone hyperplasia.
9. CT and MRI examination scan confirm the size, shape, and location of the bulged disc and its relation to the nerve tissue.

Differential Diagnosis

1. *Tumors* A tumor is suspected if the patient has persistent lumbago and body pain in the night that is not eased after symptomatic treatment, and if the patient has shown significant weight loss. Lumbar X-rays, CT and MRI scans, and myelography are helpful in confirming the diagnosis.
2. *Lumbar pyogenic infection* Severe low back pain, movement disorders, abscess formation, and paraplegia may occur. Increased WBC counts and ERS rates, positive blood germi culture.
3. *Lumbar spine tuberculosis* Continuous or intermittent lumbar pain, movement dysfunction of the lumbar vertebrae, forced protective flattened posture of the waist. Accompanying symptoms may also include fever, anemia, weight loss, afternoon hot flashes, and night sweats. X-rays reveal visible vertebral destruction, disc space narrowing, and abscess of the major psoas.

Treatment

Conditions Where Tui Na is Applicable

1. Initial onset, younger patients with relatively short disease course.
2. Signs and symptoms are relatively moderate despite the long duration of the disease.
3. No strict indications for surgery.

Contraindicated Conditions For Tui Na

1. Large centralized disc herniation.
2. Patients suffering from severe hypertension, heart disease, diabetes, and other systemic diseases or serious skin diseases.

1. *Treatment principles* changing the relationship between the protruded nucleus pulposus and the oppressed nerve tissue.
2. *Commonly used maneuvers* rolling, pressure kneading, point pressing, grasping, oblique pulling, foulage, scrubbing, fomentation, and passive movement of the waist and legs.

3. *Commonly used acupoints and areas* *āshìxué*, *shènshū* (BL 23), *jūliào* (GB 29), *huántiào* (GB 30), *chéngfú* (BL 36), *yīnmén* (BL 37), *wěizhōng* (BL 40), *yánglíngquán* (GB 34), *kūnlún* (BL 60), *jiěxī* (ST 41), and the affected waist and leg areas.
4. *Operational methods*
   a. The patient is prone with the practitioner standing on the affected side. Start from the waist and use the rolling maneuver along the bladder meridians, passing the gluteal area, posterior of the thigh and calf, getting down to the Achilles tendon, back and forth two to three times, with the focus on the waist for about five minutes.
   b. Apply pressing or point pressing on *āshìxué*, *shènshū*, *dàchángshū* and *huántiào*; then, apply palm-heel pressure kneading and rolling alternately on the ipsilateral lumbar muscles for two to three minutes. The first two steps are designed to loosen up spasms of the waist muscles.
   c. Put cushions under the chest and hips, to allow some space between the abdomen and the treatment table. Ask the patient to relax, overlap the hands on the herniated disc of the lumbosacral area, and apply downwards intense pressing by following the rhythm of the patient's breathing (see Figure 155). Repeat the maneuver five to ten times, depending on the patient's tolerance level.
   d. Remove the cushions and ask the patient to lieprone. Apply light pressure kneading with the palm-heel on the waist, followed by point pressing or intense pressing on *chéngfú*, *yīnmén*, *wěizhōng*, and *chéngshān* (BL 57) for a minute or two.

   Now, have the patient lie with the ipsilateral side up, with the practitioner facing the patient. Place one hand on the posterior

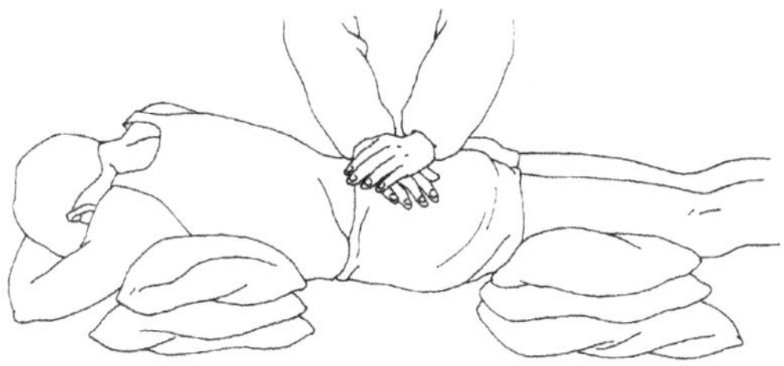

Figure 155 Waist intense pressing with cushions underneath

shoulder, and the elbow of the other arm on the hip area. Now, apply opposite forces to make the lumbar vertebrae slightly rotate; this maneuver is called oblique pulling (see Figure 144 on page). The result of this maneuver is to move the affected nerve root and alter the location of protruded material. Therefore, whether the maneuver is used correctly and properly is one of the key factors in treating lumbar disc herniation with tui na therapy

Now continue with the rest of the steps:

e. The patient is supine with the practitioner standing on the affected side. Apply the rolling or palm-heel maneuver on the posterior and lateral thigh, antero lateral leg, and dorsum of the foot respectively top-down and back and forth for three to five minutes.

f. Apply finger kneading on *fēngshì* (GB 31), *yánglíngquán*, *kūnlún,* and *jiěxī*, followed by passive straight leg lifting (see Figure 156) for one to three times depending on the tolerance of the patient. Next, apply grasping to the gluteal muscles, *wěizhōng,* and *chéngshān*, followed with foulage and shaking of the lower limbs to end the treatment.

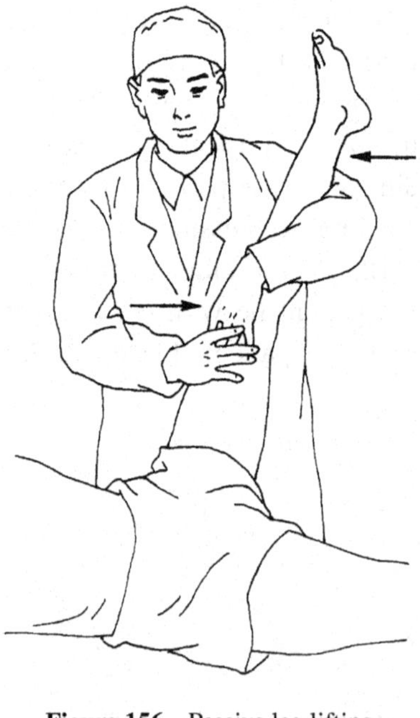

Figure 156 Passive leg lifting

g. For those with severe lumbago, add waist scrubbing and fomentation. However, it is not necessary to do it at every session.
h. Upon completion of the whole tui na session, ask the patient to lie supine and rest for ten to 20 minutes with a cushion underneath the waist. The appropriate height of the cushion is ten to 15 cm. The purpose of this procedure is to help regenerate the physiological curvature. For those who cannot lie supine, do not use a cushion the first time, but save it for the future depending on the progress of the treatment.

Self-Preventional Methods

Same as that for the third lumbar transverse process syndrome on page.

Precautions

1. Avoid physical labor, and bending and weight-bearing activities using the waist.
2. Sleep on a hard bed. Use a low back protector to support the waist. Avoid exposure to cold.
3. Move slowly when you get up. First slowly sit up, then leave the bed.
4. Be persistent with back muscle exercises.
5. Surgical treatment may be considered if conservative treatment does not work in six months.

Everyday Exercises

1. What is lumbar disc herniation? What are the two major symptoms?
2. Remember the scope of indications and contraindications of using tui na to treat lumbar disc herniation.
3. How would you apply tui na in treating lumbar disc herniation?
4. What are the precautions you need to take note of for this condition?

Day 2

ANKYLOSING SPONDYLITIS

Ankylosing spondylitis is mainly a progressive chronic inflammatory disease attacking the spine, eventually affecting the entire spine and leading to rigidity of the spine with round back deformity. The traditional name of the disease in Chinese medicine is "turtle back insanity."Older biomedical names of the disease include rheumatoid spondylitis, spinal rheumatoid arthritis, and central type rheumatoid arthritis. Most patients are male, and the most common age of onset is 20 to 30 years old.

The exact cause of the disease is not yet clear; it may relate to the following factors:

1. *Infections* It is associated with chronic urogenital or pelvic infections that spread to the spine and sacroiliac joints through the lymphatic pathways and the spinal venous system. It can also spread to the body and cause systemic disease, such as fever, and weight loss through blood circulation.
2. *Genetic factors* The incidence of this disease in patients with relatives also affected is a few dozen times higher than in patients with no family history of the disease; many cases are monozygotic twins with onset at the same time. The incidence in different ethnic groups also varies: the proportion of North American Indians having the disease is between 27/1000 and 63/1000, compared to only 2/1000 in Africans. The incidence ratio in white and black residents in the United States is 9.4 to 1.

Clinical Manifestations

1. Early stages: lower back pain and stiffness, especially morning stiffness; may be accompanied by a typical sciatica; limited squatting ability and hip movement; most patients initially would have the sacroiliac joint involved, and later the symptoms progress upwards until the whole spine is rigid. The disease may also have

other systemic symptoms such as weight loss, fatigue, night sweats, and unexplained fever.

2. Late stages: rigidity of most of, or the entire, spine with a fixed round back deformity; restricted lateral rotation of the head and neck; limited movement of thoracic expansion with constricted chest pain, obstructed breath, chest depression, and significantly reduced vital capacity. The round back deformity causes decreased volume of the chest and abdomen cavities, and dysfunction of the heart, lung and digestive system. Patients may experience palpitations, shortness of breath, fatigue, and sweating when engaging in even minimal physical activity. The hips are often involved, showing hip ankylosis with difficulties of walking, squatting, and climbing or going down the stairs.
3. Stiffness, pain, tenderness, percussion pain, and limited mobility on the sacroiliac joints or diseased spinal segment; flattened thorax, the thoracic expansion ability being below 2.5 cm; mild flexion deformity of both hips with positive results in FABER, pelvic separation and pelvic crush tests. Walking difficulties with typical signs described in the *Inner Classic*: "the protrusion of the buttock is more than that of heel of the foot, and the height of the spine surpasses the head."
4. Increased ESR and HLA-B27 positive.
5. X-ray examinations show narrowing of the sacroiliac joint spaces, visible superfluous ligaments, and bamboo-like change in the lumbar spine.

Diagnosis and Differentiation

Key Diagnostic Criteria

1. Persistent pain in the back and waist, stiffness not relieved with rest of three months.
2. Limited range of thoracic expansion: equivalent to that of the fourth inter costal space; the difference between the contraction and expansion of the thorax is less than 2.5 cm at maximal voluntary ventilation.
3. The spine movement is significantly restricted.
4. X-ray examination shows a typical sign of change of bilateral or unilateral sacroiliac joint.

Differential Diagnosis

1. *Osteitis condensansilii* This condition is more common in women who have borne two or more children; it only affects the ilia with circumscribed, even increased bone density, smooth edge, and clear boundary from normal bones and does not affect the joint.
2. *Sacroiliac joint tuberculosis* There is often unilateral joint damage, accompanied by systemic symptoms of tuberculosis sera.
3. *Degenerative spondylitis* This condition is more common in patients over the age of 40; X-rays reveal vertebral hyperplasia and no superfluous ligament; normal ESR.

Treatment

Tui na is effective for early ankylosing spondylitis, and can alleviate pain, help to restore motor function to the spine and hips, reduce stiffness, and prevent or delay abnormal development of the round back deformity. However, once the formation of bony ankylosis is complete, tui na would not be much of a help.

1. *Treatment principles* unblocking meridians and collaterals, smoothening and benefiting vertebrae.
2. *Commonly used maneuvers* rolling, palm-heel pressure kneading, acupressure, grasping, finger kneading, scrubbing, plucking, and passive movements of the spine and hips.
3. *Commonly used acupoints and areas* *píshū* (BL 20), *wèishū* (BL 21), *shènshū* (BL 23), *mìngmén* (DU 4), *bāliào* (BL 31 to 34), *huántiào* (GB 30), *zúsānlǐ* (ST 36), *yánglíngquán* (GB 34), *xuánzhōng* (GB 39), *dànzhōng* (RN 17), the back, the lumbosacral area, and the hips.
4. *Operational methods*
   a. The patient is prone, with the practitioner standing to his or her side. First, use brisk palm-heel kneading on the back, top-down to the sacroiliac area and both hips for one or two minutes to make the area adapt to the treatment and prevent it from being tense. Next, apply rolling on both the sacrospinal muscles, then the thoracic, lumbar, sacral, and both sides of the iliac area. The two maneuvers

can be used alternately. The power of the manipulation must penetrate to a deeper level of sacrospinal muscles in order for them to loosen up. While working on the hips, combine passive internal rotation, external rotation (see Figure 157), and extension of the hips. The above procedure should last for about ten minutes.

b. Apply finger kneading and acupressure on points of *du mai* and back *shu* points for three to five minutes. Some main points may include *fèishū* (BL 13), *géshū, píshū, wèishū, sānjiāoshū* (BL 22), *shènshū, dàzhuī* (DU 14), *shēnzhù* (DU 12), *zhìyáng* (DU 9), *jīnsuō* (DU 8), *mìngmén, yāoyángguān* (DU 3), *bāliào,* and *huántiào.*

c. Keeping the same position, perform top-down plucking for three to five minutes along the sacrospinal muscles with the focus on the affected site. The maneuver can improve the circulation of the sacrospinal muscles, relieve stiffness, and restore muscular tensility.

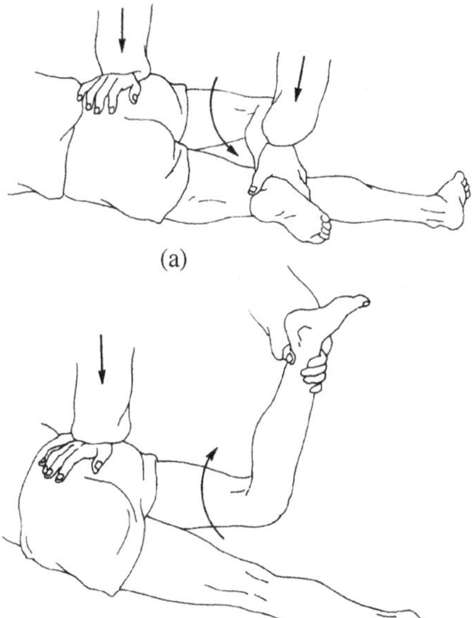

(a) 内旋	-	Internal Rotation
(b) 外旋	-	External Rotation

Figure 157 Passive hip rotation

d. The patient is prone, with the practitioner standing to the left of the patient. Apply unilateral chest stretching and spinal pressing (see Figure 158). Use your left hand to support the patient's front part of the right shoulder for posterior extension, and use your right palm to apply intense pressing on the thoracic spinous processes of the patient. When both hands work coordinately at the same time, the thoracic spine receives passive expansion with unilateral chest stretching. Then the right palm can move down one section after another and perform the same operation with the coordination of the left hand along the thoracic spine until the passive stretching is done for the entire right side of the chest. Conversely, stand at the patient's right side, and apply the same maneuver to the entire left side of the chest. The method effectively improves the rib-vertebral joint movement.
e. The patient remains in prone position with the practitioner standing at the patient's right side. Apply passive posterior extension of the lumbar, lumbosacral, sacroiliac, and hip joints (see Figure 159) by using your right hand to perform downward pressing on lumbar, lumbosacral, sacroiliac, and hip joints successively while your left hand holds one or both legs of the patient to perform passive posterior extension. Both hands should exert forces concurrently to complete the action and restore the motor function of the waist and hips.
f. Next, apply scrubbing along the *du mai* and both sides of the bladder meridian, in the order of thoracic, lumbar, and sacroiliac segments

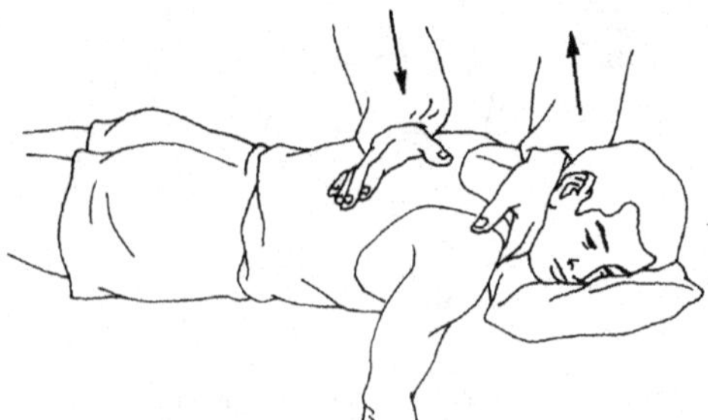

Figure 158 Unilateral chest stretching and spinal pressing

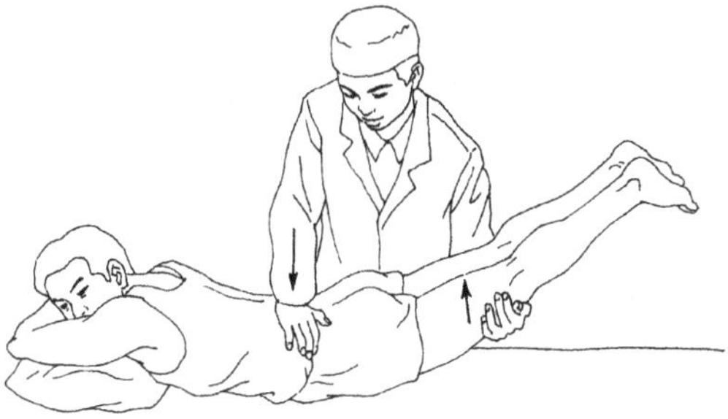

Figure 159 Passive posterior extension of the lumbar, lumbosacral, sacroiliac, and hip joints

until the patient feels the frictional heat. The penetration of heat relieves the pain. Fomentation can be used in addition to the manual operation, with the focus on the sacroiliac and lumbosacral areas.

g. The patient is supine with the practitioner standing at the affected side. Apply rolling on the anterior thigh, vastus medialis, and vastus-lateralis, coordinating with passive hip abduction, internal rotation, external rotation, flexion, and flexion rotation. Then, perform grasping on the vastus adductor and posterior vastus muscles, *wěizhōng* (BL 40), and *chéngshān* (BL 57); and finger-kneading *zúsānlǐ*, *yánglíngquán*, and *xuánzhōng* for about five minutes. Apply the same manipulation on the other hip.
h. The purpose of the next maneuver is to expand the chest and stretch the spine (see Figure 160). The patient should sit with hands clasped to hold the occipital area of the head, with the practitioner standing behind the patient. Use one knee to support the thoracic spinous process of the patient, and both hands to hold the patient's elbows. First, push the patient's elbow forward with both hands, so that the patient's body bends toward the front, and ask the patient to breathe out (see Figure 160a). Then, with the knee supporting the thoracic spinous process, pull the patient's elbows backwards to make them hyper extended as far as possible. At the same time, ask the patient to breathe in to increase the expansion level of the chest (see Figure 160b). Perform the operation twice or three times. The method can improve thoracic expansion and lung capacity.

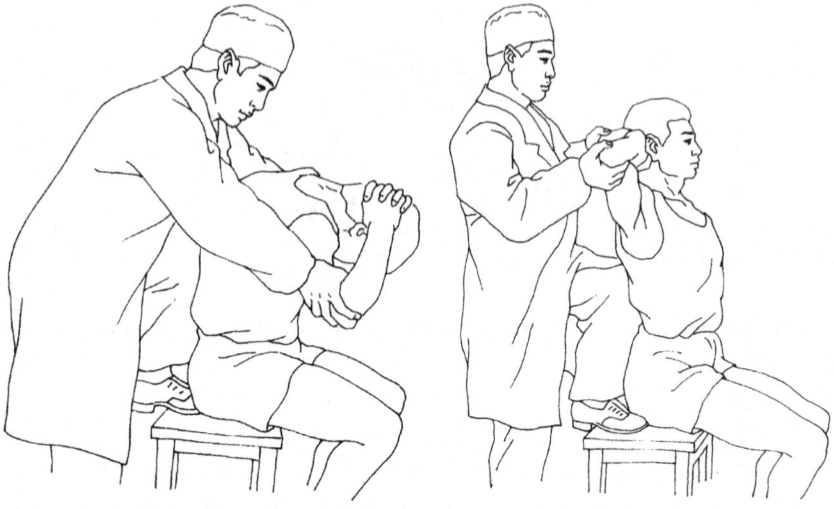

(a) (b)

Figure 160 Chest expansion and spinal stretching

i. Lastly, end the treatment with finger kneading on *dànzhōng*, pressure kneading on the sternum, and grasping *jiānjǐng* (GB 21).

Self-Preventional Methods

1. Apply finger kneading on *dànzhōng* and all intercostal spaces.
2. Perform deep breathing exercise in conjunction with thoracic expansion exercise.
3. Apply kneading on the lower abdomen with the entire palm for three minutes. Then, apply finger kneading on *zúsānlǐ* for a minute.
4. Use the palm to scrub the lumbar and sacroiliac area until it feels warm.

Precautions

1. Try to follow the normal routine in your daily life.
2. Be perseverant in doing exercises of thoracic expansion, deep breathing, and squatting.

3. Be persistent in sleeping supine on a hard-board bed and use a low pillow.
4. Stay on a diet of balanced nutrition.
5. Stay warm.

Everyday Exercises

1. What is ankylosing spondylitis?
2. How would one complete the manipulation of unilateral chest stretching and spinal pressing?
3. What are the passive hip movements?

Day 3

JUVENILE KYPHOSIS

This condition is seen in young people aged 12 to 18, and characterized by a round back deformity, affecting more boys than girls. In 1921, Dr. Scheuermann first reported that the disease was the lesion of the vertebral epiphy seal cartilage, and described its X-ray signs. As the result, the disease is also known as osteochondrosis of the vertebral epiphy seal plates, or Scheuermann's disease.

The predilection sites of the disease are the lower thoracic and upper lumbar spine, especially T10 through L1where the physiological posterior protrusions are obvious and carry a lot of weight. The cause of the disorder is not yet very clear. Generally, it is due to immature young people participating in intensive manual labor, especially weight-bearing work, or unreasonable overloaded exercises, causing oppression to the disc tissue and irregular epiphy seal plate fractures on the upper or lower corner of the vertebral body, a form of aseptic necrosis. Eventually, it will lead to the "wedging" shape of the vertebrae, causing kyphosis. (See Figure 161.)

Clinical Manifestations

1. The main manifestation is mid-level back pain with fatigue that worsens after doing manual labor or weight-bearing activities, that is alleviated after rest, and that is not related to climate change. Over time, there will be a round back deformity. When the deformity is fully developed, mid-level back pain is spontaneously relieved.
2. There is tenderness and percussion pain on the diseased spinous process; thora columbo spinal deformity results due to arc-shaped posterior protrusion.
3. X-rays provide the main evidence for diagnosing the disease, especially with its lateral view. The X-ray signs are as follows:
   a. Vertebra lepiphyses are poorly developed, sub-divided, irregular, and of higher density.

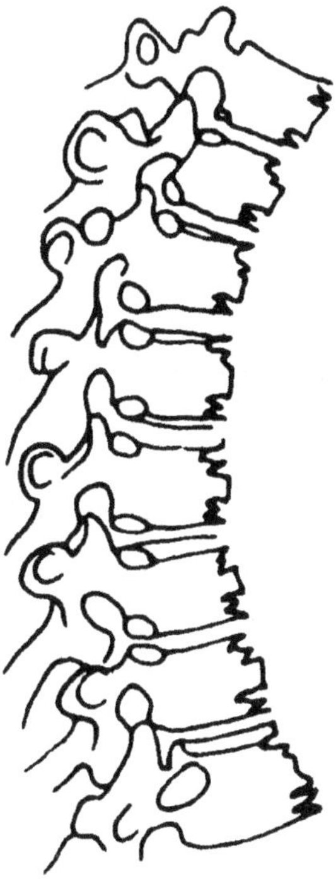

Figure 161 X-ray signs of osteochondrosis of vertebral epiphyseal plates

b. Increased kyphosis results in cylindrical arc-shaped thoracic and lumbar vertebrae.
c. There may be multiple vertebrae with wedge-shaped changes.
d. Inter vertebral disc spaces are narrowed.

Diagnosis and Differentiation

Key Diagnostic Criteria

1. 12 to 18-year-old adolescents with a history of heavy physical labor involving oppression to the shoulders.
2. Mid to low back pain with fatigue that is relieved after rest.
3. Round back kyphosis of the spine.
4. X-rays reveal signs of juvenile kyphosis.

Differential Diagnosis

1. *Spinal tuberculosis* This is more common in young people, while extra pulmonary tuberculosis is more common in children. It is often accompanied by systemic symptoms including low-grade fever, night sweats, fatigue, weight loss, and anemia. In addition, there are movement disorders of the spine and forced posture, with multiple vertebral bodies affected. X-rays would show para vertebral or psoas abscess, and the destruction and necrosis of bones are often obvious.
2. *Pyogenic vertebral osteomyelitis* This is more common in adults, and occurs especially in the lumbar spine. It has an acute onset, often accompanied with high fever, chills, sharp back pain, limited spinal activities, and local percussion pain. There is an increased level of leukocytes and ESR with positive blood culture. X-rays can detect destruction of the bone and narrowed discs of the affected vertebrae.

Treatment

1. *Treatment principles* fortifying the spleen and kidney, strengthening bones and muscles, and relieving back pain.
2. *Commonly used maneuvers* rolling, palm-heel pressure kneading, double-finger kneading, spinal pressing, spinal pinching, scrubbing, and passive movement method.
3. *Commonly used acupoints and areas píshū* (BL 20), *wèishū* (BL 21), *sānjiāoshū* (BL 22), *shènshū* (BL 23), *yāoyángguān* (DU 3), *wěizhōng* (BL 40), *yánglíngquán* (GB 34), *xuánzhōng* (GB 39), the back *shu* points of the waist and the sacrospinal muscles.
4. *Operational methods*:
   a. The patient is prone, with the practitioner standing at the left. Apply rolling and palm-heel pressure kneading along both sides of the sacro-spinal muscles alternately in top-down order, with the focus on the thoracic and lumbar regions. Repeat for about five to eight minutes.
   b. Keeping the above position, apply the rolling maneuver on sacrospinal muscles and switch to spinal pressing while reaching the thoracolumbar spines with obvious posterior. Apply spinal pressing

with overlapped palms on top of the affected area, slowly pressing down. Tailor the amount of force used to the patient's tolerance level. Generally, it can be done three to ten times.

c. Apply unilateral chest stretching and spinal pressing on the upper thoracic segment of the spine, and passive posterior lumbar extension to the lower thoracic spine. For detailed operations, refer to the treatment section of ankylosing spondylitis on page.
d. Apply double-finger kneading on the back *shu* points with the focus on *píshū*, *wèishū*, *sānjiāoshū,* and *shènshū*, one minute per acupoint, preferably to obtain a soreness *de*-qi sensation. Then, apply finger kneading on *yāoyángguān*, *wěizhōng*, *yánglíngquán,* and *xuánzhōng* for a total of two minutes.
e. Apply the spinal pinching method and start from the sacrococcygeal region, past the lumbosacral, lumbar, and thoracic segments, and all the way up to the cervicothoracic area. Focus more on the thoracic and lumbar regions. The manipulation can be enhanced with the use of "triple-pinching plus one lifting" or intense pressing on back *shu* points.
f. Apply scrubbing on the thoracolumbar portion of *du mai* and the bladder meridian until frictional heat is felt. End the operation with foulage on the back.

Self-Preventional Methods

1. Apply fist kneading on the back: make a loose fist and use the dorsum of the metacarpophalangeal joint to pressure knead the thoracolumbar region of the back.
2. Apply finger kneading on *yánglíngquán* and *xuánzhōng*, for one to two minutes on each acu point.

Precautions

1. Adolescents at the physical development stage should avoid heavy manual labor.
2. Immediately cease weight-bearing activities involving the spine when a patient is suspected of the disease.

3. Engage in exercises enhancing the back muscles and chest expansion. Sleep supine on a hard bed.
4. If necessary, wear a steel vest, TLSO brace, or Milwaukee brace.

Everyday Exercises

1. What is juvenile kyphosis?
2. Try to memorize the self-preventional methods and precautions for juvenile kyphosis.

Day 4

SPONDYLOLYSIS AND SPONDYLOLISTHESIS

The anatomic area between the arches of two vertebral articular processes is called pars interarticularis. A defect or fracture of the pars inter articularisis known as spondylolysis, pars fracture, or spondyloschisis. Spondylolysis can be either unilateral or bilateral. In case it is unilateral, it could easily lead to the torsion of the vertebral body. If it is bilateral, the upper vertebral body of the detached area would slip forward, causing spondylolisthesis. L5 and L4 are the most commonly affected vertebrae of this condition.

Spondylolysisis mainly congenital, occurring during the embryonic development process, as the result of an ossification disorder of the spine, leading to a defective pars interarticularis. External factors such as trauma and strain can then exacerbate the development of the disease.

From a biomechanical perspective, the fifth lumbar vertebra takes a lot of strain. If the area encounters trauma, it would cause the pars interarticularis to be fractured. When the individual bends forward, the inclination above the sacra increases, and the center of gravity moves forward, leading to greater force on the pars interarticularis. Moreover, when the lumbar vertebrae are hyperextended, the L4 articular process would directly compress the pars of L5. As a result, damage of the pars interarticularis occurs owing to the clamping force of the adjacent superior and inferior articulations (see Figure 162).

Clinical Manifestations

1. The disorder is more common in adults between the ages of 30 to 45, affecting more men than women.
2. Continuous or intermittent low back pain is the most common symptom; sometimes it only occurs while pressed, while bearing excessive weights, or during physical activities. Most of the pain is limited to the lower waist; some may radiate to the gluteal and sacrococcygeal regions or even the lower extremities. Some patients have unilateral or bilateral sciatica, while a few have severe lower limb muscle weakness,

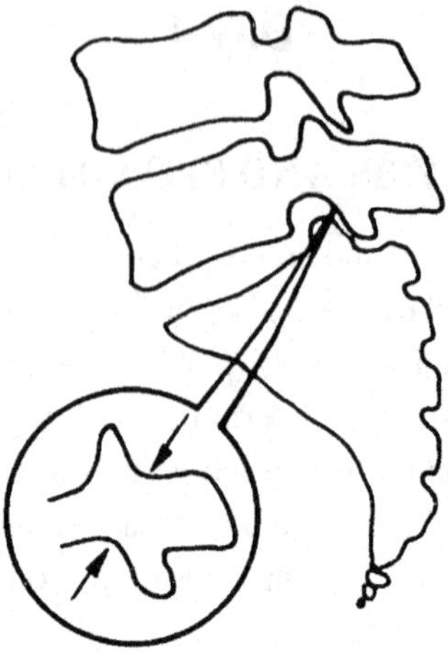

Figure 162 Weight-bearing on pars interarticularis of L5

muscle disuse atrophy, hypoalgesia, and even symptoms related to neurothlipsis of the caudaequina.

3. Patients with simple spondylolysis or mild spondylolisthesis generally do not show positive signs for the disorders. A significant increase of physiological lumbar curvature can only be visible when the slippage is apparent. A ladder-shaped object can be felt upon palpation over the diseased spinous process, accompanied by local muscle spasms and limited range of motion.
4. X-ray examinations can diagnose spondylolysis and spondylolisthesis. Commonly used lumbar radiography positions are anterior, lateral, and paired left-and-right oblique.
   a. *Anterior radiograph* There is difficulty in showing the condition with a lower than expected positive rate.
   b. *Lateral radiograph* Visible fractures can be seen at the pars with the width related to the degree of spondylolisthesis. The greater the slippage, the clearer the crack. If we draw grids on the graph dividing the sacral surface into four equal parts, one grid of forward shift of the upper vertebral edge represents Grade I slippage, while two grids are equal to Grade II slippage. This is the so-called method of four-degree spondylolisthesis classification (see Figure 163).

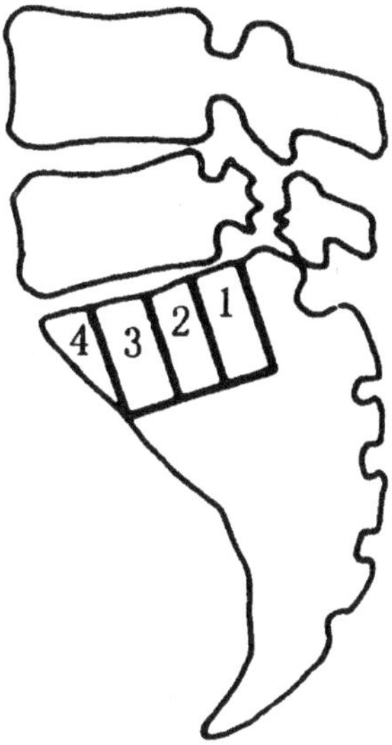

Figure 163 Four-degree spondylolisthesis classification

c. *Oblique radiograph* This is the best position to show the entire view of the fracture in diagnosing spondylolysis. Where spondylolysis exists, a strip-shaped crack can be seen at the pars interarticularis. The projection of a normal vertebral arch adnexa is shaped like a dog. The "dog head" is the ipsilateral transverse process while the "ear" is the superior articular process. The longitudinal section of the pedicle of the vertebral arch is shaped like a dog's eye and the pars interarticularis looks like its neck. If there is a fracture of the pars interarticularis, i.e., spondylolysis, it looks as if a dog is wearing a necklace. (See Figure 164.)

Diagnosis

An X-ray examination can confirm the diagnosis.

Treatment

Tui na is only used in simple spondylolysis and Grade I or II spondylolisthesis without obvious sign of neurothlipsis. Avoid rough manipulations,

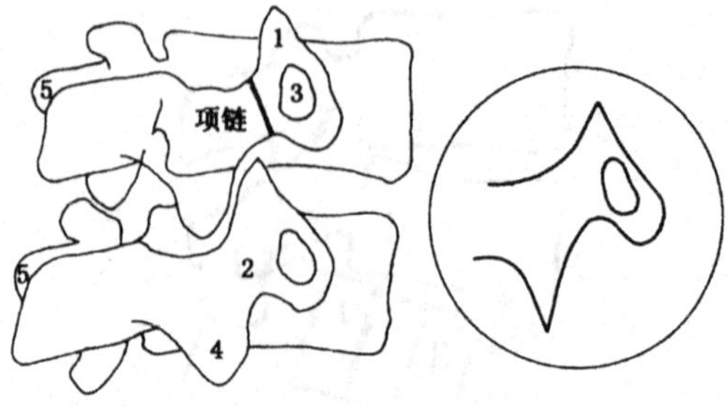

Figure 164 Oblique view of lumbar vertebrae

1. Superior Articular Process 2. Pars Interarticularis
3. Pedicle of the Vertebral Arch 4. Inferior Articular Process

intense pressing maneuvers on the waist, and posterior extension maneuvers. Tui na is not recommended for severe spondylolisthesis with obvious symptoms of neurothlipsis or that of the caudaequina. Patients with this condition should seek surgical treatment.

1. *Treatment principles* harmonizing *ying* qi, unblocking the vessels, easing the spasms, and relieving pain.
2. *Commonly used maneuvers* rolling, palm-heel pressure kneading, finger kneading, scrubbing, grasping, and passive flexion of lumbosacral, knee, and hip joints.
3. *Commonly used acupoints and areas shènshū* (BL 23), *guānyuánshū* (BL 26), *xiǎochángshū* (BL 27), *shàngliào* (BL 31), *cìliào* (BL 32), *wěizhōng*(BL 40), and the lumbosacral region.
4. *Operational methods*:
   a. The patient is prone,with the practitioner standing to his or her side. Apply rolling or palm-heel kneading with moderate force on both sides of sacrospinal muscles at the lumbosacral segment to loosen up the spasms of the muscles. Do this for about eight minutes.
   b. Perform double-finger kneading on *shènshū*, *guānyuánshū*, *xiǎochángshū*, *shàngliào*, and *cìliào*, for one minute per acupoint. For those with disseminating pain affecting the gluteal and thigh, apply the maneuver on these areas. If there is sciatica, refer to the treatment section for lumbar disc herniation on page .

c. Next, apply scrubbing on the lumbosacral region until the heat is felt, then apply kneading on *wěizhōng* 30 to 50 times.
d. Have the patient change to a supine position. Put a pillow under the sacrum of the patient. Stand at the patient's feet. Hold the patient's knees with both hands and perform passive flexion for both hips and knees to their largest extent to make the pelvis tilt to the back and decrease the degree of slippage (see Figure 165). Another method is to apply side to side swaying to relax deep lumbosacral muscles and ligaments, then apply passive flexion of both hips and knees. Alternately use the two methods five to ten times.
e. Finally, apply grasping on *wěizhōng* and shaking the lower limbs to end the treatment.

Self-Preventional Methods

1. Do sit-up exercises: lie supine, then slowly sit up. This is originally an exercise of the abdominal muscles. It is used here because while sitting up, the lumbar spine will shift posteriorly.
2. Another helpful exercise is rolling with knees held (see Figure 166). Lie supine and use both hands to hold both knees. Perform forward and backward rolling along the longitudinal axis of the spine. Ask someone to help and complete the exercise if you cannot do it alone initially.

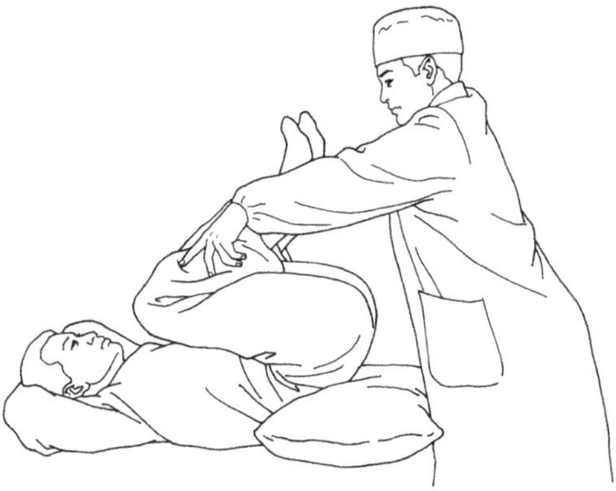

Figure 165 Passive hip and knee flexion with pillow underneath of sacrums

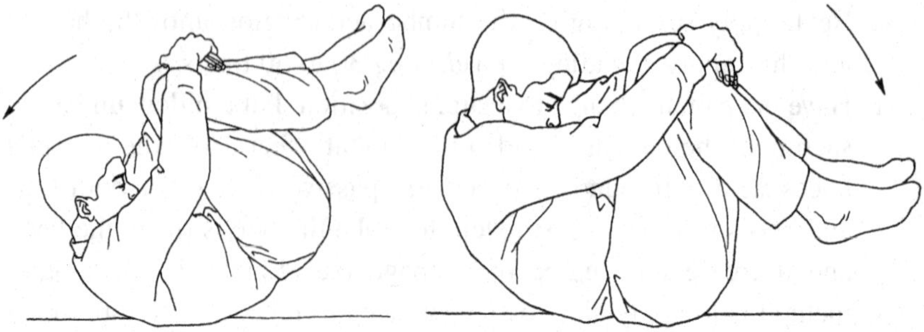

Figure 166 Rolling with knees held

3. Reduce weight-bearing activities involving the waist.
4. Wear a waist protector.
5. Surgical treatment may be considered if symptoms are severe with apparent slippage, neurothlipsis, and unsuccessful conservative therapy.

Everyday Exercises

1. Look at an oblique lumbar X-ray film and point out the pars interarticularis.
2. What is the four-degree classification of spondylolisthesis?
3. What are the self-preventional measures for this disease?

Day 5

LUMBAR SPINAL STENOSIS

Lumbar spinal stenosis, also known as lumbar spinal stenosis syndrome, refers to a series of clinical symptoms caused by the narrowing and deforming of the lumbar spinal canal, the nerve root canal, and intervertebral foramen due to changes of the lumbar vertebral bone and fibrous tube, leading to neurothlipsis of the caudaequina or nerve root. It is one of the common causes of chronic low back pain.

The causes of the disorder fall into two broad categories. The first one is congenital or developmental lumbar spinal stenosis, an abnormality that occurs at the early development stage. The anteroposterior and transverse diameters of the lumbar spinal canal are both smaller than those in a normally developed one. The narrowing throughout the canal is even and consistent. The second cause is postnatal, and include lumbar degenerative changes, spondylolisthesis, and the result of lumbar vertebral fracture, dislocation, or sequelae of spinal surgery. There are also patients with both existing congenital spinal stenosis and slight degenerative changes of the spine, which lead to obvious symptoms.

Clinical Manifestations

1. The disorder has a slow onset with a progressively aggravating tendency, is more common in middle-aged men, and has the main symptoms of distension and soreness of the waist,leg pains, and intermittent claudication.
2. The pain of the lower back and legs has a recurrent tendency, and is mostly bilateral. In some patients, the pain is unilateral, while in others the pain alternates between the two legs. The patient often experiences pain, numbness, and fatigue on the distal limbs that worsen with standing or walking, and are alleviated with squatting, sitting, and rest.
3. Walking for even a few hundred meters or less will give rise to symptoms such as numbness, heaviness, and distension and weakness of the

legs, symptoms that are reduced with rest. However, when the patient continues to walk after the rest, symptoms can recur. Such a walking disorder is known as intermittent claudication, which is a very important diagnostic evidence of the disease.

4. The disease has only a few positive physical signs. The following methods may help in the diagnostic process:
   a. Standing and posterior extension test: the patient stands with the doctor supporting the back. The patient is told to bend backwards in order to increase the elongation of the lumbar spine. The test is positive, if, when holding the position for about ten seconds, there is pain, distension, and numbness on the ipsilateral hip, as well as leg pain. Mostly, the patient does not have paraspinal tenderness and radiating pain affecting the lower limb.
   b. Some patients may experience a diminished or disappeared feeling when a pin is used to scratch the lateral side of the ipsilateral calf; there is muscle weakness or atrophy mainly at the anterior tibialis often with diminished or disappeared reflex of the Achilles tendon.c.
   c. A few patients may suffer from dysuria.
   d. A lumbar X-ray examination is the easiest and most convenient way to find out the left-to-right and anteroposterior diameters of the spinal canal (see Figure 167). If the left-to-right spinal canal diameter is less than 2.5 cm and that of the anteroposterior one less than 1.5 cm, and the clinical manifestations match, then lumbar spinal stenosis should be considered.
   e. Myelography and CT scans can provide a more definite diagnosis of the disease.

Diagnosis and Differentiation

Key Diagnostic Criteria

1. Chronic waist and leg pain in middle-aged patients, with symptoms on the distal lower limbs and intermittent claudication.
2. The disorder is confirmed by lumbar X-rays, myelography, and CT scans.

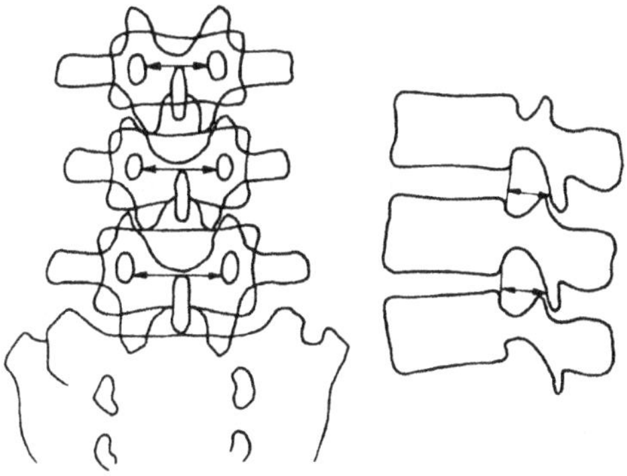

1. 正位片，椎管左右径测量	-	Anteroposterior radiograph: to measure left-to-right diameter
2. 侧位片，椎管前后径测量	-	Lateral radiograph: to measure anteroposterior diameter measurement

Figure 167 Measuring methods of left-to-right and anteroposterior diameter of the spinal canal

Differential Diagnosis

1. *Lumbar disc herniation* This condition usually affects only a single limb and compresses a specific nerve root; when the abdominal pressure increases, the ipsilateral limb can have paroxysmal aggravation; there are no signs of intermittent claudication; there is paraspinal tenderness with pain radiating to the ipsilateral limb; there are limitations in passing the straight leg raise test and there is positive result for the enhanced straight leg raise test.
2. *Caudaequina tumors* The patient suffers significant night pain, saddle area numbness, fecal and urine incontinence, and positioning signs of caudaequina. X-rays and myelography can help to get a more definite diagnosis.

Treatment

1. *Treatment principles* invigorating blood, resolving stasis, unblocking collaterals, and relieving pain.

2. *Commonly used maneuvers* rolling, pressure kneading, grasping, scrubbing, shaking, and passive movements of the lower extremity.
3. *Commonly used acupoints and areas*: *yāoyángguān* (DU 3), *shènshū* (BL 23), *dàchángshū* (BL 25), *huántiào* (GB 30), *fēngshì* (GB 31), *wěizhōng* (BL 40), *yánglíngquán* (GB 34), *kūnlún* (BL 60), and the waist and leg areas.
4. *Operational methods*
   a. The patient is prone, with the clinician standing at the affected side. First, apply rolling and palm-heel pressure kneading on the lumbar area along the bladder meridian to reach the buttock, thigh, popliteal fossa, and all the way down to the posterior of the lower leg, up and down and back and forth several times, with the focus on the lumbosacral region for about ten minutes.
   b. Apply pressure kneading on *yāoyángguān*, *shènshū,* and *dàchángshū,* for a minute per acupoint, followed by palm-heel pressure kneading on the lower waist for three to five minutes. Avoid squeezing and passive backwards extension of the waist.Violent stimulation is also forbidden.
   c. Perform scrubbing on the *du mai* and bladder meridian at the lumbar region until the heat can be felt. Local fomentation can also be used.
   d. Apply rolling or palm-heel pressure kneading on the anterolateral thigh and shank, up and down and back and forth for about five minutes, with the focus on the anterolateral shank. Then, apply intense pressing on *bìguān* (ST 31), *fútù* (ST 32), and *xuèhǎi* (SP 10), for five to ten times for each acupoint. Apply finger-kneading on *yánglíngquán*, *zúsānlǐ* (ST 36), *xuánzhōng* (GB 39), *kūnlún*, and *jiěxī* (ST 41) for one minute per acupoint, and grasping on *wěizhōng* and *chéngshān* (BL 57).
   e. *Femoral artery compression method* Continue with the patient in the supine position. Overlap the thumbs and place them on where the femoral artery pulsates, i.e., the anterior proximal part of the thigh in the center of the groin. Press it lightly and gradually increase the pressure, until the blood supply of the ipsilateral limb temporarily stops. Now, rapidly take off your hands so that the blood supply to the lower limb suddenly increases, forcing the

blood vessels of the ipsilateral limb to dilate and achieve the therapeutic purpose.

f. Lastly, perform passive flexion and extension on the lower limb for five to ten times, and shake them to end the treatment.
g. If both lower extremities have symptoms, bilateral treatment is required.

Self-Preventional Methods

1. Use both palms to rub and scrub bilateral *yāoyǎn* (EX-B 7).
2. Apply finger kneading on bilateral *zúsānlǐ*, *xuánzhōng*, and *yánglíngquán*.

Precautions

1. When the waist and leg pain is severe, take bed rest on a hard bed for a week or two in addition to the treatment.
2. Keep the waist area warm, and use a waist protector.
3. After six months of conservative treatment with no improvement, if the condition still affects normal life and work, surgical treatment may be an option.

Everyday Exercises

1. What is lumbar spinal stenosis?
2. What are the main symptoms of lumbar spinal stenosis?
3. What is intermittent claudication?

Day 6

OSTEITIS CONDENSANSILII

Osteitis condensansilii is the bone sclerosis near the edge of the iliac joint. It occurs most often in 20-to 30-year-old women of child-bearing age. A lot of patients are manual workers with jobs requiring standing for long periods of time. Often, it is unilateral, though there are a few bilateral cases.

The etiology of the disease is not very clear. It may be associated with long-term mechanical strain, pregnancy, parturition, endocrine effects, chronic pelvic inflammation, urinary tract infections, and local trauma that affect the blood supply to one or both sides of the ilium, leading to ischemic bone densification.

Clinical Manifestations

1. Chronic persistent low back pain radiating to the buttock and thigh without obvious symptoms of root pain. In females, it is exacerbated during the menstrual cycle. Exhaustion and injuries are also common factors leading to aggravated pain.
2. Some individuals have been shown to have the disorder via X-ray examination, but yet not show any subjective symptoms.
3. In clinical examination, the waist movement is usually normal with localized tenderness and muscle hypertonia near or on the sacroiliac joint. There is no positive findings in the straight leg raise and FABER test.
4. X-ray examinations show evenly distributed increased density on the iliac auricular surface of the sacroiliac joint with blurred edges and disappearance of the trabecular bone that do not affect the articular surface. The width of the lesion is 0.5 to 3.0 cm, thick, solid and white with dense signs on the radiograph. The sclerotic area can have a variety of shapes: generally triangular, crescent-shaped, and pear-shaped (see Figure 168).

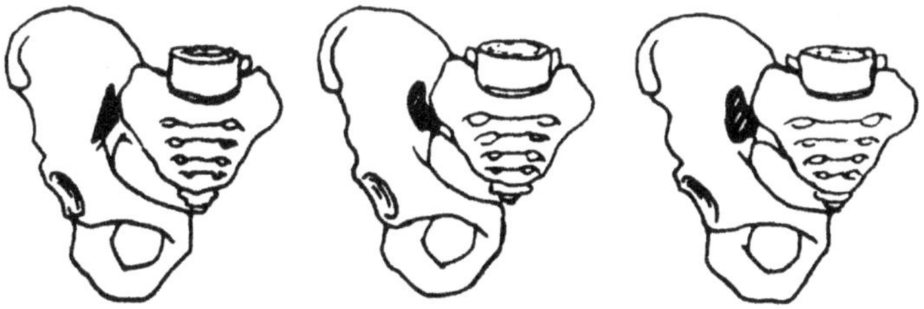

a. 三角形–Triangular b. 新月形–Crescent-shaped c. 梨形–Pear-shaped

Figure 168 Osteitis condensansilii

Diagnosis and Differentiation

Key Diagnostic Criteria

1. The disorder should be considered if a woman, especially of childbearing age, has a history of chronic, persistent, and recurrent low back pain, which is aggravated during the postpartum period.
2. X-ray examination is a reliable diagnostic aid and a CT scan is even more accurate at diagnosing the disorder.

Differential Diagnosis

1. *Tuberculous sacroiliitis* The pain is mostly unilateral. The pain is worse while walking or climbing the stairs, after sitting for a long time, or when changing position while lying supine. There are systemic symptoms such as hot flashes, night sweats, and fatigue. X-rays reveal blurred joint spaces and bone destruction, accompanied by calcification of various sizes.
2. *Ankylosing spondylitis* There is stiffness of the spine, accompanied by low back pain. X-rays show a fuzzy sacroiliac joint with irregular and jagged articular surface. In the late stages, there is trabecular bone across the joint space, forming the bony ankylosis.
3. *Metastatic tumor* The patient has a history of tumors with significant night pain. Dyscrasia exists in those who have been afflicted with the

condition for a long time. X-ray examinations show nodular or flake-shaped dense shadows on the affected area that are irregular, without a clear boundary.

Treatment

1. *Treatment principles* invigorating blood, dissolving stasis, strengthening the waist, and relieving the pain.
2. *Commonly used maneuvers* rolling, pressure kneading, and fomentation.
3. *Commonly used acupoints and areas āshìxué*, *yāoyángguān* (DU 3), *mìngmén* (DU 4), *shènshū* (BL 23), *pángguāngshū* (BL 28), *shàngliào* (BL 31), *cìliào* (BL 32), *zhìbiān* (BL 54), *jūliào* (GB 29), *wěizhōng* (BL 40), and the sacroiliac region.
4. *Operational methods*:
   a. The patient is prone, with the practitioner standing at the affected side. First, apply rolling or palm-heel kneading on the ipsilateral lumbosacrospinal muscles, passing through the sacroiliac region and the hip, and reaching the posterior side of the thigh, up and down and back and forth several times for about ten minutes, with a focus on the ipsilateral sacroiliac region and its surrounding muscles and ligaments.
   b. Apply pressure kneading on *yāoyángguān*, *mìngmén*, *shènshū*, *pángguāngshū*, *shàngliào*, *cìliào*, *zhìbiān*, and *jūliào* for a total of three minutes. Then, apply palm-heel kneading on *āshìxué* at the sacroiliac region for three to five minutes, followed by finger kneading on *wěizhōng*. The operation can strengthen the waist and kidney, and relieve low back pain.
   c. Apply scrubbing on the sacroiliac joint of the ipsilateral lower waist until the patient feels the frictional heat. End the session with fomentation on the ipsilateral sacroiliac joint.

Self-Preventional Methods

1. *Fist kneading on the sacroiliac region* Make a loose fist, and apply force using the dorsal side of the metacarpophalangeal joint to perform kneading on *āshìxué* at the sacroiliac for a minute or two.

2. *Finger kneading on kūnlún* Use the pulps of the middle fingers to apply kneading on bilateral *kūnlún* for one minute.

Precautions

1. Avoid weight-bearing activities involving the sacroiliac joint as much as possible to reduce the compression.
2. Keep the affected area warm. Physical therapies such as shortwave diathermy can be used to supplement tui na treatment.
3. Rest and sleep on a hard bed.

Everyday Exercises

1. What is osteitis condensansilii?
2. How does osteitis condensansilii look like under X-rays?

WEEK 10

Day 1

DEVELOPMENTAL LUMBOSACRAL ABNORMALITIES

Common dysplasia of the lumbosacral bones includes sacralization, lumbarization, asymmetry of the posterior joints, sacral spina bifida occulta, and dissociated spinous. Although these kinds of bone dysplasia are not necessarily the causes of low back pain, they are potential etiological causes. Even though tui na cannot eliminate development abnormalities, it can strengthen the muscular tensility and stability of the lumbosacral segment, increase blood and lymph circulation, and improve the metabolism of local tissues, thereby indirectly easing the pain of the lumbosacral region.

Sacralization and Lumbarization

Sacralization and lumbarization (see figure 169), also known as transitional vertebrae, are the most common types of dysplasia of the vertebrae among the mutual congenital spinal transitions. The occurrence rate is about 10%. These malformations can exist alone, or co-exist with other conditions such as spina bifida and neural arch hypoplasia.

Sacralization and lumbarization can cause lumbosacral pain due to the following reasons:

1. Bursitis occurs as the result of friction between the elongated transverse process and the sacral ala.
2. A false joint may be formed by the elongated transverse process and the ilium, which is prone to traumatic arthritis.

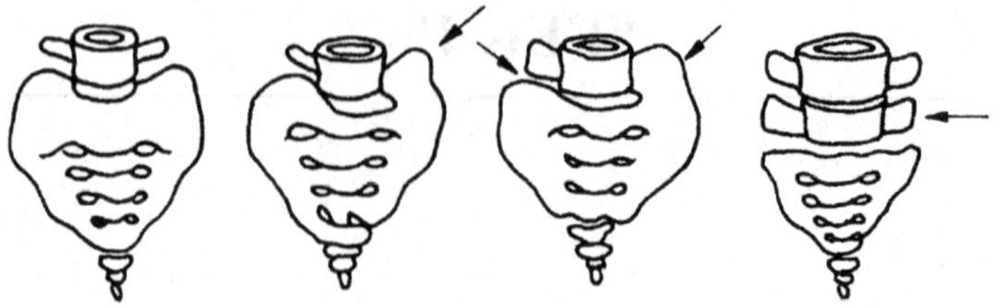

(a) (b) (c) (d)

(a) 正常 - Normal
(b) 第五腰椎单侧骶化 - Unilateral Sacralization of the Fifth Lumbar Vertebra
(c) 第五腰椎一侧骶化，一侧横突形成假关节 - Sacralization of the 5th Lumbar on One Side: the Transverse Process of One side Forms a False Articulation
(d) 第一骶椎腰化 - Lumbarization of the 1st Sacral Vertebra

Figure 169 Transitional vertebrae

3. The spaces among the elongated transverse process, ilium, and sacrum are decreased, resulting in irritation and pain to local soft tissues, including the ligament and fascia.

The low back pain of transitional vertebrae is similar to that of osteoarthritis. Since the ipsilateral side is locked, the pain is more intense in unilateral lumbar sacralization than in bilateral ones owing to increased activities and tendency of traumatic arthritis on the contralateral side. The pain is generally obvious after laborious work or exercise, and eases after rest. In addition, sacralization can lead to the loss of dynamic equilibrium and increase the burden on L4 and L5 discs, resulting in degenerative changes of the discs, disc tissues, and facet joints.

Lumbarization, on the other hand, reduces the tensility of the sacrospinal and intervertebral ligaments and weakens the stability of the spine, causing chronic lumbosacral pain.

Spina Bifida Occulta

Spina bifida, also known as vertebral arch split or vertebral lamina split, is a spinal defect and deformity caused by insufficient chondrification or ossification during the embryonic period, leading to incomplete fusion of the two sides of the posterior spinal arch. The disorder is often accompanied by dysplasia of the spinal cord. According to whether tissues inside the spinal cord protrude out or not, it is divided into two categories: spina bifida occulta and spina bifida cystica. The latter requires neurosurgical correction, therefore, we will only deal with spina bifida occulta in this book.

Spina bifida occulta affects mostly L5 through S2, with the rear side of the backbone being completely split, or just a narrow gap, which may be even or uneven. Clinically, there may be lamina deformation with short, detached, or missing spinous processes. Since spinous processes and laminas are important attachment sites of muscles and ligaments, the disease decreases the adhesion capacity for certain muscles and ligaments, weakening the stability of the lumbosacral spine and resulting in chronic lower back pain.

Clinically, there is a three-degree grading system for lumbosacral spina bifida occulta based on X-ray findings: (a) normal, (b) grade I, (c) grade II, and (d) grade III (see Figure 170).

In someone suffering from spina bifida occulta, there are fibrous tissue covering the spinal cord. In those without missing meninges or myelomeningocele, generally there is no low back pain. However, due to decreased or lack of adhesion of the local muscles and ligaments, the stability of the lumbosacral spine is weakened, resulting in chronic strain, leading to low back pain. If there are detached spinous processes, patients often

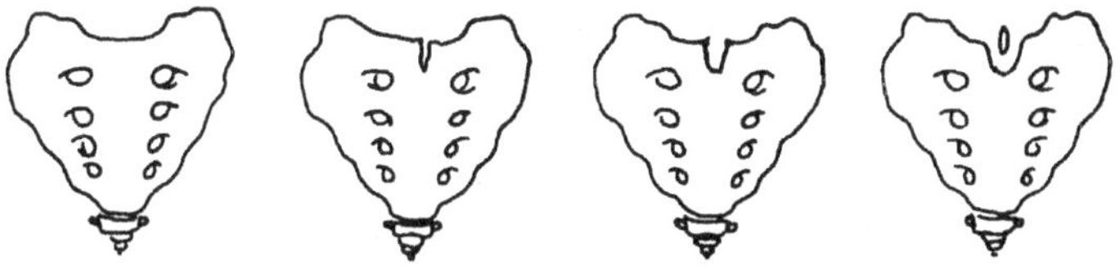

(a) (b) (c) (d)

Figure 170 Sacral Spina Bifida Occulta

(a) Normal
(b) Grade I: hypoplasia of the spinous processes; there is a very narrow slit between the laminas of both sides.
(c) Grade II: there are missing spinous processes and the laminas of both sides are clearly separated.
(d) Grade III: the spinous processes and the majority of lamina are missing; the distance between the two sides of the lamina is more than half of the spinal canal width; often accompanied by detached spinous processes.

experience a transient dura pain when the dural sac is stimulated by the spinous process while bending their waists. The skin of the diseased area often has sparse and short hair, thick clustered long hair, pigmentation, or tenderness.

Treatment

The above two disorders are examples of congenital lumbosacral dysplasia. The majority of patients do not have symptoms and there is no need to be treated. Patients with chronic low back pain can choose tui na therapy to enhance muscle tensility, promote the stability of the lumbosacral region, and relieve low back pain.

1. *Commonly used maneuvers* rolling, palm-heel kneading, finger kneading, and scrubbing.
2. *Commonly used acupoints and areas yāo yáng guān* (DU 3), *shèn shū* (BL 23), *guān yuán shū* (BL 26), *xiǎo cháng shū* (BL 27), *páng guāng shū* (BL 28), *ā shì xué*, *chéng shān* (BL 57), *yáng líng quán* (GB 34), *xuán zhōng* (GB 39), *du mai,* and sacrospinal muscles.
3. *Operational methods*
   a. The patient is prone, with the practitioner standing on one side of the patient. First, apply rolling and palm-heel kneading along the bilateral sacrospinal muscles of the lumbosacral regions. The amount of stimulation should not be overwhelming, and it can combine and alternate with finger-kneading on acupoints of the bladder meridians for ten to 15 minutes. Apply finger-kneading on *yāo yáng guān* and *ā shì xué*. Next, use scrubbing on *du mai* and the bladder meridians top-down until the patient feels the heat. Without any passive movement, the whole set of the procedures serves as the main manipulation in treating the problem, can invigorate blood, strengthen the waist and enhance the tensility of the sacrospinal muscles.
   b. The patient remains supine with the healer standing to his or her side. Perform finger kneading on bilateral *wěi zhōng* (BL 40), *yáng líng quán,* and *xuán zhōng* for three to five minutes. This procedure relieves lumbago and strengthens the tendons and bones.

Self-Preventional Methods

1. Do more exercises involving the back extensors to enhance the stability of the lumbosacral region. For specific details, refer to the related content of The Third Lumbar Transverse Process Syndrome in Week Eight.
2. Keep the lumbosacral area warm and prevent waist injury.

Everyday Exercises

1. What are transitional vertebrae?
2. What is spina bifida occulta?

Day 2

SUPERIOR CLUNEAL NERVE INJURY

The superior cluneal nerve is a cutaneous branch composed of the posterolateral branches from L1 to L3 spinal nerves. It comes out from the edge of the sacrospinal muscle, passes through the iliac crest and distributes at the skin of the gluteal area (see Figure 171).

The branches of the nerve distribute on the fascia surface of the low back, travel toward the inferolateral side and form the superior cluneal neurovascular bundle. Then, they pass over the iliac crest and enter into the superior gluteal part of lobulated adipose tissue. When they reache the edge of the belly of the gluteus maximus muscle, they appear as a lobular structure along with the layered adipose tissue. At the same time, the

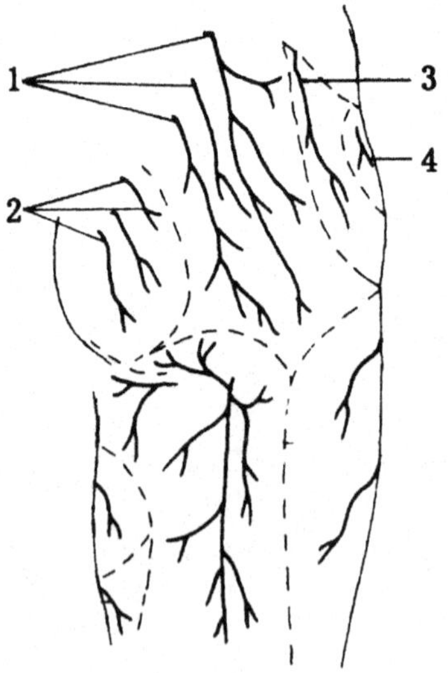

(a)	□臀上皮神经	-	Superior cluneal nerve
(b)	□臀中皮神经	-	Medial cluneal nerve
(c)	□闭孔神经	-	Obturator nerve
(d)	□股神经前皮支	-	Anterior cutaneous branch of fomeral nerve

Figure 171 Distribution area of cutaneous nerves on hips and thighs

superior cluneal nerve entering this area divides into many fine branches to innervate the corresponding portions of the gluteal fascia and skin.

If soft tissues are compressed or injured from traction on the anatomical location of the superior cluneal nerve, there will be neurothlipsis or referred pain (see Figure 172). Sometimes the fiber directions of the back and the gluteal fascia are not consistent, so the neurovascular bundle may be damaged when the body moves around. Other factors causing injury to the nerve are developmental defects associated with the valgus of the iliac crest.

The basic pathology of the disease is the increased internal pressure of the superior cluneal neurovascular bundle, causing neurothlipsis that leads to venous obstruction and pain of the gluteal area. In turn, it contributes to the increased tension of the soft tissue of that area, forming a vicious circle.

Clinical Manifestations

1. Tearing pain in the ipsilateral buttock which is unbearable in the acute phase, even affecting the waist movement.
2. Limping gait and diffusing pain in the posterolateral side of the ipsilateral thigh.
3. Touching pain and referred cutaneous pain on the upper portion of the ipsilateral hip where the superior cluneal nerve distributes.
4. Tenderness and tight cord-like knots formed by subcutaneous soft tissues at the inward side, three to five centimeters inferior to the highest point of the iliac crest. This is because the cutaneous nerve gets thicker owing to the disease.

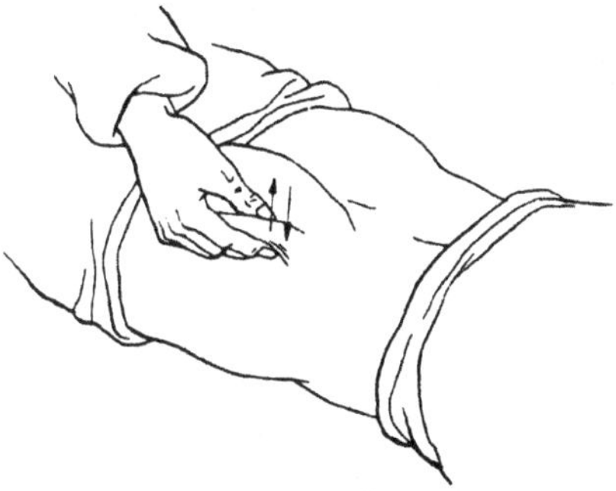

Figure 172 Touching and referred cutaneous pain of the superior cluneal nerve

Diagnosis and Differentiation

Diagnosis

The diagnosis of the condition mainly depends on the clinical manifestations such as local pain, touching pain, tenderness, referred cutaneous pain and palpable cord-like subcutaneous knots.

Differential Diagnosis

The condition often needs to be differentiated from a number of other conditions.

1. *Superior gluteal neuralgia* The superior gluteal nerve is composed of the anterior rami of L5 to S1. It travels between, and supplies, the gluteus medius and gluteus minimus. Clinically, the pain and tenderness associated with this condition is relatively deeper, and there is no referred cutaneous pain.
2. *Piriformis syndrome* In addition to gluteal pain, there is obvious lower extremity pain. In a physical examination, the straight leg raise test reveals restricted movement. Especially in piriformis tension test, there is the significant positive sign.

Treatment

1. *Treatment principles* soothing tendons, resolving knots, invigorating blood, and unblocking collaterals.
2. *Commonly used maneuvers* pressure kneading, plucking, finger kneading, scrubbing, and fomentation.
3. *Commonly used acupoints and areas ā shì xué, huán tiào* (GB 30), *wěi zhōng* (BL 40).
4. *Operational methods*
    a. The patient is prone, with the practitioner standing at the affected side. Apply palm-heel pressure kneading on the gluteal area for five to eight minutes. The stimulation does not require much physical force since the main purpose is to improve local blood and lymph circulation, reduce internal pressure of the neurovascular bundle, and eliminate the compression.

b. Apply plucking vertically on the neurovascular bundle inferior to the iliac crest to resolve knots and unblock collaterals. Combine the operation with finger-kneading on *ā shì xué, huán tiào,* and *wěi zhōng* for about five minutes.
c. You may perform the two procedures alternately three to five times.
d. Lastly, apply scrubbing along the path of the neurovascular bundle until the patient feels the heat. Local fomentation can also be used in conjunction with the manual operation.

Self-Preventional Methods

1. Use the entire palm to perform pressure kneading over the superior cluneal nerve for three to five minutes.
2. Apply self-plucking over the affected neurovascular area for five to ten times.

Precautions

1. Keep the affected area warm to improve the blood supply.
2. Avoid muscle strain of the waist and hip to reduce increased tension of the soft tissue.

CATATONIA FASCIA LATA

The fascia lata, the body's thickest fascia, is located in the upper antero-lateral thigh. Since its lateral part contains tendon fibers of the tensor fascia lata at about the upper and middle 1/3 of the vastus lateralis, it is particularly thick and shaped like a wide and flat ribbon. This part is the so-called iliotibial tract (see Figure 173), which goes down and ends at the lateral tibial condyle.

Catatonia fascia lata, also known as snapping hip, occurs because when the fascia lata is tense, activities such as hip flexion, adduction, or internal rotation follow. As a result, repeated friction will cause thickening of the posterior margin of the iliotibial tract or the anterior edge of the gluteus maximus tendon. In addition, trochanteric bursitis can occur with repeated stimulation of thickened tissues. The tension of the fascia lata can also cause forward rotation of the pelvis, increased physiological protrusion of the lumbar vertebrae, and a widened lumbosacral angle. (See Figures 174 and 175.)

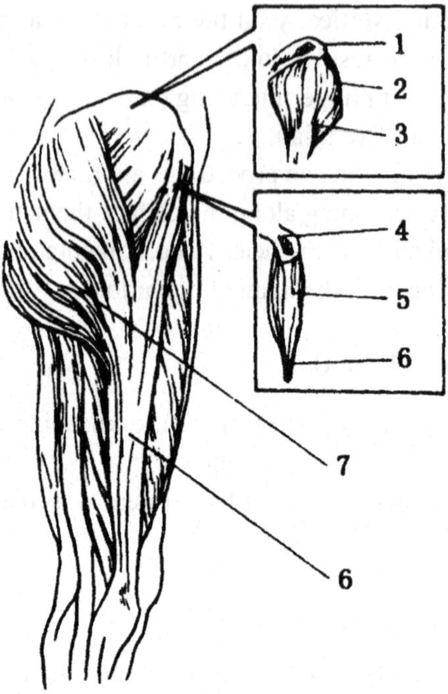

Figure 173 Tensor fascia lata muscle and the Iliotibial tract

1. Iliac Crest 2. Gluteus Medius Fascia 3. Gluteal Muscle 4. Anterior Superior Iliac Spine 5. Tensor Fascia Lata 6. Iliotibial Tract 7. Gluteus Maximus

Clinical Manifestations

1. *Snapping and discomfort of the exterior articulation* Whenever the hip is flexing, adducting, or rotating internally, thickened tissue of the posterior edge of the iliotibial tract or anterior edge of the gluteus maximus tendon will slide over the greater trochanter processes, causing a snap. At the same time, a thick and tight fiber can be palpated or even seen on the body surface of a slim patient, sliding back and forth on the greater trochanter.

   Generally, patients do not feel the pain but there is subjective discomfort of the hip. If there is secondary bursitis, localized pain may present.
2. *Chronic lower back pain* Due to increased lumbosacral angle, the weight-bearing center of the waist moves from the anterior of the

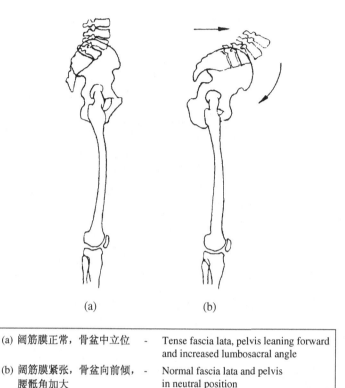

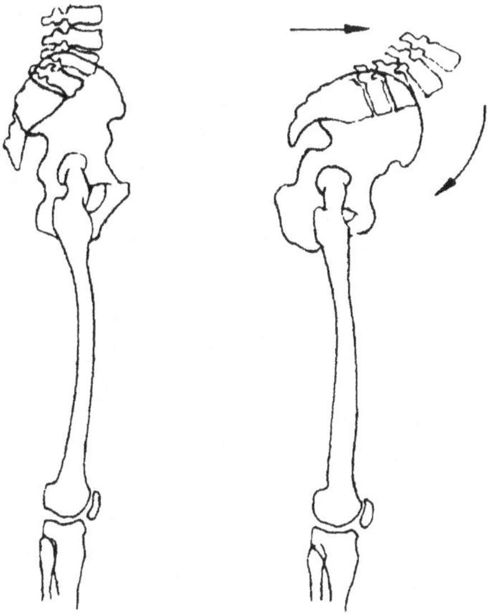

(a) (b)

(a) 阔筋膜正常，骨盆中立位	-	Tense fascia lata, pelvis leaning forward and increased lumbosacral angle
(b) 阔筋膜紧张，骨盆向前倾，腰骶角加大	-	Normal fascia lata and pelvis in neutral position

Figure 174 Relationship of the fascia lata and the pelvis

vertebrae backwards to the articular process, making the posterior lumbosacral joint prone to chronic injury.

3. *Positive iliotibial band contracture test result* For details, refer to this test under the topic Examination of the Lower Extremities in Week Two.

Diagnosis and Differentiation

1. Snapping and discomfort on the ipsilateral hip with a palpable tense fibrous band.
2. Positive for iliotibial band contracture test.
3. Hip X-ray excludes bone and joint lesions.
4. Clinically, an extra-articular snap should be differentiated from an intra-articular one. Intra-articular snap is mainly a result of the friction

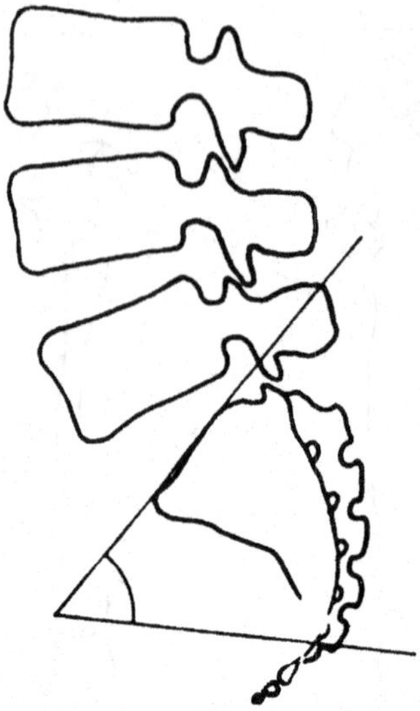

Figure 175 Increased lumbosacral angle

of the femoral head and superior part of the acetabulum. Hip X-rays can identify the location of the lesion.

Treatment

1. *Treatment principles* soothing the tendons, resolving spasms, smoothening and benefiting the joints.
2. *Commonly used maneuvers* palm-heel kneading, plucking, grasping, scrubbing, and fomentation.
3. *Commonly used acupoints and areas jū liào* (GB 29), *huán tiào* (GB 30), *fēng shì* (GB 31), *yáng líng quán* (GB 34), *wěi zhōng* (BL 40), lumbosacral area, hips, and vastus lateralis.
4. *Operational methods*

   a. The patient is prone, with the practitioner standing at the affected side. Apply palm-heel kneading on both sides of the lumbosacral spinal muscles with more focus on the ipsilateral side, and gradually transition to the ipsilateral buttock. Work on the area up and down and back and forth for three to five minutes, then apply pressure kneading on *wěi zhōng* for a minute.

b. Ask the patient to lie on his contralateral side. Apply palm-heel kneading on the ipsilateral side, starting from the fascia lata and the iliotibial band and going down to the knee, up-and-down and back-and-forth for five to eight minutes. At the same time, combine the operation with passive hip flexion and extension. Then, perform plucking along the iliotibial tract top-down and back and forth (see Figure 176). Next, apply intense pressing to *jū liào*, *huán tiào*, *fēng shì*, and *yáng líng quán*.
c. Have the patient supine. Apply palm-heel kneading along the anterior superior iliac spine, tensor fascia lata, anterior proximal of the thigh, vastus lateralis, and all the way down to the knee joint, top-down and back and forth for five to eight minutes. The operation should be combined with passive hip external rotation (see Figure 177). Then, apply plucking to the tensor fascia lata of the anterior superior iliac spine and the tense fascia at the greater trochanter.
d. Finally, apply scrubbing on the affected area until the patient feels the heat. In addition, fomentation may be applied on the greater trochanter.

Precautions

1. For patients with low back pain, exercise the abdominal muscles more to reduce the lumbosacral angle.
2. While the patient is supine, use a pillow underneath the popliteal fossa, making the knees lightly bent, iliotibial tract relaxed, and

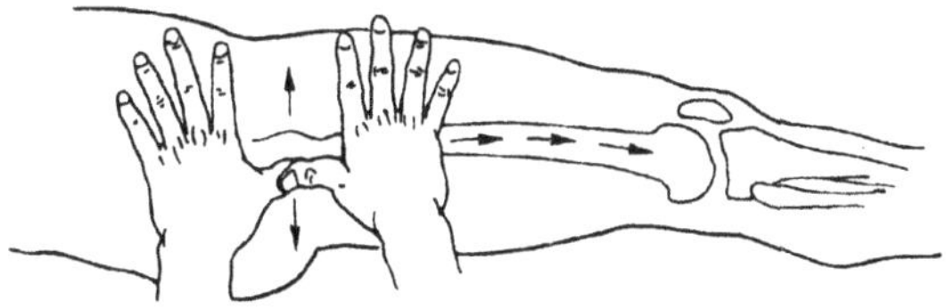

Figure 176 Plucking on the iliotibial tract

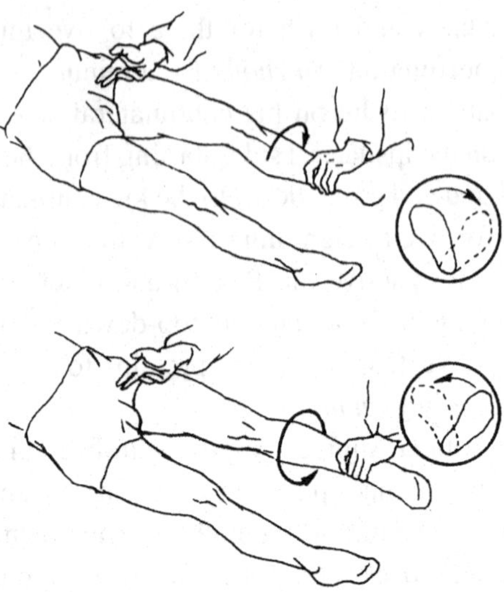

Figure 177 Rolling, and internal and external hip rotation

lumbosacral angle reduced, so that the psoas muscle can be at a complete resting status.

Everyday Exercises

1. Are the superior cluneal nerve and the the superior gluteal nerve the same thing? What are the main criteria to distinguish them?
2. What are the basic pathological changes of superior cluneal neuralgia?
3. What is the fascia lata?
4. What are the two categories of snapping hip? Which category does catatonia fascia lata belong to, and what are the clinical manifestations?

Day 3

PIRIFORMIS SYNDROME

The piriformis muscle originates from the lateral side of the anterior sacral foramina of S2, S3, and S4 in front of the sacrum at the interior side of the pelvis. It goes downwards and outwards, passes through the greater sciatic foramen, and reaches the hip. As the supinator of the hip, its tendon ends at the greater trochanter.

The superior gluteal nerve and superior gluteal blood vessels pass above the piriformis, while the inferior gluteal nerve and inferior gluteal blood vessels pass below it. The sciatic nerve is slightly lateral to it. Therefore, any variations, spasms, inflammation, or edema of the piriformis can result in neurothlipsis of the sciatic nerve.

The anatomic variations of the piriformis (see Figure 178) is an important factor causing the condition. Because of the variations, the muscle is vulnerable to stimuli such as trauma and inflammation, causing piriformis contracture and constriction of the sciatic nerve. As a result, there will be circulatory disturbance of the nutrient vessels supporting the sciatic nerve, producing pathological changes including arterial insufficiency and venous obstruction. Furthermore, after the piriformis is stimulated by factors such as inflammation, there will be local adhesion of the sciatic nerve, leading to decreased space and increased tension of the nerve.

Clinical Manifestations

The pain is mainly located on the ipsilateral buttock and sciatica. It is intensified after exposure to cold and increased activities such as walking, or when abdominal pressure increases due to coughing and bowel movement. In addition, there will be pain on the posterolateral lower leg radiating to the foot. Bed rest will alleviate the symptoms.

Diagnosis and Differentiation

Key Diagnostic Criteria

1. Sciatica symptoms of the unilateral hip and lower limb.
2. Limited movement with straight leg raising test, positive piriformis tension test.

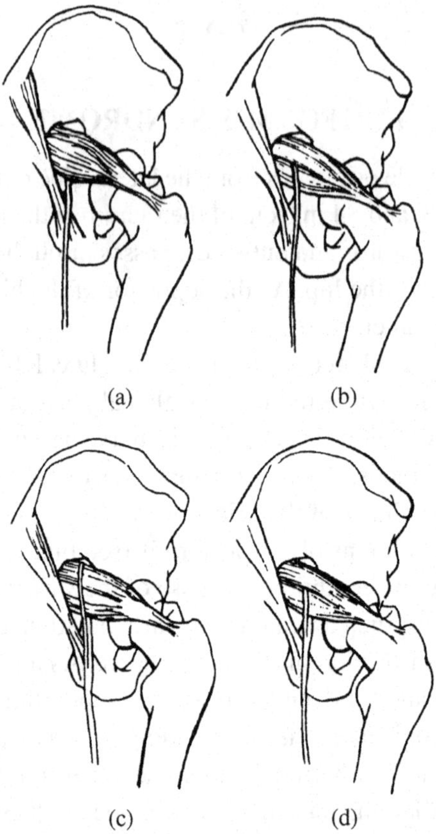

(a) 从梨状肌下缘穿出约占60%	-	About 60% passes underneath of the inferior margin of the piriformis
(b) 从梨状肌中穿出约占30%	-	About 30% transverses from the middle of the piriformis
(c) 从梨状肌上下缘穿出占9.7%	-	9.7% comes out from the inferior and superior margin of the piriformis
(d) 从梨状肌下缘及中间穿出占0.7%	-	0.7% comes out from the inferior margin and middle of the piriformis

Figure 178 The Relationship between the sciatic nerve and the piriformis

3. Deep tenderness of the surface projection of the piriformis site (see Figure 179).
4. Exclusion of diseases of the joints.

Differential Diagonosis

See Table 19 for the differential diagnosis between piriformis syndrome and lumbar disc herniation.

Treatment

1. *Treatment principles* sparsing tendon spasms, resolving blood stasis, and unblocking meridians.
2. *Commonly used maneuvers* palm-heel kneading, intense pressing, finger-kneading, plucking, scrubbing, and fomentation.
3. *Commonly used acupoints and areas cì liào* (BL 32), *zhōng liào* (BL 33), *xià liào* (BL 34), *huán tiào* (GB 30), *yīn mén* (BL 37), *wěi*

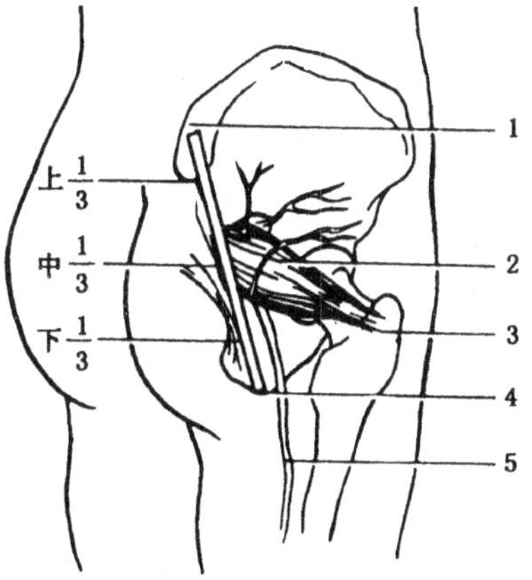

1. 髂后上棘	-	Posterosuperior Iliac Spine
2. 梨状肌	-	The Piriformis
3. 大转子	-	The Greater Trochanter
4. 坐骨结节	-	Ischial Tuberosity
5. 坐骨神经	-	Sciatic Nerve

Figure 179 Surface projection of the piriformis

Table 19 Main differential manifestations of piriformis syndrome and lumbar disc herniation

Name of Condition	Main Location of the Pain	Tenderness and Radiating Pain	Impact of Abdominal Pressure	Piriformis Tension Test	Piriformis Block
Piriformis syndrome	Hip pain and sciatica	Deep tenderness of the hip; sciatica is not significant	Not significant	Positive	Relieves
Lumbar disc herniation	Lumbago and sciatica	Paraspinal tenderness with ipsilateral radiating pain	Significant	Negative	Does not relieve

zhōng (BL 40), *yáng líng quán* (GB 34), the gluteal area, posterior thigh, and lateral calf.

4. *Operational methods*

   Generally, the tension of the gluteus maximus in most patients increases due to obvious sciatica upon occurrence of the injury on the piriformis muscle, which is located deep in the gluteus maximus. The tightness of the gluteus maximus makes it difficult to perform tui na. In order to have the manipulation effect to reach deeply located piriformis, we must first relieve the spasm of the gluteus maximus muscle.

   a. The first step is to relax the gluteal muscles. The patient should be in a prone position with the ipsilateral hip and lower limbs relaxed, and the practitioner standing at the affected side. First, apply palm-heel pressure kneading on the gluteal area with moderate, slow, and gentle stimulus in order to relax the hip muscles and improve the local blood supply and backflow. Then, apply the same maneuver on the rear side of the thigh and calf, back and forth for three to five minutes. Next, apply finger-kneading on *wěi zhōng*, *chéng shān* (BL 57) and *kūn lún* (BL 60).
   b. After the gluteal muscles are relaxed, apply intense pressing and plucking on the surface projection area of the piriformis. Start with

mild stimulation and gradually increase the force, and avoid the resistance of the gluteus maximus. The direction of plucking should be vertical to the piriformis. This operation can relieve spasms of the piriformis, resolve blood stasis, and unblock meridians, which form the core of the treatment. The healer may combine palm-heel pressure kneading, intense pressing, and plucking, and use them alternately for five to eight minutes. In addition, to avoid the resistance of the gluteus maximus, have the knee flexed, and apply passive internal and external rotation of the hip (see Figure 180) to improve the treatment effect.

c. Apply scrubbing on the surface projection area of the piriformis following its direction until the patient feels the heat of the friction. For patients with severe pain, local fomentation may be used as well.

Self-Preventional Methods

1. Apply fomentation on ipsilateral hip.
2. Use the pulp of the finger to apply the kneading maneuver on *yáng líng quán* and *kūn lún*.

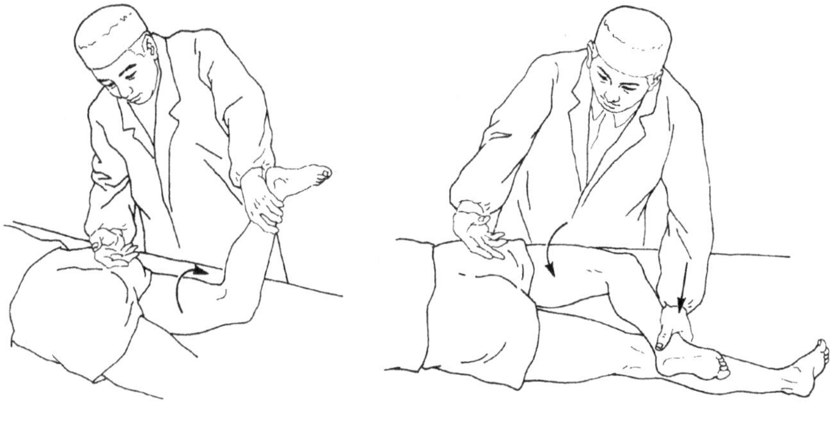

(a) (b)

(a) 内旋	-	Internal Rotation
(b) 外旋	-	External Rotation

Figure 180 Internal and External Hip Rotation in Prone Position

Precautions

1. Keep the ipsilateral limb warm, take more rest, and reduce physical activities.
2. If conservative treatment is ineffective, seek surgical probing procedures to resolve the cause of the problem.

Everyday Exercises

1. Where is the piriformis located? How would you determine its surface projection?
2. How do you differentiate piriformis syndrome from lumbar disc herniation?
3. How would you treat piriformis syndrome with tui na therapy?

Day 4

SUPRAPATELLAR BURSA HEMATOMA

Suprapatellar bursa (see Figure 181) is the largest bursa of the knee, located above the patella basal and deep surface of the quadriceps. Normally the wider opening of it connects with the synovial capsule of the knee, so that it can also be seen as part of the complete synovial bursa. It plays an important role in maintaining the functions of knee flexion and extension. If the knee encounters a traumatic injury, it would result in bleeding of the suprapatellar bursa and a hematoma may form (see Figure 182).

Clinical Manifestations

In addition to pain and significantly limited activities, acute injury of the knee would immediately result in a crescent-shaped swelling at the edge of the patella with local tenderness and fluctuations.

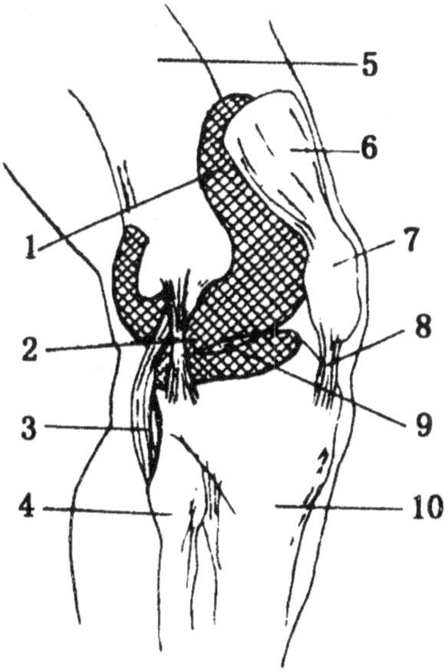

Figure 181 The Joint of the right knee (lateral view)

1. Suprapatellar Bursa 2. Lateral Collateral Ligament 3. Popliteal Tendon 4. Fibula 5. Femur 6. Quadriceps 7. Patella 8. Patellar Tendon 9. Lateral Meniscus 10. Tibia

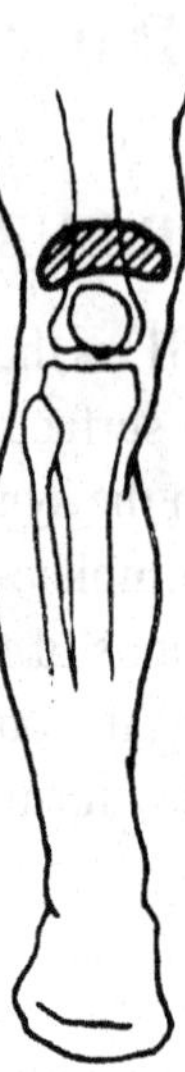

Figure 182 External view of suprapatellar bursa hematoma

Table 20 Main differential manifestations of suprapatellar bursa hematoma and traumatic synovitis

Name of Condition	Post-traumatic Hematoma Bleeding Time	Swelling	Floating Patella Test	Local Skin Temperature
Suprapatellar bursa hematoma	Immediately	Limited to the suprapatellar margin	Negative	Normal
Traumatic synovitis	Generally, a few hours after the injury	The entire knee	Positive	May increase

Diagnosis and Differentiation

This condition is not difficult to diagnose based on the history of recent trauma and clinical manifestations. It should be differentiated from traumatic synovitis (see Table 20).

A knee fracture needs to be considered if the post-traumatic lower limb of the patient shows these signs and symptoms:

1. The patient cannot stand and walk normally.
2. There is local deformity and movements are abnormal movements.
3. Physical examination detects bony crepitus and signs of vertical limb percussion. A positive percussion sign is as follows: when the limb straightens, the examiner uses the fist to lightly tap the heel of the patient; the transitivity percussion pain on the site of the fracture indicates a positive result, which can be confirmed with X-rays.

Treatment

1. *Treatment principles* resolving knots, dissolving swelling, removing blood stasis, and relieving pain.
2. *Commonly used maneuvers* pressure kneading, intense pressing, and passive flexion and extension of the knee.
3. *Commonly used acupoints and areas bì guān* (ST 31), *fú tù* (ST 32), *jiě xī* (ST 41), patellar bursa, and quadriceps.
4. *Operation methods*
    a. The patient is supine, with the practitioner standing on the affected side. Apply pressure kneading on both ends of the affected site with the focus on *bì guān*, *fú tù*, *jiě xī,* and the quadriceps for two to three minutes. This is the preparation technique.
    b. Then, using one hand with the thumb and index finger separated, clamp the superior margin of the suprapatellar bursa hematoma, and get ready for the pressing. Use the other hand to grip the ipsilateral ankle to be prepared for calf stretching (see Figure 183). Apply forces with both hand concurrently, hyperextending and fully flexing the knee rapidly, followed by slowly straightening it (see Figure 184).
    c. In the course of the treatment, a crisp sound can often be heard with the disappearance of the suprapatellar bursa hematoma, and there will be significantly reduced knee pain.
    d. *Care after tui na manipulation* First of all, immobilize the knee, and avoid weight-bearing forces. This can be done by using hard

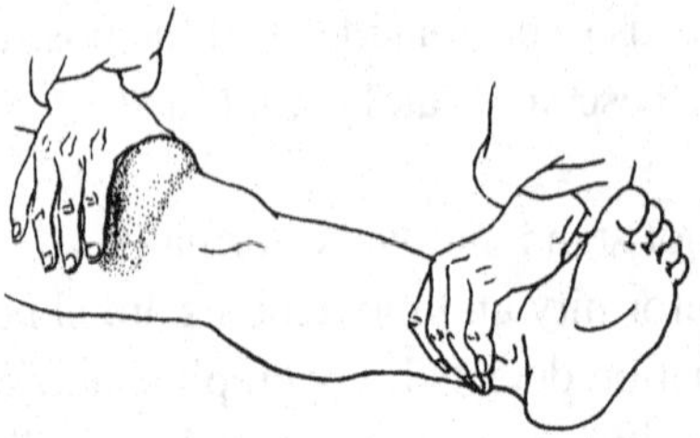

Figure 183 Thumb web pressing the superior edge of the suprapatellar bursa hematoma

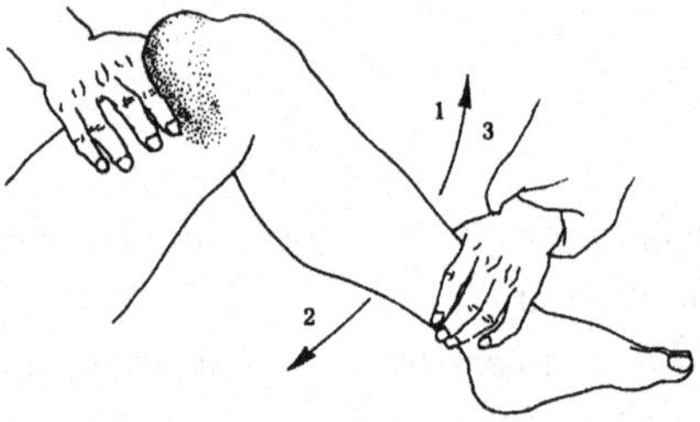

Figure 184 Treatment maneuvers for suprapatellar bursa hematoma

cardboard to fix both sides of the knee and leaving it for seven to ten days. During this period, topical medication such as Stasis-n'-Pain Resolver plaster can be used on the affected area to reduce exudation of the local tissue and prevent further bleeding. In addition, encourage the patient to do exercises of quadriceps stretching and contracture without bearing weight while lying down. Local herbal fumigation can be used in conjunction with it. If the exercise can be done for five minutes every hour, quadriceps atrophy can be avoided while reducing the incidence of adhesions and improving the functional recovery of the knee.

Precautions

1. The differentiation must be correct. Avoid medical malpractice due to mistakenly diagnosing traumatic synovitis or knee fracture as suprapatellar bursa hematoma.

2. Once the diagnosis is confirmed for suprapatellar bursa hematoma, the manipulations should be accurate without hesitance, but they must not be reckless. Avoid repeated passive knee flexion and extension.
3. When the hematoma is eliminated with manual operation, it is only half way done. The fourth item under the treatment section is an essential component in dealing with the condition.

KNEE MENISCUS INJURY

Knee menisci are two wedge-shaped fibrocartilage discs located between the articular surfaces of the femur and tibial bones. The medial meniscus is larger and C-shaped while the lateral meniscus is smaller and nearly an O-shape (see Figure 185). The knee menisci increase the depth of the glenoid fossa and stability of the joint. At the same time, they assist the femoral condyle to rotate against the tibial condyle to increase the flexibility of the knee. They also prevent friction, reduce shock, distribute synovial fluid, moisten the joint, and absorb heat.

When the knee is semi-flexed the meniscus may get stuck between the femoral condyle and tibial plateau due to sudden adduction, rotation, and extension; or abduction, rotation, and extension of the knee, leading to injury. If the patient's daily activities involve long periods of squatting, this may be a contributing factor, making the meniscus vulnerable to compression, resulting in injury.

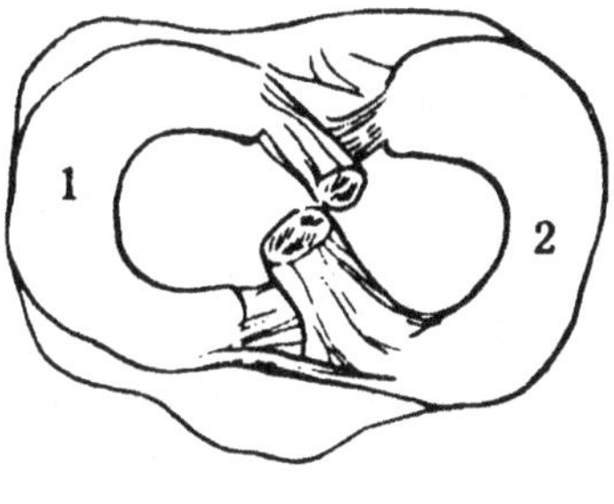

1. 内侧半月板	-	Medial Meniscus
2. 外侧半月板	-	Lateral Meniscus

Figure 185 Knee Meniscus

Clinical Manifestations

1. *Joint swelling* This is more common in the acute phase. If the injury is old, joint swelling is usually not obvious.
2. *Joint pain* There is knee pain with a certain position that disappears immediately after change in the position.
3. *Joint locking and snapping* This "joint interlocking" generally occurs while walking. When the ruptured and displaced meniscus is drifting in the joint space, it interferes with the normal activities of the knee. Sometimes, the knee is suddenly "locked" with a snapping sound of the joint and cannot move. When it happens, stay in place and slightly move the knee, and another snapping, or "unlocking", should take place, and the joint can resume its normal activities.
4. *Muscle atrophy and weakness* This involves mainly the quadriceps. Meniscus injury leads to restricted mobility of the knee. Over time, it will lead to atrophy of the muscles. The more severe the muscle atrophy, the more obvious is the weakness of the lower extremity.
5. *Sense of instability of the joint* The affected knee often has an unstable feeling while walking, especially on an uneven road, and going up or down the stairs.

A physical examination will reveal ipsilateral joint space tenderness. Most patients will show a positive result for the McMurry test while some patients will show a positive result for the Apley grind test and hyperextension test.

Diagnosis and Differentiation

Diagnosis A history of knee trauma with clinical manifestations of the five symptoms described above, combined with tenderness in the joint space, as well as positive results for McMurry test, Apley grind test, and hyperextension test, can be used to diagnose knee meniscus injury. In addition, arthrography, especially knee arthroscopy, is a more valuable tool to locate the damage caused by the condition.

Differential Diagnosis

1. *Knee fracture* When fractures occur, there is obvious swelling, pain, movement disorder, appearance of deformity, bony crepitus, and positive signs of lower limb vertical percussion. An X-ray examination is able to make a clear diagnosis.
2. *Meniscal cysts* These are more common on the lateral side of the knee with local swelling and persistent pain. Lumps can be palpated at the joint space of the knee; these lumps are more prominent with the knee extended and disappear or shrink with the knee flexed.

Treatment

1. *Treatment principles* fortifying muscles, unblocking collaterals, and smoothening and benefiting joints.
2. *Commonly used maneuvers* finger kneading, palm-heel kneading, grasping, scrubbing, fomentation, and appropriate amount of passive flexion and extension of the joint.
3. *Commonly used acupoints and areas fú tù* (ST 32), *xuè hǎi* (SP 10), *xī yǎn* (EX-LE 5), *yáng líng quán* (GB 34), *wěi zhōng* (BL 40), quadriceps, proximal lateral side of the calf.
4. *Operational methods*

   a. The patient is supine, with the practitioner sitting at the affected side. First, apply palm-heel pressure kneading and grasping alternately on the quadriceps for five to eight minutes. This maneuver enhances the tensility of the quadriceps to prevent it from atrophy, and maintains the stability of the knee.
   b. Apply finger-kneading on *fú tù*, *xuè hǎi*, *yáng líng quán,* and *xī yǎn* of the ipsilateral meniscus for about ten minutes, with the focus on *xī yǎn*. Be careful not to damage the skin during the treatment. This maneuver can promote blood circulation and tissue metabolism.
   c. Apply grasping the four-sea points and *wěi zhōng*, followed by scrubbing the ipsilateral joint space using the hypothenar until the patient feels the heat. You may also apply passive knee flexion and extension gently in small amplitudes. Finally, end the treatment with moist fomentation.

Self-Preventional Methods

1. *Be persistent with quadriceps exercises* You may choose one of the following two exercises:
   • *Bare-handed exercise* Choose a standing, sitting or lying position. There is no special equipment or facilities required. The key is to be perseverant. Stretch the lower leg to its utmost extent with quadriceps contracted to its maximum. Then, slowly relax the lower extremities until the quadriceps feels sore. Take a short break and repeat.
   • *Weight-bearing exercise* Sit and place a sandbag or rice bag that is one to three kilograms on the ipsilateral dorsum of the foot. Then repeat the same procedure as in the bare-handed exercise.
2. *Self tui na* Apply finger kneading on *xuè hǎi* and *xī yǎn*, one minute per acupoint. Appropriately increase the operation time on *xī yǎn*.

Precautions

1. Do not repetitively perform the McMurry test during tui na treatment to avoid further damage of the meniscus.
2. Do more functional exercises for the quadriceps to improve the stability of the knee.
3. Avoid knee injury, and use knee pads to protect the knees.

Everyday Exercises

1. Describe the diagnosis and differential diagnosis of suprapatellar bursa hematoma.
2. What are the clinical precautions in treating suprapatellar bursa hematoma using tui na?
3. What is the meniscus, and what are its functions?
4. What are the main symptoms of knee meniscus injury?
5. How would a person exercise the quadriceps?

Day 5

MEDIAL COLLATERAL LIGAMENT INJURY

The medial collateral ligament (see Figure 186), also known as the tibial collateral ligament, starts from the medial femoral epicondyle, and ends at the medial epicondyle of the tibia. It is more vulnerable to trauma during daily activities and exercises comparing to other ligaments such as the lateral collateral and cruciate ligaments of the knee.

Medial collateral ligament injury often occurs as the shank suddenly abducts with the knee slightly flexed. In strenuous exercises such as when playing soccer and basketball, improper movements or external forces directly on the lateral knee joint make the joint abduct, leading to medial collateral ligament injury.

The severity of ligament damage depends on the strength of the external force. If it is milder, only part of the ligament fiber tears. In more serious cases, complete rupture of the ligament can occur in conjunction with meniscus or cruciate ligament injury.

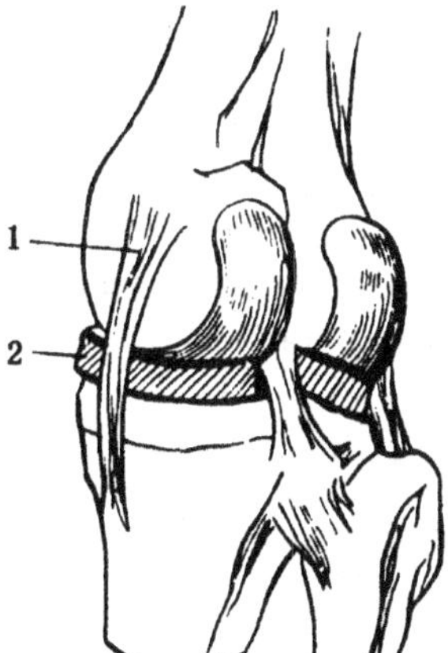

1. 内侧副韧带	-	Medial Collateral Ligament
2. 内侧半月板	-	Medial Meniscus

Figure 186 Medial Collateral Ligament

Clinical Manifestations

1. Obvious medial side swelling, bruises, pain, and reduced joint mobility of the affected knee.
2. If there is also meniscus or cruciate ligament injury, there would be intra-articular bleeding, interlocking symptoms, and a tearing sensation within the joint, causing lax joint immediately and loss of its stability.
3. On the site where the ligament adheres, there will be swelling and tenderness. A lateral push to the affected knee will cause medial knee pain, a sense of loosening, and increased gap. All of these are positive signs of medial collateral ligament injury. Refer to the associated sections in Examination of the Lower Extremities in Week Two for details.

Diagnosis and Differentiation

The diagnosis of this condition is generally not difficult. Based on the patient's clinical history of knee injury, and local signs and symptoms, a correct diagnosis can be made. However, precautionary measures must be taken, such as taking anteroposterior and lateral X-rays of the knee to rule out fractures. In addition, complications of meniscus and cruciate ligament injury also need to be ruled out, because tui na therapy cannot be used to treat these conditions.

Treatment

Tui na for medial collateral ligament injury is applicable only to treat partial fiber breakage, twists, sprains, and contusions of the ligament.

1. *Treatment principles*
   a. *Acute phase*: stopping bleeding, resolving swelling, harmonizing *ying* (营) level and relieving pain.
   b. *Chronic phase*: soothing tendons and unblocking collaterals.
2. *Commonly used maneuvers* ice *an mo*, palm-heel kneading, finger kneading, grasping, and fomentation.
3. *Commonly used acupoints and areas xuè hăi* (SP 10), *ā shì xué*, *yīn líng quán* (SP 9), and medial aspect of the knee.

4. *Operational methods*
   a. Ice *an mo* is the method of using ice in medical massage. It is not only applicable to medial collateral ligament injury, but also to acute contusion of the soft tissues while the swelling is obvious. The method is as follows:

      - Choose round-edged and suitable-sized ice cubes, wrap these in a cloth, and place it on the site of the medial collateral ligament for a gentle and slow *an mo*. Replace it when it is about to melt. The operation should last for ten to 20 minutes, one to three times on the day that the injury occurs.
      - Ice induces vasoconstriction that rapidly and effectively controls bleeding and oozing of the injury site, while relieving pain at the same time. Upon completing the ice treatment, dress and immobilize the site with an elastic bandage at once, then elevate the wounded limb. When the bleeding stops, tui na therapy should be used at the earliest date.

   b. For patients without immediate damage and local bleeding tendency, or for those whose bleeding has been stopped after ice *an mo*, follow these steps to treat the affected area:

      - The patient is supine, with the practitioner sitting or standing on the affected side. Apply palm-heel kneading on the quadriceps for three to five minutes. This maneuver can be used as both the basic technique and an important step to maintain proper muscle tensility of the quadriceps, creating a positive effect on restoring the functions of the knee.
      - With the patient in the same position, apply finger kneading on *xuè hǎi*, *ā shì xué*, *yīn líng quán,* and the medial collateral ligament for eight to ten minutes. This is the principal method to treat the condition. The manipulation should be gentle, avoiding passive movement. At the beginning of the manipulation, there may be some pain. On the other hand, it is a great way for the hematoma to dissipate and be absorbed, which is beneficial for the repairing process of the damaged tissue to take place.
      - If it is necessary, apply scrubbing and fomentation at the site of the injured medial collateral ligament.

Precautions

1. Immobilize the affected knee, avoid weight-bearing forces involving the knee for four to six weeks, and try not to flex the knee.
2. After the bleeding caused by the acute injury stops, start quadriceps functional exercises.
3. Passive joint movement is prohibited while treating this condition using tui na.
4. If the ligament is completely broken or complicated by other injuries, seek surgical treatment as early as possible.
5. Use knee pads to protect the knee.

TIBIAL TUBERCLE EPIPHYSITIS

The tibial tubercle is a bony prominence located at the anterior of the knee and proximal to the tibia. Tibial tubercle epiphysitis is an aseptic inflammation caused by trauma or strain, and tends to occur in adolescents.

Clinical Manifestations

1. The condition is characterized by pain and swelling of the tibial tubercle.
2. Strenuous activity may aggravate the already obvious pain while kneeling down.
3. The disease course is long with slow recovery, and it is self-limiting.
4. There is no redness of the skin, subjective hot sensation, and obvious joint dysfunction on the affected site.
5. There is limited tenderness of the tibial tuberosity. Although there is swelling, the color is normal and the skin temperature is not high.

Diagnosis and Differentiation

1. This condition occurs most often in adolescents. There is localized pain, tenderness, swelling, and acute inflammation on the tibial tubercle, but there is no redness of the skin and subjective hot sensation.

2. X-ray examinations show soft tissue swelling anterior to the tibial tuberosity. The tuberosity may consist of multiple cracked segments (see Figure 187), while the shadowed patellar tendon area may have visible irregular calcification.
3. The condition should be differentiated from avulsion fracture of the tibial tubercle that has a history of trauma as well as strong traction of the quadriceps tendon. X-rays of the latter would find a displaced tibial tubercle epiphysis.

Treatment

1. *Treatment principles* removing blood stasis and relieving pain.
2. *Commonly used maneuvers* finger-kneading, smearing, scrubbing, grasping, and fomentation.
3. *Commonly used acupoints and areas ā shì xué, yáng líng quán* (GB 34), *xuán zhōng* (GB 39), *wěi zhōng* (BL 40), the distal side of the quadriceps and proximal part of the crus.
4. *Operational methods*

   a. The patient is supine, with the practitioner sitting on the affected side. First, apply palm-heel kneading at the distal aspect of the

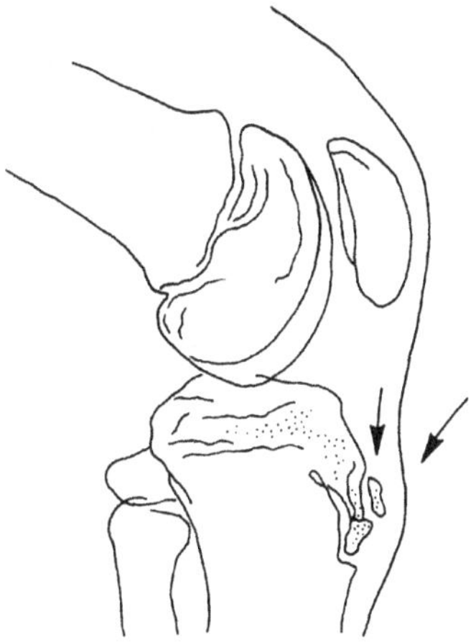

Figure 187 Tibial tubercle cracks

quadriceps and gradually transition down along the patellar tendon to the tibial tubercle, up and down and back and forth for three to five minutes.

b. Finger-kneading on *xuè hăi* (SP 10), *ā shì xué*, *yáng líng quán,* and *xuán zhōng*. Focus on *ā shì xué,* doubling your efforts compared with the other acupoints. The operation should last for five to eight minutes. Then, apply smearing along the tibial crest for 20 to 30 times from top to bottom.

c. End the treatment with grasping on *wĕi zhōng*, scrubbing on the tibial tuberosity, and fomentation on the local area.

Precautions

1. It is better to immobilize the affected limb.
2. Avoid strenuous physical exercise, such as soccer and jogging.
3. When there is severe pain, your physician may offer a local injection containing combined agents of 5 mg dexamethasone with 1% lidocaine at 2 ml.

Everyday Exercises

1. What is ice *an mo*? Under what circumstance can this be an option?
2. What are the precautions for medial collateral ligament injury?
3. What are the main clinical manifestations of tibial tubercle epiphysitis?
4. What are the precautions that need to be taken for adolescents suffering tibial tubercle epiphysitis?

Day 6

TARSAL TUNNEL SYNDROME

The tarsal tunnel is the bone-fiber sheath posteroinferior to the medial malleolus, a retinaculum structured with the calcaneus, talus, and flexor (see Figure 188). This structure encapsules the flexor longus tendon, flexor digitorum longus tendon, posterior tibial tendon, posterior tibial vein, and posterior tibial nerve. When the posterior tibial nerve is compressed, it results in a group of symptoms marked by plantar pain called tarsal tunnel syndrome.

Due to heavy weight-carrying and involvement of frequent activities, the ankles are prone to acute and chronic injury. The malunion of a fractured ankle joint or other injuries would cause symptoms like aseptic tendon inflammation, hyperemia, and edema, further leading to tarsal canal stenosis. As a result, the increased pressure in the tube can compress and stimulate the tibial neurons to trigger the occurrence of tarsal tunnel syndrome.

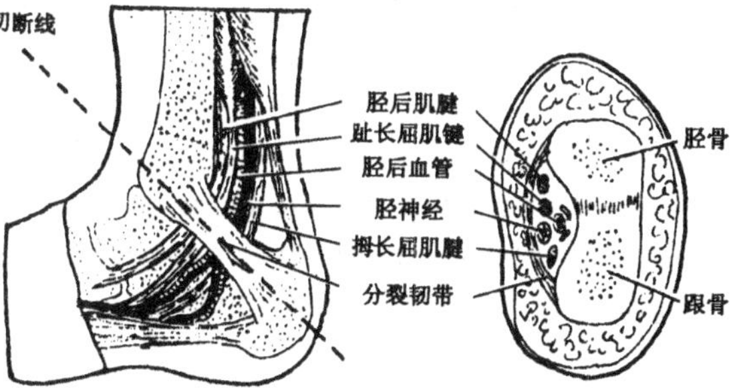

切断线	-	anatomy section line	拇长屈肌腱	-	flexor pollicis longus tendon
胫后肌腱	-	posterior tibial tendon	分裂韧带	-	ligamenta laciniatum
趾长屈肌腱	-	digitorum longus tendon	胫骨	-	tibia
胫后血管	-	posterior tibial vessels	跟骨	-	calcaneus
胫神经	-	tibial nerve			

Figure 188 Structure of the tarsal tunnel

Clinical Manifestations

1. Burning pain from the toes that extends along the medial side of the foot to the pelma and is worse at night or while walking. It may radiate to the knee.
2. Sympathetic dystrophy symptoms such as dry skin and falling hair of the toes.
3. Plantar skin hypoesthesia.
4. The pricking pain of the pelma increases while tapping on the retinaculum of the ankle flexor, which is a positive Tinel's sign.

Diagnosis

1. The diagnosis is based on the clinical manifestations of the disease, such as burning pain of the pelma and a positive Tinel's sign.
2. An electromyography (EMG) is quite helpful in diagnosing the problem, with diagnostic significance such as decreased conduction velocity and an extended latent period.
3. Ankle X-rays usually show up normal. At the same time, X-rays will be able to determine if there is the occurrence of malunion of bone fracture or deformed bone disease.

Treatment

1. *Treatment principles* soothing tendons and unblocking meridians.
2. *Commonly used maneuvers* finger-kneading, intense pressing, twiddling, grasping, scrubbing, passive joint movement, and fomentation.
3. *Commonly used acupoints and areas sān yīn jiāo* (SP 6), *tài xī* (KI 3), *shāng qiū* (SP 5), *jiě xī* (ST 41), *gōng sūn* (SP 4), *yǒng quán* (KI 1), *ā shì xué*, the medial malleolus area, pelma, and toes.
4. *Operational methods:*
   a. The patient is supine, with the practitioner sitting on the side of the affected foot. First, flex the lower leg and apply gentle grasping on the calf muscles from the proximal to the distal part for three to five times. Then, apply finger-kneading on *sān yīn jiāo*, *tài xī*, *jiě*

xī, *shāng qiū*, and *gōng sūn*, for one minute per acupoint. Use the line connecting *sān yīn jiāo*, *tài xī*, and *shāng qiū* as the treatment axis and put more focus on finger kneading on these points. At the same time, coordinate the manipulations with passive flexion and extension, varus and valgus of the ankle.

b. Slightly abduct and externally rotate the ipsilateral limb and flex the crus to make the center of the sole facing up. With thumbs overlapped, apply intense pressing following the direction of the heel to the toe, and from the medial to the lateral aspect (see Figure 189) for five to eight minutes. Put more focus to stimulate *yǒng quán* and *ā shì xué*. Then, apply twiddling on each toe two to three times.
c. The last step starts with scrubbing on the foot, especially the treatment axis of *shāng qiū*, *tài xī*, and *sān yīn jiāo*. End the treatment with moist fomentation to the medial malleolus and the bottom of the affected foot.

Self-Preventional Methods

1. Apply finger kneading on the treatment axis of *shāng qiū*, *tài xī*, and *sān yīn jiāo*, twice to three times a day, and three to five minutes each time.
2. Apply herbal fumigation on the affected foot.

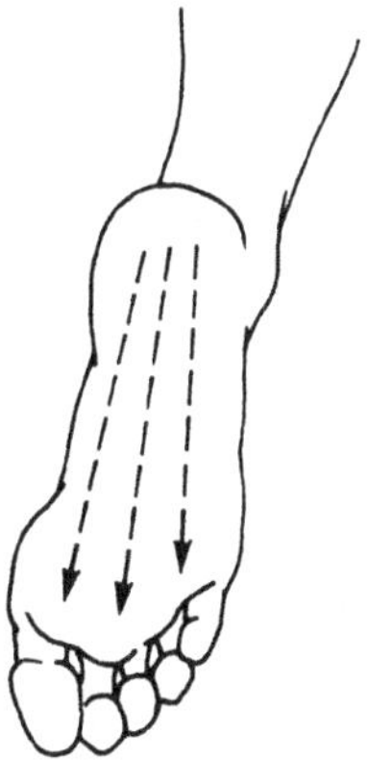

Figure 189 Intense pressing of the foot

Precautions

1. Use an ankle pad to protect the ankle. It can keep it warm and maintain the stability of the ankle joint at the same time.
2. For people with serious symptoms and unsuccessful conservative treatment, surgical treatment may be considered.

Everyday Exercises

1. What is tarsal tunnel syndrome?
2. How would you treat tarsal tunnel syndrome using tui na?

CALCANODYNIA

Calcanodynia is characterized by pain on the plantar side of the heel. Calcanodynia is one kind of bone degeneration. Since the plantar fascia adhering to the calcaneal tuberosity is under long-term traction and stimulation, there may be chronic injury, degeneration, chronic inflammation, and hyperplasia of the calcaneus bone, causing heel pain. In Chinese medical practice, it is believed that the condition is caused by liver and kidney deficiency.

Clinical Manifestations

1. Heel pain that increases with walking or weight-bearing, and decreases with rest.
2. Apparent tenderness at the bottom of the heel on the medial aspect of the calcaneal tuberosity.
3. Lateral X-rays of the calcaneus show a spur or thickening of the periosteum.

Diagnosis

1. The condition is seen mostly in middle-aged people; there is pain on the medial plantar side of heel with obvious tenderness.
2. Lateral X-rays of the calcaneus may provide evidence for the diagnosis. However, it cannot be used as the only diagnostic measure of the disease since many people with heel spurs do not feel any pain.

Treatment

1. *Treatment principles* smoothening tendons, invigorating blood, removing stasis, and relieving pain.
2. *Commonly used maneuvers*: finger-kneading, intense pressing, grasping, scrubbing, and fomentation.
3. *Commonly used acupoints and areas chéng shān* (BL 57), *sān yīn jiāo* (SP 6), *tài xī* (KI 3), *yǒng quán* (KI 1), *ā shì xué*, the medial malleolus, and the bottom of the heel.
4. *Operational methods*
   a. The patient is supine, with the practitioner sitting on the affected side of the patient. Using your left and right hand alternately, flex the patient's crus and perform grasping on the distal side of the triceps surae and the Achilles tendon with gentle force three to five times. Then, apply finger-kneading on *chéng shān*, *sān yīn jiāo,* and *tài xī*, one minute for each acupoint.
   b. Slightly abduct and externally rotate the affected limb, flex the leg, and make the sole face up. With both thumbs overlapped, apply intense pressing on the bottom of the heel from the back forward using lateral force. Focus on *ā shì xué* points, doubling the manipulation time. At the same time, supplement the operation with pressure kneading to ease the pain. The step should total up to five to six minutes. Apply finger kneading on *yǒng quán* with moderate amount of stimulation for about a minute.
   c. Apply scrubbing on the bottom of the foot until it feels warm. Finally, end the treatment with fomentation on the bottom of the heel.

Self-Preventional Methods

1. Perform finger kneading on *tài xī* and *yǒng quán*, one minute on each acupoint, twice to three times a day.
2. Apply intense pressing on *ā shì xué* and surrounding points for about two minutes, twice to three times a day.
3. Use a Chinese herbal decoction to wash the affected area by soaking the heel in the liquid once daily. You may add 30 to 50 ml vinegar to the decoction.

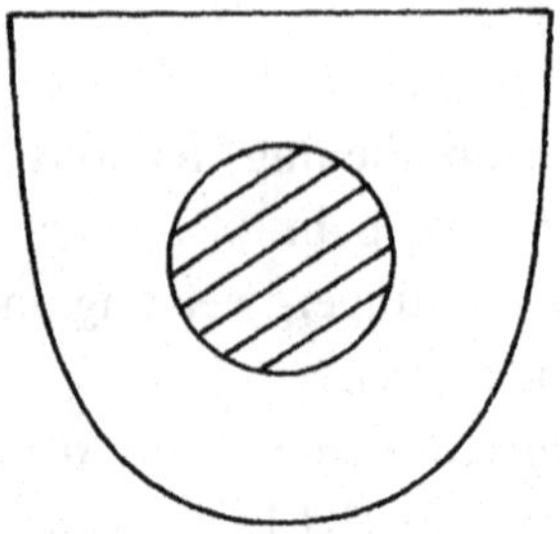

Figure 190 Sponge heel pad

Precautions

1. Wear soft-soled or flat-heeled shoes.
2. Reduce weight-bearing activities involving the affected foot.
3. Place a sponge heel pad inside the shoe (see Figure 190) to reduce local compression. You can fashion your own pad using a piece of sponge 1 to 1.3 cm thick. First, fit it to a hoof-shaped heel pad that can fit in the back of the shoe. Then, cut a small round hole in the middle of the sponge so that it will cover where the heel spur is located.

Everyday Exercises

1. What is calcanodynia?
2. What is the function of a sponge heel pad? How would you make one?

WEEK 11

Day 1

RHEUMATOID ARTHRITIS

Rheumatoid arthritis, a systemic autoimmune disease with its main characteristic of chronic symmetry polyarthritis, can cause severe deformities. The etiology of this disease is still not very clear. Most scholars believe that it is an autoimmune disease with joint synovitis due to certain infections. In the early stages, the symptoms are migratory pain and dysfunction of affected joints. It is recurrent, and in its late stages, symptoms include joint stiffness, deformity, and loss of function, accompanied by atrophy of bones and skeletal muscle. About 80% of patients experience the first onset of rheumatoid arthritis between the ages of 20 to 45 years old, with the disease affecting mainly young and middle-aged women. In Chinese medical practice, it is believed that rheumatoid arthritis is within the scope of the bone *bì* pattern.

Clinical Manifestations

1. *Insidious and slow onset in the majority of patients* Prior to the appearance of symptoms in the joints, initially patients would have prodromal symptoms including fatigue, weakness, loss of appetite, muscle aches, numbness of hands and feet, and unexplained low grade fever. Following that, local symptoms would show up, such as joint pain, morning stiffness, swelling, and local rise of body temperature. At the same time, there are systemic symptoms, including irregular fever, weight loss, increased pulse, and anemia.

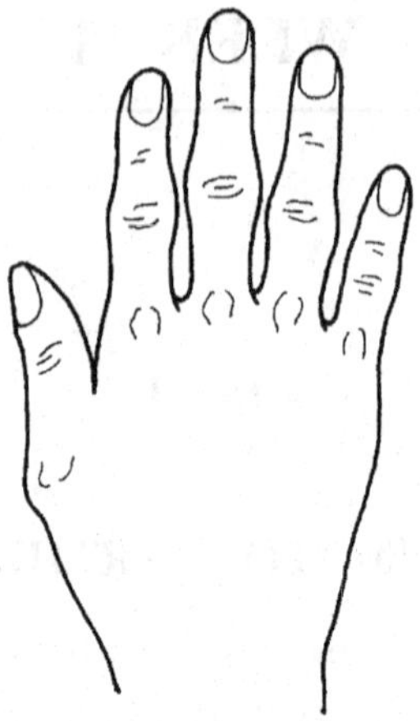

Figure 191 Fusiform swelling of interphalangeal joints

2. *Multiple joints involved* First, the disease may start with only one or two joints involved, the pain being often migratory. Afterwards, it develops into symmetric polyarthritis. It often starts in the small joints of distal limbs, most commonly the interphalangeal joints, showing a fusiform enlargement (see Figure 191). Then, it progresses gradually to the metacarpophalangeal joints, toes, wrists, knees, elbows, ankles, shoulders, and hips. Morning stiffness, also known as morning ankylosis, is another important symptom of the disease.
3. *Slow onset with progressive development* Attacks and remission occur alternately. The course of the disease can be several years to several decades. Eventually, there will be extremely limited joints activities, and even deformities. Knees, elbows, fingers, and wrists are fixed in flexion status while the fingers often show lateral subluxation at the metacarpophalangeal joints, forming a characteristic deformity of ulnar deviation (see Figure 192). At this stage, patients need assistance to perform normal daily activities such as dressing, eating, and turning over. If multiple joints are affected, the patient is forced to stay in bed.
4. *Laboratory tests*
   a. Generally, the majority of the patients would have anemia with an increased erythrocyte sedimentation rate (ESR), this being an indicator of the disease at the active stage.

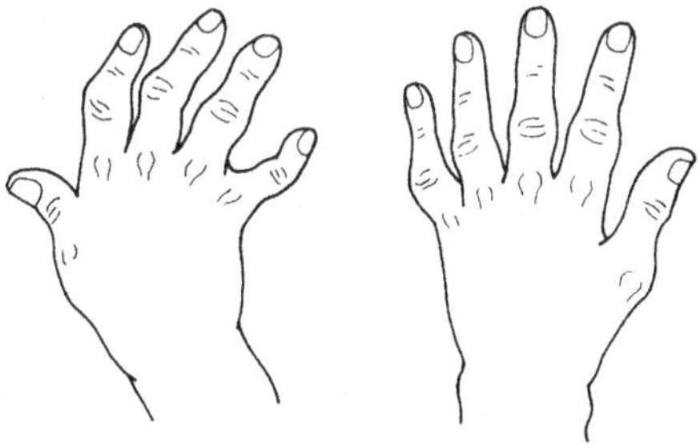

Figure 192 Rheumatoid hands

b. The rheumatoid factor test or the rheumatoid arthritis latex test is positive.
c. In the early stage, X-rays show only soft tissue swelling. Then, there is osteoporosis, joint space narrowing, joint edge erosion, and cystic destruction of bones. In the late stage, the joint space disappears, and joint deformity and ankylosis occur.

Diagnosis and Differentiation

Key Diagnostic Criteria

1. History of morning stiffness.
2. Migratory multiple joint pain, often symmetrical and recurrent.
3. Swollen spindle-shaped metacarpophalangeal and proximal interphalangeal joints.
4. Anemia and elevated ESR.
5. X-rays reveal signs of rheumatoid arthritis (RA) joints.
6. Positive for rheumatoid factor.

Differential Diagnosis

1. *Rheumatic arthritis* This disease is more common in children, with a rapid onset and high fever, mainly involving large joints. There are no joint deformities after the onset, but the disease can damage the heart. There is a rapid and significant response to salicylic acid preparations (aspirin).

2. *Tuberculous arthritis* This disease may be associated with other types of tuberculosis. It mostly affects a single joint, and is negative for rheumatoid factor test.
3. *Hyperplasia osteoarthritis* This disease has a slow onset, and occurs mostly in people over 40 years of age. It generally affects weight-bearing joints such as knees, hips, and the spine. There is no migratory joint pain or systemic symptoms; ESR is normal; and rheumatoid factor test result is negative. X-rays show signs of bone hyperplasia.

Treatment

1. *Treatment principles* Fortifying the liver and kidney, strengthening tendons and bones, unblocking qi and blood, and benefiting joints.
2. *Commonly used maneuvers* Finger kneading, spinal pinching, grasping, twiddling, smearing, rotating, scrubbing, and passive joint movements.
3. *Commonly used acupoints and areas*: *gé shū* (BL 17), *gān shū* (BL 18), *pí shū* (BL 20), *wèi shū* (BL 21), *shèn shū* (BL 23), *jiān sān xuè*, *qŭ chí* (LI 11), *wài guān* (SJ 5), *yáng chí* (SJ 4), *yáng xī* (LI 5), *hé gŭ* (LI 4), *hòu xī* (SI 3), *xuè hăi* (SP 10), *yáng líng quán* (GB 34), *zú sān lĭ* (ST 36), *xuán zhōng* (GB 39), *kūn lún* (BL 60), *jiě xī* (ST 41), *yŏng quán* (KI 1), and affected limbs.
4. *Operational methods*
   We will mainly discuss the operation on the hands and feet.

   Operational methods for rheumatoid hands

   a. The patient is prone, with the practitioner standing to the left of the patient. Apply finger kneading to back-*shu* points with the focus alternating amongst *gé shū*, *gān shū*, *pí shū*, *wèi shū,* and *shèn shū* until the soreness *de*-qi sensation is felt on each acupoint. Apply scrubbing on the bladder meridians along the mid-back area. Apply spinal pinching three to five times starting from the sacrococcygeal region up to the cervicothoracic area. These maneuvers total up to about five minutes.
   b. The patient changes to the supine position, with the practitioner sitting at the ipsilateral side. First, apply palm-heel pressure kneading

alternately between the volar and dorsal side of the ipsilateral forearm, transitioning with the direction from the proximal side to the distal wrist. Then, apply grasping on the radial and ulnar forearm muscles, finger kneading on *wài guān*, *yáng chí,* and *dà líng*, coordinating with clockwise and counter-clockwise passive wrist movements such as flexion, extension, radial deviation, and ulnar deviation.

c. Apply scrubbing on the dorsal and palmar sides of the wrist until the frictional heat is felt. Apply grasping on *hé gŭ*, and twiddling and smearing on the metacarpophalangeal joints and the proximal and distal interphalangeal joints. At the same time, coordinate with the passive flexion of various small joints and rotation of metacarpophalangeal joints. Lastly, apply finger kneading on the palmar and dorsal sides of the interosseous muscles. Steps (a) and (b) total up to about ten minutes.

Operational methods for rheumatoid feet

a. The patient is supine, with the practitioner sitting at the ipsilateral side. Apply pale-heel pressure kneading on the tibialis anterior muscle from the proximal aspect to the distal side to reach the dorsum of the foot. Ask the patient to slightly flex the lower limbs, and use both hands alternately to apply grasping on the gastrocnemius and gradually transition to the Achilles tendon. Repeat the operation top-down a few times.
b. Perform finger kneading on *yáng líng quán*, *zú sān lĭ*, *xuán zhōng*, *kūn lún*, *tài xī,* and *jiě xī,* and coordinate with the passive ankle flexion, extension, varus, and valgus. Apply scrubbing to the dorsum of the foot until the heat is felt. Apply finger kneading on the dorsum of the foot, medial and lateral malleolus, and the intrinsic muscles of the dorsum side of the metatarsal gap. Apply twiddling, smearing, and rotation on the toe joints. Apply plantar pressing method (refer to the section on Tarsal Tunnel Syndrome in Day Six of Week 10 for details.) Steps (a) and (b) should last for about ten minutes.
c. After completion of tui na, apply fomentation on the affected hands and feet.

Self-preventional Methods

1. Apply rubbing on the lower abdomen for three to five minutes and kneading on both sides of *zú sān lǐ* for one minute, twice a day.
2. Apply herbal fumigation to the affected joints once a day.

Precautions

1. Persevere with regularly exercises of all the joints involved within the limit of tolerable joint pain, one to three times a day, a few minutes to ten minutes each time.
2. Adherence to comprehensive and early treatment improves the efficacy.
3. Keep warm and avoid exhaustion to reduce the chance of recurrence.
4. Increase dietary intake of protein, carbohydrate, and various vitamins.

Everyday Exercises

1. What is rheumatoid arthritis? How does it differ from rheumatic arthritis?
2. How would you describe the typical deformity of a rheumatoid hand?
3. Describe the operational procedures in treating rheumatoid hands using tui na.

Day 2

HEMIPLEGIA

Hemiplegia refers to paralysis of one side of the body, and is the most common type of paralysis. Hemiplegia has many causes, with cerebrovascular and brainstem vascular diseases at the top of the list, followed by brain trauma, brain tumor, and encephalitis. According to the site of injury, it can be divided into cortical, subcortical, internal capsular, brainstem, and spinal hemiplegia.

Clinically, tui na is used in the sequelae of cerebrovascular diseases belonging to two major categories: hemorrhagic and ischemic. The former is mainly cerebral hemorrhage while the latter is mostly cerebral infarction. In tui na, hemorrhagic and ischemic cerebrovascular diseases are handled very differently in their early stages. On the other hand, the sequelae of both (i.e., hemiplegia) are the same. Therefore, tui na treatment is the same for all stroke sequelae.

In Chinese medical practice, the common names for hemiplegia are *piān kū*, literally meaning "unilateral withering" and *bàn shēn bú suí*, meaning "dysfunction of one side of the body." In Chinese medical etiology, the disease reveals a serious imbalance of the yin-yang of *zang-fu* organs, and disorder of qi and blood circulating. It is coupled with yin deficiency of the lower trunk, and hyperactive liver-yang affecting the head. Consequently, blood inverses with the counter-flow of qi, mingles with phlegm and internal fire, and causes blood rushing into the brain, obstructing the heart *shen*, and trespassing the meridians and vessels. As the result, qi and blood are not able to nourish the body owing to deficient healthy qi complicated by blood stasis blocking the meridians, leading to hemiplegia.

Clinical Manifestations

1. *Unilateral paralysis affecting the body* The paralysis is usually more obvious on extensors of the arm and flexors of the leg with increased muscle tension. Therefore, with the upper limb flexed and lower limb straightened, the patient often swings the affected leg and makes a half circle while walking, which is referred as the mowing gait.

2. *Facial paralysis* There is centralized facial paralysis, i.e., the upper half of the facial muscles are normal or with very mild paralysis of a short duration, which soon returns to normal.
3. *Unilateral sensory disturbance* This is most obvious at the distal aspect of the affected body.
4. *Other concomitant symptoms* These include distal edema, dry and dull skin, desquamation, dry and brittle body hair that is easy to come off, and nail depression and deformation. In the late stages, there is muscle atrophy.
5. *Major characteristics during physical examination*
   a. Distal hypoesthesia.
   b. Decreased muscle strength with increased muscle tension, and resistance of affected limbs during passive movements.
   c. Change in nervous reflexes: disappearance of superficial reflections of the paralyzed side such as abdominal reflex and cremasteric reflex; hyperreflexia of deep reflections of the affected side such as those of the biceps, triceps tendon, patellar tendon, and Achilles tendon, often accompanied by patellar and ankle clonus; and pathological reflexes such as positive Babinski and Hoffmann signs.

Diagnosis

There is a history of cerebrovascular accident with signs and symptoms of unilateral paralysis on the same side of the upper and lower body.

Treatment

Tui na can only be applied after the patient has been rescued from a cerebrovascular emergency, and is in a stable condition with normal blood pressure and vital signs; there will then be no danger in performing tui na.

1. *Treatment principles* invigorating blood, resolving stasis, dredging meridians, unblocking collaterals, and revitalizing the body.
2. *Commonly used maneuvers* intense pressing, finger and thenar kneading, smearing, grasping, scattering sweeping, rotating, foulage, shaking, twiddling, scrubbing, and passive joint movement.

3. *Commonly used acupoints and areas*
   - *Head, face and neck*: *bǎi huì* (DU 20), *sì shén cōng* (EX-HN 1), *jīng míng* (BL 1), *tài yáng* (EX-HN 5), *jiá chē* (ST 6), *dì cāng* (ST 4), *yíng xiāng* (LI 20), *fēng chí* (GB 20) and *fēng fǔ* (DU 16), the orbicularis, orbicularis oris muscle, and facial muscles.
   - *Back*: back-*shu* points and acupoints along *du mai*.
   - *Upper limbs*: *jiān sān xuè*, *qǔ chí* (LI 11), *hé gǔ* (LI 4), *wài guān* (SJ 5) and extensors of the arm.
   - *Lower limbs*: *huán tiào* (GB 30), *bì guān* (ST 31), *fú tù* (ST 32), *xuè hǎi* (SP 10), *fēng shì* (GB 31), *chéng fú* (BL 36), *yīn mén* (BL 37), *wěi zhōng* (BL 40), *chéng shān* (BL 57), *kūn lún* (BL 60), *jiě xī* (ST 41), and lower limb flexors.
4. *Operational methods*:

   a. Start with the patient in the prone position. If he or she is not able to lie prone or remain in the position for an extended period of time, get the patient to lie on the contralateral side. The practitioner should stand at the affected side. Apply palm-heel pressure kneading in the following order: *jiān jǐng* (GB 21), back of the shoulder, upper back, the sacrospinal muscles, and the lumbosacral region; work up and down several times with pressure kneading on the sacrospinal muscles.
   b. Apply intense pressing on the back-*shu* points. Put more focus on *gé shū* (BL 17), *gān shū* (BL 18), *sān jiāo shū* (BL 22), *shèn shū* (BL 23), and *du mai* acupoints such as *dà zhuī* (DU 14), *jīn suō* (DU 8), and *yāo yáng guān* (DU 3), for a total of up to about five minutes.
   c. Apply palm-heel pressure kneading on the ipsilateral buttock with intense pressing on acupoints such as *huán tiào* and *jū liào* (GB 29), and combine with passive internal and external rotation of the hips. See details in the relevant section of treating piriformis syndrome in Week 10.
   d. Apply intense pressing on *chéng fú*, *yīn mén*, *wěi zhōng*, and *chéng shān*, and palm-heal pressure kneading on the posterior thigh, popliteal fossa, and calf flexors. Next, focus on grasping and twiddling the Achilles tendon and passive dorsiflexion of the ankle (see Figure 193). Steps (c) and (d) should total up to about five to six minutes.

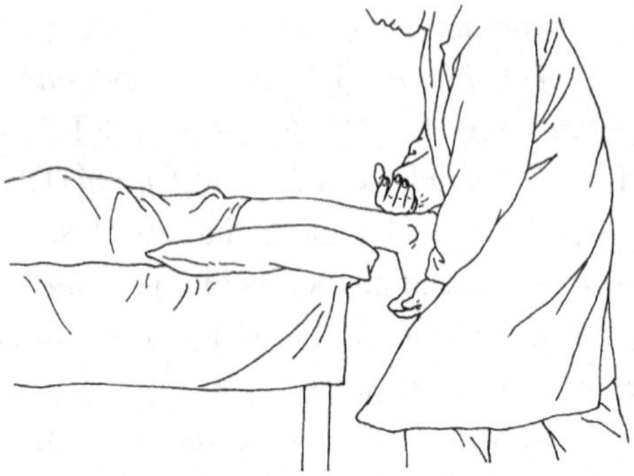

Figure 193 Passive ankle dorsiflexion in prone position

e. Shift the patient to a supine position, with the practitioner standing at the affected side. Apply palm-heel pressure kneading on the deltoid muscle, finger-kneading *jiān sān xuè*, and grasping the deltoid, biceps, and triceps, with more focus on the triceps. This procedure can be coordinated with passive shoulder abduction, external rotation, internal rotation, adduction, and forward flexion. Refer to the treatment section in Week Six for shoulder periarthritis.
f. Apply finger kneading on *qŭ chí* and *shŏu sān lĭ* (LI 10), grasping on both the radial and ulnar aspects of the forearm muscles, and coordinating with passive flexion and extension of the elbow.
g. Apply finger kneading on *wài guān* and *yáng chí* (SJ 4), grasping on *hé gŭ*, and pressure kneading on the thenar and hypothenar muscles. Afterwards, apply finger kneading on the palmar and dorsal sides of the interosseous muscles, combining passive movements of wrist flexion and extension, ulnar and radial deviation. Next, apply twiddling, smearing, and rotating on the metacarpophalangeal and interphalangeal joints. Steps (e) to (g) should last for about five minutes.
h. Apply palm-heel pressure kneading on the anterior, posterior, and medial aspects of the thigh followed by intense pressing on *bì guān*, *fú tù*, *fēng shì*, and *xuè hăi*, grasping on the quadriceps and muscles on the posterior side of the thigh and adductors. Coordinate these maneuvers with passive hip flexion and extension. See the relevant sections in treating ankylosing spondylitis in Week Nine.

i. Apply palm-heel pressure kneading on the patella, finger kneading on *xī yǎn* (EX-LE 5), *yáng líng quán* (GB 34), *zú sān lǐ* (ST 36), *xuán zhōng* (GB 39), *tài xī* (KI 3), and *kūn lún*, and grasping on the gastrocnemius, combined with passive knee flexion and extension. Apply finger kneading on *jiě xī*, *yǒng quán* (KI 1), and the interosseous muscles, smearing and twiddling on the toes, and rotating the ankle and toes. Step (h) and (i) should last for a total of five to six minutes.

j. Lastly, apply smearing on the forehead, scattering sweeping on both tempora, pressure kneading on *bǎi huì* and *sì shén cōng*, and grasping on *fēng chí* to end the treatment. If there is facial paralysis, refer to the treatment section for this condition.

Self-Preventional Methods

Try exercise the paralyzed joints one after another within your physical ability, and avoid being too tired.

Precautions

1. Maintain emotional stability and do not get irritable.
2. Avoid tobacco, alcohol, spicy food, and high-fat and greasy foods. Do not eat animal organs.
3. Live to a regular and reasonable schedule, balance work and rest, and maintain bowels open.
4. Be confident while fighting the disease, and adhere to the treatment and self-exercises.
5. For patients who need long-term bed rest, avoid pneumonia, pressure sores, and urinary tract inflammation.

Everyday Exercises

1. What is hemiplegia?
2. What are the common factors causing hemiplegia?
3. What are some things that a hemiplegiac patient need to pay attention to?

Day 3

ASTHMA

Asthma is a condition characterized by reversible airway spasms and stenosis with increased bronchial reactivity through neurohumoral feedback triggered by allergens or non-allergic factors. Typical clinical manifestations include paroxysmal expiratory wheezing and breathing difficulty that can last from several minutes to several hours, and is alleviated after receiving treatment; asthma is sometimes self-limiting. In severe cases, the symptoms can last for several days to several weeks, or there may be repeated episodes. Its long-term, recurrent disease course can often lead to complications such as chronic bronchitis and emphysema. Asthma can occur at any age with more than half of onsets before the age of 12 years. The incidence rates of adult men and women are roughly the same.

In Chinese medical practice, the name for asthma is *xiào chuǎn*. *Xiào* means wheezing while *chuǎn* can be translated to mean panting or labored breathing. It is also known as *shàng qì*, meaning abnormal rising of qi. Medical professionals in the past once divided the disease into two categories. *Orthodox Medicine Science* (*Yī Xué Zhèng Chuán*, 医学正传) states that "*chuǎn* is to describe the breathing, [while] *xiào* gets the name from its sound (喘以气息言，哮以声响名)." However, it is often difficult to completely distinguish *xiào* and *chuǎn* clinically. For example, in the same patient, it seems like panting if the onset is mild while in a severe attack, the patient would be wheezing. At the same time, the etiology and disease mechanisms of *xiào* and *chuǎn*, from the point of view of Chinese medical practice, are basically the same. Therefore, they will be discussed as one topic.

The etiology and pathogenesis of the disease are not yet fully understood. However, genetic and allergic constitutions are greatly associated with the disease. Most patients have a history of infantile eczema, allergic rhinitis, and allergies to certain foods and drugs. In some cases though, there is no family member or close relative having a history of allergies.

Clinical Manifestations

Prior to the onset of exogenous or allergic asthma, the patient may experience nasal and throat itching, sneezing, chest tightness, and coughing, often induced by inhaling pollen, organic dust, and cold air. In endogenous or infection-induced asthma, the attack can be triggered by upper respiratory tract infection. Drugs such as aspirin, indomethacin, and propranolol can also induce the attack, while exercise is another trigger. The typical manifestations are sudden breathing difficulties and extensive wheezing of the lungs. Labored breathing can be alleviated in a few minutes or hours followed by spitting up a large amount of sticky sputum. Some patients may have irritable coughs as the main symptom. Last but not least, a patient is experiencing status asthmaticus if the following situations exist: a regular treatment is ineffective, there is extreme difficulty in breathing, the asthma attack lasts for more than 24 hours, and there is irritability, disturbance of consciousness, sweating, and cyanosis.

Diagnosis and Differentiation

Diagnosis

The diagnosis is fairly simple. The majority of patients have a history of recurrent episodes of bronchial asthma attack accompanied by expiratory dyspnea and pulmonary wheezing in general. The asthma attack can be alleviated with a bronchial antispasmodic agent.

Differential Diagnosis

1. *Cardiac asthma* Patients have a history of hypertension, coronary heart disease, or mitral stenosis and other symptoms; there may be frothy hemoptysis sputum; moist rales can be heard on the bottom of both lungs; chest X-rays detect cardiac enlargement and pulmonary congestion.
2. *Lung cancer* There is often a lack of predisposing factors for the breathing difficulty in patients. Symptoms usually become severe

progressively. Patients with lung cancer do not show a significant response to bronchodilators. Their sputum is bloody with cancer cells detected in it. CT scans and fiber bronchoscopy can be used in further differential diagnosis.

Treatment

First, determine if the disease shows an excess or a deficiency pattern. If, during an asthma attack there is phlegm blocking the airways with the lung qi failing to descending, it reveals an exopathogenic excess pattern. On the other hand, if the disease is recurrent, leading to depleted qi and yin and gradual deficiency of the lung, spleen and kidney, it is then a foundational deficient pattern. In treating asthma, tui na is mainly used in its remission phase. With the combination of qi gong and tui na manipulations, the patient can boost qi, fortify the spleen, and strengthen the kidney, leading to the improvement of the overall physical condition and immune function.

1. *Treatment principles*: boosting qi, fortifying the spleen, and strengthening the kidney.
2. *Commonly used maneuvers* scrubbing, finger kneading, rubbing, and grasping.
3. *Commonly used acupoints and areas dìng chuǎn* (EX-B 1), *fèi shū* (BL 13), *pí shū* (BL 20), *shèn shū* (BL 23), *mìng mén* (DU 4), *zhōng fǔ* (LU 1), *yún mén* (LU 2), *nèi guān* (PC 6), *yú jì* (LU 10), *zú sān lǐ* (ST 36), *fēng lóng* (ST 40), the chest, and the hypochondria.
4. *Operational methods*

   Basic operations

   a. The patient is supine, with the clinician sitting to the patient's right. First, apply finger-rubbing on both sides of *zhōng fǔ* and *yún mén* under the subclavian fossa to promote the flow of lung qi for one to two minutes each side. Then, apply finger-kneading on *dàn zhōng* (RN 17) to loosen the chest and rectify qi for one to two minutes. Apply thenar-kneading on *qì hǎi* (RN 6) and *guān yuán* (RN 4) on the lower abdomen to warm and supplement kidney qi for three to five minutes to end the operation of the chest and abdomen.

b. With the position of the patient remaining unchanged, use finger-kneading on both *nèi guān* for one minute to loosen the chest and resolve agitation, then on both *zú sān lǐ* for about a minute or two in order to fortify the spleen.
c. Ask the patient to sit, with the practitioner standing to the lateral or rear side. Apply double-finger kneading on *dìng chuǎn*, *fèi shū*, *pí shū*, *shèn shū*, and *mìng mén*, one to two minutes per acupoint. This manipulation calms labored breathing, fortifies the spleen, and strengthens the kidney. then, use the hypothenar as the focal point and apply scrubbing on the hypochondria with a top-down order repeatedly, followed by horizontal scrubbing on *shèn shū* and *mìng mén* until the frictional heat is felt.
d. For a patient with labored breathing, add finger-kneading on the bilateral *yú jì* until the soreness *de*-qi sensation is achieved; start gently and gradually increase the force, depending on the tolerance range of the patient. In addition, the same bilateral finger-kneading manipulation can also be used on *fēng lóng*. Lastly, you may enhance the operation on *dìng chuǎn* and *fèi shū* with bilateral finger-kneading.

Self-Preventional Methods

1. Apply finger-kneading on *nèi guān*, *yú jì*, *zú sān lǐ*, *fēng long,* and so on, one to two minutes per acupoint until the *de*-qi sensation is felt.
2. Apply finger-rubbing on *zhōng fǔ*, *yún mén*, *dàn zhōng,* and so forth, one to two minutes per acupoint.
3. Apply finger-kneading on every intercostal space, and scrubbing on the hypochondria.
4. Be persevering with costal and abdominal breathing exercises.

Precautions

1. Remove inducing factors to reduce the opportunity of the onset of an attack.

2. Put more emphasis on comprehensive treatment during the remission period.
3. Improve immunity to diseases. Receive desensitization and bacterination.
4. Pay attention to the impact of the climate, avoid exposure to cold, keep warm, and avoid exterior inducing factors.
5. Avoid tobacco, alcohol, and greasy, sour, spicy, fishy, and odorous food.
6. Avoid overwork and emotional stimulations.

Everyday Exercises

1. What is asthma?
2. How should tui na treatment be carried out at the remission stage of asthma?
3. Memorize the self-preventative measures and precautions for asthma.

PERSISTENT HICCUPS

Hiccups are caused by inverse qi rushing upwards, resulting in short and frequently repeated sounds from the throat that cannot be controlled. In ancient literature, it is referred to as *yuě* (哕) or *yuě nì* (哕逆). Hiccups can vary in terms of severity. If a bout of hiccups is occasional, mostly it is mild and disappears on its own. It can also be stopped by stimulating the nose to induce a sneeze, making a sudden noise to intimidate the sufferer, or holding the breath for a while.

However, when it is persistent and cannot be stopped, then we need to give appropriate treatment to relieve it after determining if it is of cold, heat, deficiency, or excess pattern. If hiccups appear in the severe stage of acute or chronic diseases, it is a harbinger of the patient's condition turning critical, entering a so-called stage of "failure of the stomach earth (土败胃绝)." When it happens, the prognosis is poor, so the healthcare worker should pay close attention to such patients.

In Chinese medical practice, the fundamental etiology of hiccups is inversed stomach qi affecting the diaphragm. The root causes leading to disharmony of the stomach and its failure to descend its qi may include interior accumulation of cold qi, excessive interior dryness and heat, stagnant qi with blockage of phlegm, and deficiency of qi and blood.

In addition, if the lung fails to disperse and raise qi, it could also contribute to the onset of hiccups.

Clinical Manifestations

1. *Accumulation of cold qi* The sound of the hiccups is deep, slow and strong; there is discomfort of the epigastric area that can be reduced with heat, and aggravated with cold; other symptoms include an absence of thirst, a white tongue coating, and a slow or moderate pulse.
2. *Dryness and heat in the stomach* The sound of hiccups is loud, continuous, powerful, and rushing up; the sufferer has a desire for cold drinks, and has a red face, yellow tongue coating, and rapid pulse.
3. *Qi stagnation with phlegm blockage* The hiccups are continuous with distension and tightness of the hypochondria; the onset is related to gloom or exasperation; the hiccups are slightly alleviated when the sufferer is in a good mood; other symptoms include dizziness, vertigo; a thin greasy tongue coating, and a slippery pulse.
4. *Qi and blood deficiency* The sound of the hiccups is low and weak; the sufferer has a pale face, a pale tongue with white coating, and a weak thready pulse; the hands and feet are not warm.

Diagnosis

The diagnosis of hiccups is mainly based on its clinical manifestations, which is fairly clear.

Treatment

1. *Treatment principles* harmonizing the stomach, descending qi, calming hiccups.
   a. With stomach coldness: warming the center to dispel coldness.
   b. With stomach heat: draining the heat and unblocking the bowels.
   c. With qi stagnation and phlegm blockage: descending qi and transforming phlegm.
   d. With qi and blood deficiency: warming and fortifying the spleen and stomach.

2. *Commonly used maneuvers* pressing, rubbing, kneading, scrubbing, point pressing.
3. *Commonly used acupoints and areas* *quē pén* (ST 12), *tiān tū* (RN 22), *dàn zhōng* (RN 17), *zhōng wǎn* (RN 12), *zhāng mén* (LR 13), *qī mén* (LR 14), *gé shū* (BL 17), *wèi shū* (BL 21), and *nèi guān* (PC 6).
4. *Operational methods*

   Basic operations

   a. The patient is supine, with the practitioner sitting at the right side. Use the tip of the middle finger to apply pressure kneading on *quē pén*, one minute each side, until the patient feels the soreness *de*-qi sensation. Apply pressure kneading on *tiān tū* for half a minute followed by kneading and rubbing *dàn zhōng*, one minutes for each acupoint. All three points can comfort the chest and descend inverse qi.
   b. Apply kneading on *zhōng wǎn* and rubbing on both sides of *zhāng mén* and *qī mén*, each acupoint for a minute or two. Apply finger kneading on both sides of *nèi guan*.
   c. Have the patient change to a sitting position, with the practitioner standing at the back. Apply double-finger kneading to boths side of *gé shū* and *wèi shū*, for a minute per acupoint. It is better to get the soreness *de*-qi sensation. Lastly, perform scrubbing on the back and the hypochondria.

   Supplementing operations

   a. *With stomach coldness* Reinforce the kneading maneuver on *zhōng wǎn*, preferably until the patient feels the warmth at the epigastric area. Also, apply horizontal scrubbing on *wèi shū* until the patient feels the frictional heat.
   b. *With stomach heat* Apply pressing or point pressing on *shàng liào* (BL 31), *cì liào* (BL 32), and *yǒng quán* (KI 1), preferably until the patient gets the soreness *de*-qi feeling.
   c. *With qi stagnation and phlegm blockage* Apply rubbing on *zhōng fǔ* (LU 1) and *yún mén* (LU 2); reinforce kneading or rubbing on *zhāng mén* and *qī mén*. In addition, apply pressure kneading on *fēng lóng* (ST 40).

d. *With qi and blood deficiency* Apply knead-rubbing on *qì hǎi* (RN 6) and *guān yuán* (RN 4), spinal pinching, and pressure kneading on *nèi guān* and *zú sān lǐ* (ST 36).
e. *Frequent hiccups* Reinforce point or intense pressing on *gé shū* and *wèi shū*.

Precautions

1. Eat less raw, cold, acidic, and hot food.
2. Maintain emotional tranquility.

Everyday Exercises

1. How should tui na be performed for asthma in its remission period?
2. Memorize the self-preventional methods and precautions for asthma.
3. What are the fundamental causes of hiccups?
4. What are the basic tui na operations in treating hiccups?

Day 4

FACIAL *AN MO*

Facial *an mo*, also known as facial bathing in Chinese, can clean up the surface secretions and dead epithelial cells of the skin, improve its breathing ability, and promote blood circulation of the head and face. Furthermore, the operation regulates the secretion of sweat and sebaceous glands, smoothens and moistens the facial skin, enhances its elasticity, and delays its aging. It is a great way to refresh the memory, relieve tiredness of the eyes, and improve the appearance.

Facial *an mo* can be self-administered, or performed by another person. There are three commonly used facial *an mo* maneuvers.

Facial *An Mo* on Striped Muscles

Follow the direction of the skin striae and muscles (see Figures 194 and 195) and apply finger-kneading maneuver on the face (see Figure 196).

1. *Forehead* Use the pulps of middle fingers to apply finger-kneading with a spiral circular motion on the skin, starting from the center of the forehead and transitioning toward both sides of the temples where *tài yáng* (EX-HN 5) is located. Repeat the operation five to eight times.

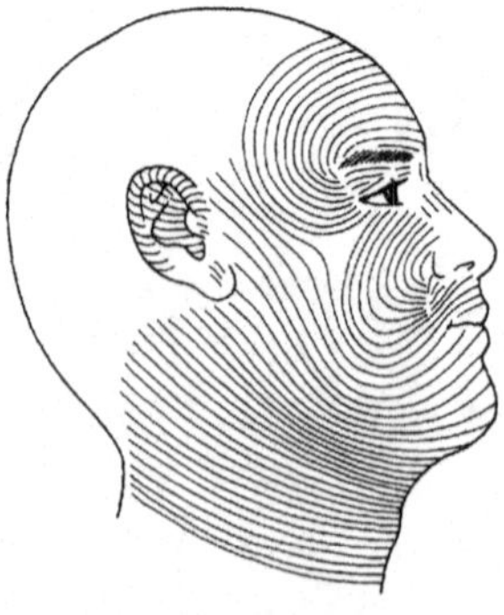

Figure 194 Skin striae

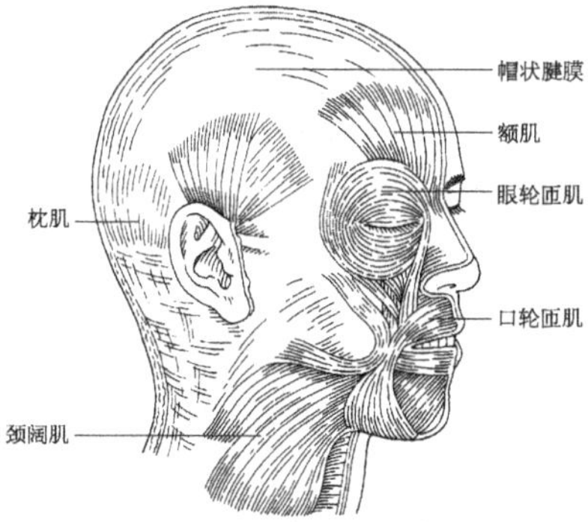

枕肌	-	occipitalis
颈阔肌	-	platysma
帽状腱膜	-	galea aponeurotica
额肌	-	frontalis
眼轮匝肌	-	orbicularis oculi
口轮匝肌	-	orbicularis oris

Figure 195 Facial and head muscles

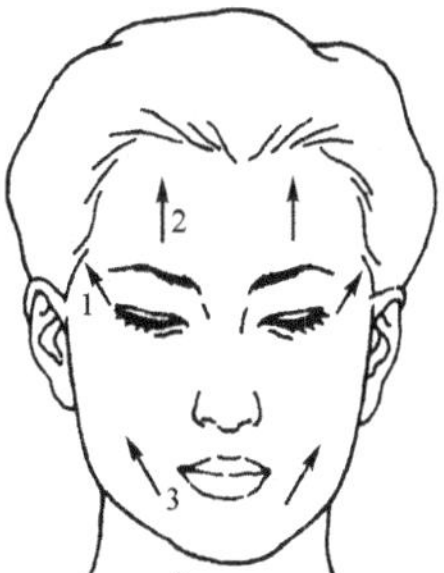

Figure 196 Finger kneading maneuver

2. *Cheeks* Apply finger-kneading using the pulps of the index, middle, and ring fingers with a spiral circular motion. Start from the corners of the mouth, gradually moving to the cheek, then the outer canthus. The bottom-up operation needs to be repeated five to eight times.
3. *Nasal area* Apply pressure rubbing with the middle fingers, up and down between both wings of the nose and the nasion three to five times.

4. *Mandibles* Rub in a spiral circular motion from the mandibular angle to the front lobe on both sides five to eight times.
5. *Orbital area* Use the pulps of the middle finger to rub around the edge of the orbits in a spiral circular motion four to five times. Avoid the eyes.
6. *Around the lips* Operate around the upper and lower lips with a spiral circular motion four to five times in a clockwise direction.

Acupressure Method

Figure 197 shows the facial acupoints.

1. Apply acupressure on *yìn táng* (EX-HN 3), *shén tíng* (GV 24), *tóu wéi* (ST 8), and *tài yáng* (EX-HN 5). Start with gentle force, gradually increase the intensity, and then decrease it. Each acupoint should be pressed four to five times.
2. Apply acupressure on *cuán zhú* (BL 2), *jīng míng* (BL 1), *yú yāo* (EX-HN 4), *sī zhú kōng* (SJ 23), *tóng zǐ liáo* (GB 1), *chéng qì* (ST 1), and *sì bái* (ST 2). The force of the operation should be gentle initially, and gradually increased and decreased. Each acupoint should be pressed four to five times.
3. Use both palms to perform lift-smearing of the skin around the eyes while the middle finger pulls up both canthi four to five times (see Figure 198).

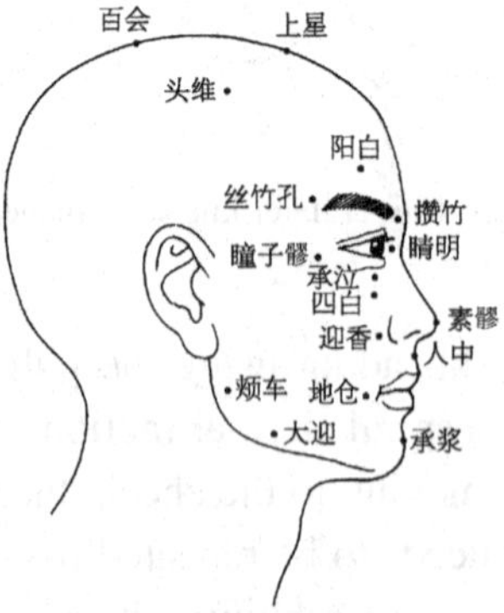

Figure 197 Facial acupoints

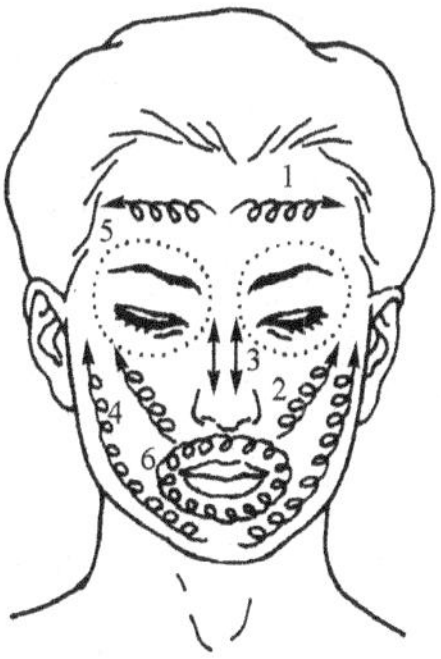

1. 提拉眼角	-	Lift-pulling the Canthi
2. 拉摸额头	-	Lift-smearing the Forehead
3. □提拉下颌	-	Lift-pulling the Lower Cheeks

Figure 198 Facial lift-pulling maneuver

4. Carry out the lift-smearing maneuver on the forehead four to five times.
5. Apply point pressing on *kǒu hé liáo* (LI 19) three to five times and finger kneading between the wings of the nose to the nasion back and forth for three to five times.
6. Apply point pressing on *chéng jiāng* (RN 24), *dì cāng* (ST 4), *jiá chē* (ST 6), and *quán liào* (SI 18). The manipulation should be gentle to start with, and gradually increased and decreased. Each acupoint should be pressed four to five times.
7. Apply finger kneading on the chin from the front toward the back, four to five times, and apply lift-pulling on the chin four to five times.
8. Apply pinch kneading on the helix of both ears twice to three times from top to bottom, and apply pinching foulage on the ears four to five times.

Loose Patting

With the wrist relaxed, use the finger pulp as the focal point and loosely pat the skin of the head and face to make the facial skin tight and elastic. This maneuver uses the power of the wrist and should be gentle and continuous. The upper eyelid should not be patted while the eyebrow area can be patted with the tip of the middle finger. On the lower eyelid, the orbitae is the site receiving the manipulation.

The following is the sequence of loose patting: right forehead → left forehead → left cheekbone → left cheek → left chin → right chin → right cheek → right cheekbone → right forehead. Repeat the sequence three or four times.

Eye: first, apply loose tapping on both eyebrows, and then on the lower orbitae.

Lips: first, apply loose tapping above the upper lips, and then the lower lips.

Loose patting and tapping on facial areas should be from the center to both sides.

Precautions

1. Facial *an mo* should be gentle, stable, and rhythmic.
2. The main maneuver of facial *an mo* is using the pulps of the middle and ring fingers of both hands to slide on the surface of the face.
3. The intensity of the force should be light to avoid the skin looking wrinkled while being pushed.
4. If the person wears makeup, use makeup removal cream or lotion on cotton swabs to remove the makeup. Then, use facial cleanser to clean the forehead, nose, cheeks, chins, ears, and neck. Next, wash the cleanser off, and remove excessive water with a dry towel or facial tissue. Lastly, facial *an mo* can be carried out.

Everyday Exercises

1. Learn the basic principles of facial *an mo* operations.
2. Learn the main points of the three operations of facial *an mo*.

Day 5

PEDIATRIC TUI NA

Pediatric tui na is an important component of Chinese medical massage. Its basic techniques and clinical applications have some unique characteristics.

Subject 1 – Overview

Physiological Characteristics of Children

Small children are rapidly growing. On the other hand, their *zang-fu* organs are delicate while their physiques and qi are not sufficient enough. From birth, children experience continuous growth, becoming stronger every day. According to an ancient saying, children in this rapid development stage is said to have "body of pure yang (纯阳之体)." However, another ancient saying is that, just like tender buds, children have "tender and insufficient yang, tender and underdeveloped yin (稚阳未充，稚阴未长)." This means children are not yet competent in either the materialistic or physiological functions, so that they need special care.

Pathological Characteristics of Children

In children, diseases have the pathological manifestations of acute onset, drastic fluctuations; and rapid recovery with the correct treatment. Children are prone to the six external pathogens and internal damage due to an improper diet because of their fragile constitution and immature physical functions, inability to add or reduce clothes, and inability control their diet. They usually cannot tolerate a sudden strong stimulus and are easily panic-stricken. In addition, any congenital deficiency or acquired disorders can often cause developmental disorders, including the five retardations and five debilities defined in traditional Chinese medicine. Moreover, because of the poor immunity of children, they are especially susceptible to measles, mumps, whooping cough, and other infectious diseases. When they get sick, the symptoms are often more severe than in adults, and can include high fever, seizures, and convulsions. If they contract a wind-cold pathogen, it could easily lead to pneumonia, labored breathing, and coughing. In general, pediatric illnesses are often acute with rapid and diverse changes, and may be complicated by otherr serious diseases and symptoms. At the same time, if they get correct treatment and appropriate care in a timely manner, it is easier for them to heal, compared to adults.

Characteristics of Pattern Differentiation in Children

Very young children are incapable of explaining their disease conditions. Therefore, the inquiry has to be indirect, and may not precisely reflect the actual situation. Although older children are able to talk, often they cannot describe the situation accurately. Secondly, qi and blood of infants are not plentiful, so it is hard to take the pulse, especially when they cannot stay still and sometimes cries during the diagnostic examination. Listening and smelling can detect some problems but these methods are not comprehensive enough.

Observation is the only diagnostic method in traditional Chinese medicine that does not have restrictions and can be used in all circumstances, thus, it is highly emphasized in pediatric TCM. Besides, from the aspect of the eight-principle pattern differentiation, young children have relatively more excessive yang qi. When they contract external cold pathogen, it is easy to transform to heat and result in yang, heat, or excess patterns. The following paragraphs will highlight several characteristic pediatric diagnostic methods.

Observing Infantile Finger Venules

Finger venules refer to the visible superficial blood vessels on the radial palmar side of the index finger that can be seen in children. These vessels belong to a branch of the hand *taiyin* lung meridian. Therefore, there are similarities in terms of clinical significance between the palmar venule of the index finger and *cun kou* pulse. It is somewhat difficult to take an accurate pulse reading, as the *cun kou* pulse of infants is very short and tiny, and they may cry when their pulse is taken. On the other hand, because the skin of the finger venule area is thin and tender and easily exposed, the finger venule is a great auxiliary diagnostic method for children under the age of three.

There are three *guan* (sections) of the finger venule: *feng* (wind), qi, and *ming* (life). The section nearest the palm is *feng guan*, the proximal interphalangeal section belongs to qi *guan*, and the distal interphalangeal section pertains to *ming guan* (see Figure 199).

Methods to expose the finger venule Have the child's palm fully exposed in natural light. Use your left thumb and forefinger to hold the distal part of the index finger, and your right thumb to push a few times from its tip to the base along the radial side with moderate force. This way, the finger venule is more obvious and easy to be observed.

Content of finger venule observation The three main aspects in observing and analyzing the finger venule are color and luster, length, and depth.

1. *Color and luster* The color of a normal finger venule is light red, and it appears underneath the skin at *feng guan*. When the child is ill, bright red mostly indicates externally contracted wind-cold pattern while purplish red usually reveals heat patterns. Dark purple signifies a critical condition with blockage of blood vessels, while pallor is mostly the sign of deficiency. A dull color indicates an excess pattern, and a bluish green color is usually the sign of pain or infantile convulsions.
2. *Length* In general, a venule within the scope of *feng guan* demonstrates that the pathogen is at a superficial level and it is a minor illness.

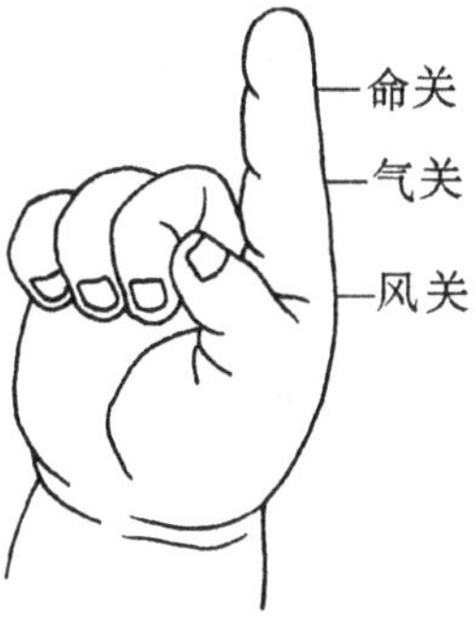

命关	-	*ming guan*
气关	-	qi *guan*
风关	-	*ming guan*

Figure 199 Three *guan* of infantile finger venule

If it extends to qi *guan*, it indicates that the pathogen has penetrated to a deeper level. When it reaches the *ming guan*, the condition is relatively severe. Lastly, when the venule goes up all the way to the finger tip next to the nail, it implies a critical condition.

3. *Depth* For those with superficial venule, the disease is of an exterior disease pattern. Otherwise, it indicates an interior pattern if it is insidious and not obvious.

In modern medicine, the way of observing the finger venule is to inspect the superficial veins on the radial side of the index finger for signs of the degree of fullness related to the venous pressure. Most children suffering heart failure and pneumonia have the venule extending toward *ming guan,* caused by increase venous pressure. The higher the venous pressure, the greater the fullness level of the veins, with the venule more extended in the direction of the fingertip. In addition, the color and luster may reflect in vivo hypoxia to some extent. The more severe hypoxia is, the higher the deoxygenated hemoglobin in the blood, resulting in more obvious purplish-blue venules. Thus, children with pneumonia and heart failure mostly show purplish-blue or purple finger venules. On the other hand, children with anemia have decreased RBCs and hemoglobin, so that their venules are light in color.

Pediatric Pulse Taking

The forearms of an infant are short, so that the *cun kou* area for pulse taking is even shorter, disallowing the three-finger method of taking the *cun, guan,* and *chi* pulses. Instead of dividing the *cun kou* into three portions, the alternative for infants is to use a finger or the thumb to determine all three section of the pulse, the so-called "determining the three *guan* with one finger" method (see Figure 200). The normal pulse of an infant is faster than that of an adult. In general, in children between the ages of one and two years old, the pulse beats six to seven times for every inhalation and exhalation cycle. The number becomes five to six times between the ages of three and six years old. As they get older, the pulse rate decreases accordingly. In pediatric pulse taking, the patterns of exterior, interior, cold, and heat are determined by superficial, deep, slow, and rapid

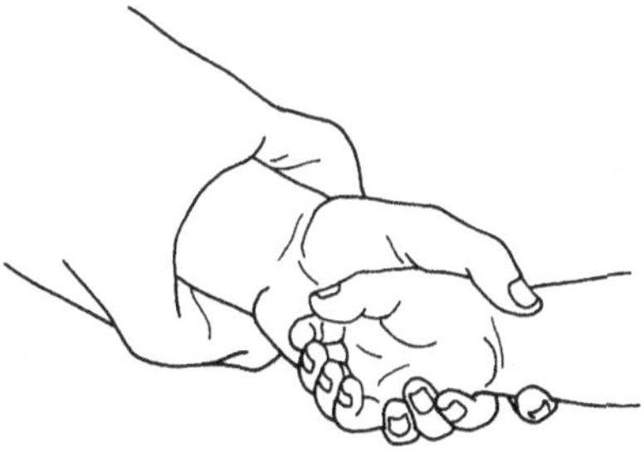

拇指直推	-	straight pushing using the thumb
食、中指直推	-	straight pushing using index and middle fingers

Figure 200 Determining the three *guan* with one finger

respectively, while powerful and powerless determine whether the pattern is excess or deficient.

1. *Superficial pulse*: can be clearly felt on the surface of the skin by placing the finger with minimal force, indicating exterior patterns.
2. *Deep pulse*: hard to feel while pressing it with minimal force. The finger needs to press down deeply to sense it, indicating interior patterns.
3. *Slow pulse*: slower than a normal child of the same age, indicating cold patterns.
4. *Rapid pulse*: faster than a normal child of the same age, indicating heat patterns.
5. *Powerful pulse*: excess patterns.
6. *Weak pulse*: deficienct patterns.

Everyday Exercises

1. Learn the physiological and pathological characteristics of small children.
2. What is infantile finger venule? What are the methods of observing and analyzing it?
3. What is the so-called "determining the three *guan* with one finger"? How would you differentiate patterns based on three *guan* venules?

Day 6

Subject 2 – Common Maneuvers in Pediatric Tui Na

Commonly used maneuvers in pediatric tui na have their own characteristics. The major maneuvers are pushing, revolving, pinching, and nailing.

Pushing

Pushing has a wide range of clinical applications in pediatric tui na. There are four types of pushing: straight pushing, disjoining pushing, joining pushing, and circling pushing.

1. *Straight pushing* Use the radial edge of the thumb or both pulps of the index and middle fingers as the focal point on the treatment area to perform one-way pushing along a straight line from point A to point B. (See Figure 201.)

   The manipulation should be light, agile and continuous as a broom sweeping the floor, preferably without making the skin turn red. The frequency needs to be between 250 and 300 times per minute. Push along a straight line and avoid skewed strokes to prevent other meridians from being affected by the operation.

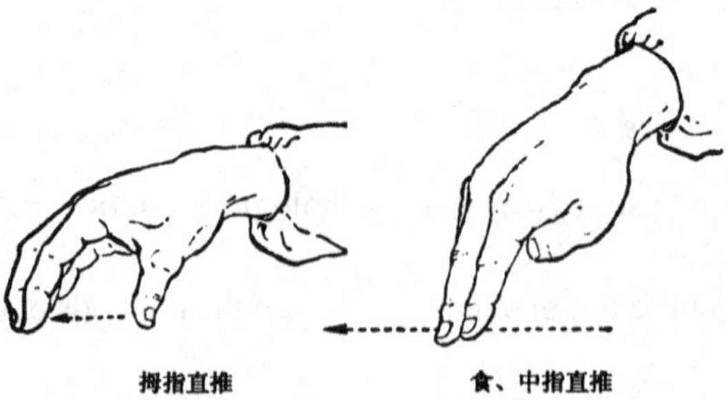

Figure 201 Straight pushing

a. *Applications*: commonly used on specific tui na points including linear points and five-meridian points.
b. *Efficacies*: clearing heat, releasing the exterior, resolving diarrhea, easing defecation, relieving restlessness, and calming the *shen* (spirit).
c. *Indications*: exogenous fever, diarrhea, constipation, panic, fright, irritability.

2. *Disjoining pushing* Use the pulps of both thumbs on the acupoint seen as the center point A, and push towards both sides of point B. This is known as the disjoining pushing or the disjoining maneuver. The force applied with both hands needs to be even, gentle, and coordinated; this maneuver is generally done for 20 to 30 minutes.

a. *Applications*: commonly used on the forehead, chest, abdomen, back, wrist, and palm.
b. *Efficacies*: rectifying qi and blood, regulating yin and yang.
c. *Indications*: fever, coughs, bloating, constipation.

3. *Joining pushing* Joining pushing, also known as joining, is the opposite of disjoining pushing; here the direction of pushing is from both sides of a symmetric point B to a center point A.

The requirements of the maneuver are the same as in disjoining but in the opposite direction.

a. *Applicable areas*: same as disjoining.
b. *Efficacies*: regulating yin and yang, rectifying qi and blood.
c. *Indications*: fever, abdominal distension, constipation.

Clinically, joining is often used in conjunction with disjoining; they are complementary to each other.

4. *Circling pushing* Place the thumb pulp on the acupoint to be treated, and perform pushing with a clockwise circular motion like this: (插入图画)

This maneuver should only affect the surface of the skin, not the subcutaneous tissues. The frequency should be 150 to 200 times per minute.

a. *Applicable areas*: mainly used on five-meridian points.
b. *Efficacies*: fortifying the spleen, harmonizing the stomach, supplementing the lung and benefiting the kidney.

c. *Indications*: deficiency of the spleen and stomach, indigestion, coughs owing to lung deficiency and other pediatric deficiencies.

Revolving

Revolving is a maneuver that applies curvy or circular pushes on the treatment site (see Figure 202). As it is a kind of pushing maneuver, some people refer to it as revolving pushing. It is also a commonly used technique in pediatric tui na.

In practice, the practitioner should place the palmar surface of the thumb or middle finger on the acupoint, and perform revolving pushing along a curvy or circular path from acupoint A to B, or around one acupoint again and again.

It looks like this (插入图画) or this (插入图画).

The revolving maneuver needs to be applied with gentle but not heavy force; friction should be created only on the surface of the skin and not move into the subcutaneous tissues. Secondly, it is appropriate to keep the frequency low, approximately 80 to 100 times per minute.

a. *Application:* on arc- or round-shaped tui na points.
b. *Efficacies*: clearing heat, relieving restlessness, soothing the chest, and rectifying qi.

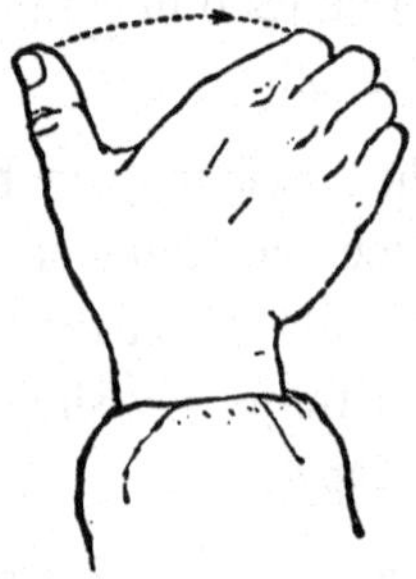

Figure 202 Revolving

Table 21 Similarities and differences between revolving and circling pushing maneuvers

	Similarities	Differences
Revolving	Both pushes in circular motions on body surface.	Bigger range of moves with lower frequency of 80 to 100 times per minute
Circling pushing	Neither drives force into subcutaneous tissues	Smaller range of moves with higher frequency of 160 to 200 times per minute

c. *Indications*: fever, chest tightness, vomiting.

Table 21 shows the similarities and differences between the revolving and circling pushing maneuvers.

Pinching

Pinching is a tui na maneuver of using the thumb and other fingers to squeeze and twiddle the treatment area symmetrically. When pinching is applied along the spine, it is called spinal pinching or pinching *jí*. Because it is a marvelous method of treating infantile malnutrition with accumulation, it is also known as the accumulation pinching method. Here we introduce two operational methods of spinal pinching (see Figure 203).

1. Make a fist with the dorsum of the middle knuckle of the index finger tightly attached to the spine of the child, and the thumb extended straight facing the radiopalmar of the middle knuckle of the index finger. Then, pinch and lift the skin, squeeze and twiddle it, and gradually move forwards with both hands operating alternately (see Figure 203a).
2. Have both wrists hanging, thumbs extending straightly to face the pulps of the index and middle fingers. Attach the pulp of one thumb closely to the spine of the child, and the other two fingers apply the force against the thumb to lift and pinch the skin on the spine. At the same time, squeeze and twiddle it with both hands alternately, and slowly move forward (see Figure 203b).

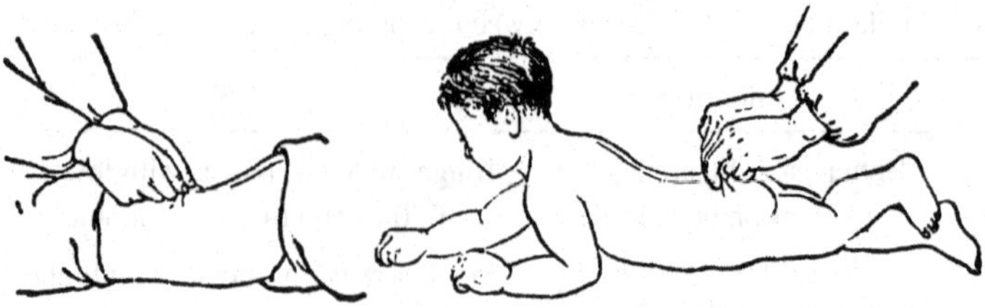

(a) (b)

Figure 203 Spinal pinching

The operation of spinal pinching usually starts from *guī wěi*, goes up along the spine, and ends at *dà zhuī* (DU 14). Repeat continuously for five to six times. Depending on the disease, if the child needs enhanced stimulation, the method of triple-pinching plus one lifting is commonly applied. That is, complete pinching the entire spine in the first round. In the second round, lift up the skin or on important acupoints such as *fèi shū* (BL 13), *pí shū* (BL 20), and *shèn shū* (BL 23) after every three forward pinches, with adequate force using both hands level. While the skin is pulled and lifted, a crisp clattering sound can be heard, which is normal and indicates the fascia being stripped.

In addition, the focal point of pinching is the whole palmar side of the thumb pulp instead of the tip of the thumb, and the skin should not be twisted at the same time. If there is too much skin being lifted and pinched, the action will be sluggish and it will be difficult to move forward. If too little skin is pinched, the skin is not easy to hold on to and slips out easily. Moreover, overly intensive force causes pain while too gentle force makes it harder to have the *de*-qi sensation.

a. *Applications*

- Commonly used for pediatric care, improving appetite, and improving physique.
- In addition to being used in pediatric tui na, spinal pinching has the same therapeutic effect in treating insomnia, neurasthenia, chronic gastrointestinal dysfunction, and lassitude in adult patients.

b. *Efficacies*: adjusting yin and yang, unblocking the meridians and collaterals, fortifying the spleen and harmonizing the stomach, promoting the circulation of qi and blood, improving the function of organs, and enhancing the body's resistance to diseases.
c. *Indications*: infantile malnutrition with accumulation, indigestion, rickets, diarrhea.

Nailing

This is the maneuver of using a thumb nail to press on the body surface of the treatment area. It is characterized by strong stimulation and focused power, and is often seen as a substitute for acupuncture needles, so that it is also known as the finger-nail puncturing maneuver. It can be used in patients with syncope during first aid.

While performing this maneuver, the thumb-nail should be perpendicular to the point being treated and the force should be firm and powerful. However, to avoid skin damage, the nail should not move in a forward-backward motion. After the application of the finger-nail pressing, kneading the area is often performed in order to ease the strong stimulation and reduce pain. The manipulation is generally performed five to six times, or when the condition is eased. It is not appropriate to prolong the operation.

a. *Applications*: head, face and sensitive pain points on hands and feet, such as *shuǐ gōu* (DU 26), *lǎo lóng,* and *shí wáng*.
b. *Efficacies*: opening the orifices, refreshing the brain, rescuing yang from its inverse escaping.
c. *Indications*: infantile convulsions, fainting, and syncope.

Everyday Exercises

1. How many pushing methods are there in pediatric tui na? How would you perform each of them?
2. What are the similarities and differences between the revolving and circling pushing maneuvers?
3. Describe the two operational methods of spinal pinching.

WEEK 12

Day 1

Subject 3 — Common Acupoints in Pediatric Tui Na

One characteristic of pediatric tui na is that, in addition to the use of acupoints of the 14 meridians and extra points, there are many specific points unique to pediatric tui na, including not only point-like acupoints, but also line-shaped points and surface areas. The second characteristic of pediatric tui na is that there are quite a number of points concentrated in both hands, as the Chinese saying goes, "in children, all vessels converge in the palms (小儿百脉汇于两掌)."

Week 12 will focus on locating pediatric tui na points (see Figures 204 and 205), methods of operation, number of times the maneuver is performed, indications, and clinical applications. The number of times indicated for a maneuver only serves as a reference guide in the clinical treatment of children aged six months to one year. It needs to be increased or decreased based on the child's age, physical strength, and disease severity.

(a)

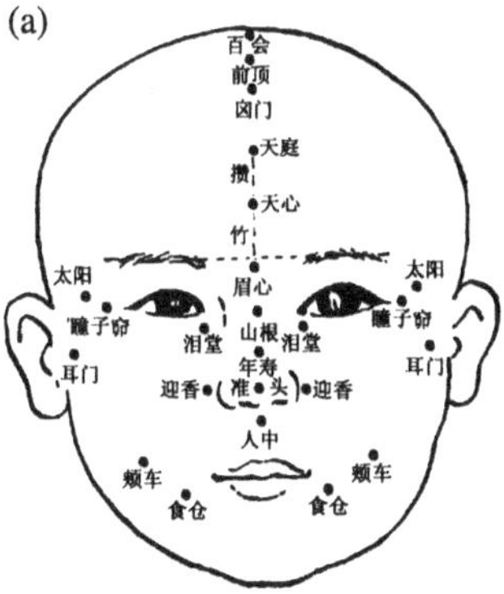

(a) Pediatric head points

百会	-	*bǎi huì*	泪堂	-	*lèi táng*
前顶	-	*qián dǐng*	瞳子髎	-	*tóng zǐ liáo*
囟门	-	*xìn mén*	耳门	-	*ěr mén*
天庭	-	*tiān tíng*	迎香	-	*yíng xiāng*
攒竹	-	*cuán zhú*	年寿(准头)	-	*nián shòu (zhǔn tóu)*
天心	-	*tiān xīn*	迎香	-	*yíng xiāng*
太阳	-	*tài yáng*	耳门	-	*ěr mén*
眉心	-	*méi xīn*	人中	-	*rén zhōng*
太阳	-	*tài yáng*	颊车	-	*jiá chē*
瞳子髎	-	*tóng zǐ liáo*	食仓	-	*shí cāng*
泪堂	-	*lèi táng*	食仓	-	*shí cāng*
山根	-	*shān gēn*	颊车	-	*jiá chē*

Figure 204 Pediatric Tui Na acupoints

(*Continued*)

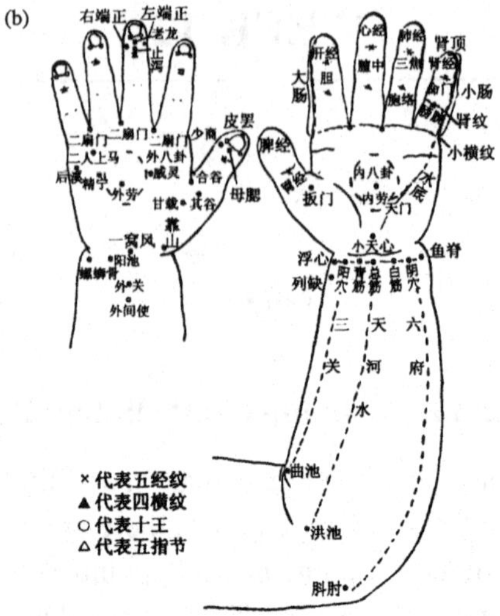

b. Pediatric hand points (dorsal side) b. Pediatric hand and arm points (palm side)

右端正	- *yòu duān zhèng*	脾经	- *pí jīng*	鱼脊	- *yú jǐ*
左端正	- *zuǒ duān zhèng*	胃经	- *wèi jīng*	三关	- *sān guān*
老龙	- *lǎo lóng*	板门	- *bǎn mén*	天河水	- *tiān hé shuǐ*
止泻	- *zhǐ xiè*	大肠	- *dà cháng*	六府	- *liù fǔ*
二扇门	- *èr shàn mén*	肝经	- *gān jīng*	曲池	- *qǔ chí*
二扇门	- *èr shàn mén*	胆	- *bǎn mén*	洪池	- *hóng chí*
二扇门	- *èr shàn mén*	心经	- *xīn jīng*	肼肘	- *jǐng zhǒu*
少商	- *shào shāng*	膻中	- *dàn zhōng*		
皮罢	- *pí bà*	内八卦	- *nèi bā guà*	Legend	
二人上马	- *èr rén shàng mǎ*	内劳	- *nèi láo*	x 代表五经纹	- *wǔ jīng* creases
外八卦	- *wài bā guà*	肺经	- *fèi jīng*	▲ 代表四横纹	- four transverse creases
母腮	- *mǔ sāi*	三焦	- *sān jiāo*	O代表十王	- *shí wáng* points
后溪	- *hòu xī*	胞络	- *bāo luò*	Δ代表五指节	- five finger knuckles
精宁	- *jīng níng*	肾顶	- *shèn dǐng*		
威灵	- *wēi líng*	肾经	- *shèn jīng*		
合谷	- *hé gǔ*	命门	- *mìng mén*		
外劳	- *wài láo*	肾纹	- *shèn wén*		
甘载	- *gān zǎi*	膀胱	- *páng guāng*		
其谷	- *qí gǔ*	小横纹	- *xiǎo héng wén*		
一窝风	- *yī wō fēng*	浮心	- *fú xīn*		
靠山	- *kào shān*	阳穴	- *yáng xué*		
螺狮骨	- *luó shī gǔ*	青筋	- *qīng jīn*		
阳池	- *yáng chí*	总筋	- *zǒng jīn*		
外关	- *wài guān*	白筋	- *bài jīn*		
外间使	- *wài jiān shǐ*	阴穴	- *yīn xué*		

Figure 204 Pediatric Tui Na acupoints

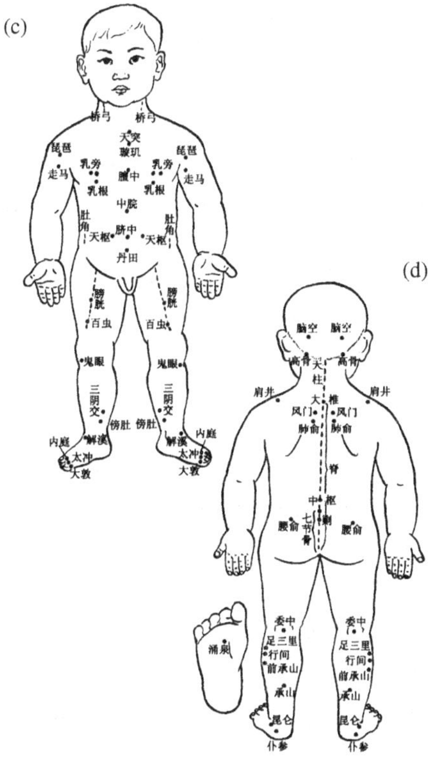

c. Front of the body							
桥弓	*qiáo gōng*	桥弓	*qiáo gōng*	天突	*tiān tū*	琵琶	*pí pá*
璇玑	*xuán jī*	琵琶	*pí pá*	走马	*zǒu mǎ*	乳旁	*rǔ páng*
膻中	*dán zhōng*	乳旁	*rǔ páng*	走马	*zǒu mǎ*	乳根	*rǔ gēn*
乳根	*rǔ gēn*	中脘	*zhōng wǎn*	肚角	*dù jiǎo*	天枢	*tiān shū*
脐中	*qí zhōng*	天枢	*tiān shū*	肚角	*dù jiǎo*	丹田	*dān tián*
膀胱	*páng guāng*	膀胱	*páng guāng*	百虫	*bǎi chóng*	百虫	*bǎi chóng*
鬼眼	*guǐ yǎn*	鬼眼	*guǐ yǎn*	三阴交	*sān yīng jiāo*	三阴交	*sān yīng jiāo*
傍肚	*bàng dù*	傍肚	*bàng dù*	解溪	*ji✈xī*	解溪	*ji✈xī*
内庭	*nèi tíng*	内庭	*nèi ting*	太冲	*tài chōng*	大敦	*dà dūn*
大敦	*dà dūn*	太冲	*tài chōng*				
d. Back of the body, sole of the foot							
脑空	*nǎo kōng*	脑空	*nǎo kōng*	高骨	*gāo gǔ*	高骨	*gāo gǔ*
天柱	*tiān zhù*	肩井	*jiān jǐng*	大椎	*dà zhuī*	肩井	*jiān jǐng*
风门	*fēng mén*	风门	*fēng mén*	肺俞	*fèi shū*	肺俞	*fèi shū*
脊	*jǐ*	中枢	*zhōng shū*	腰俞	*yāo shū*	七节骨	*qī jié gǔ*
腰俞	*yāo shū*	委中	*wěi zhōng*	委中	*wěi zhōng*	足三里	*zú sān lǐ*
足三里	*zú sān lǐ*	行间		前承山	*qián chéng shān*	前承山	*qián chéng shān*
承山	*chéng shān*	承山	*chéng shān*	昆仑	*kūn lún*	昆仑	*kūn lún*
仆参	*pú cān*	仆参	*pú cān*	涌泉	*yǒng quán*		

Figure 205 Pediatric Tui Na acupoints

When operating on the acupuncture or tui na points of a child's upper limb, there is no difference for boys or girls. Usually, it is enough to work on only one hand, commonly the left one, but you can also work on the right one. The order of pediatric tui na is generally the head, face, upper extremities, chest, belly, back, and the lower limbs. In addition, the order can be altered according to the disease suffered by the child. At the same time, a certain procedure should be followed at the end such as encountering pain sensitive points or manipulating with a high level of stimulation in order to obtain coordination of the child.

Head and Facial Acupoints

cuán zhú (*tiān mén*, 攒竹, 天门): line-shaped tui na acupoint

Location Two straight lines from between the two eyebrows to the front hairline.

Operations Using both thumbs alternately, perform bottom-up pushing straight, also known as opening *tiān mén* (the heavenly gates) (see Figure 206).

Number of times 30 to 50 times.

Indications Cold, fever, headache, listlessness, fright due to sudden disturbance.

Clinical Applications

1. As a commonly used pediatric tui na maneuver, it is often combined with pushing *kăn gōng* and kneading *tài yáng* (EX-HN 5) and can be

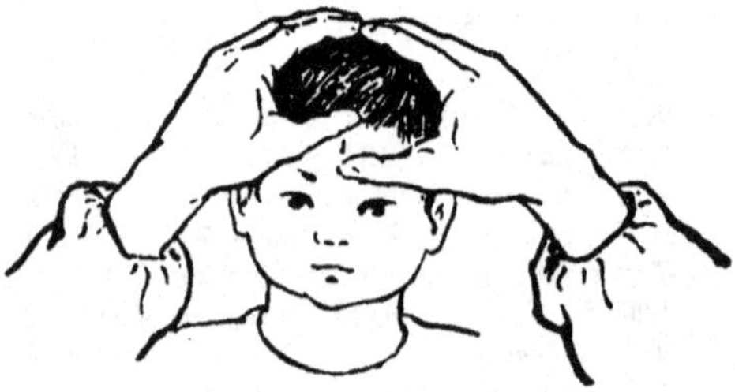

Figure 206 Pushing on *Cuán Zhú*, also known as opening *Tiān Mén*

used to treat either exterior patterns with exogenously contracted pathogens, or miscellaneous interior damage.

2. Fright owing to sudden disturbances, irritability: combine with clearing *gān jīng* and pressure kneading *bǎihuì* (DU 20).

kǎn gōng (*yīn yáng*, 坎宫, 阴阳): line-shaped point

Location Along the horizontal line from the inner ends of the eyebrows to the outer ends.

Operations Using both thumbs to perform disjoining pushing from the middle to both ends along *kǎn gōng* is known as pushing *kǎn gōng*, also known as disjoining *yīn yáng* (see Figure 207).

Number of times 30 to 50 times.

Indications Fever of exterior patterns with contracted pathogens, headache, and red eyes.

Clinical Applications

1. This is a commonly practiced techniques in pediatric tui na and can be used in both exterior pattern owing to externally contracted pathogens and miscellaneous interior damage.
2. If eyes are red and painful, it can be used in conjunction with clearing *gān jīng*, nailing *xiǎo tiān xīn,* and clearing *tiān hé shuǐ.*

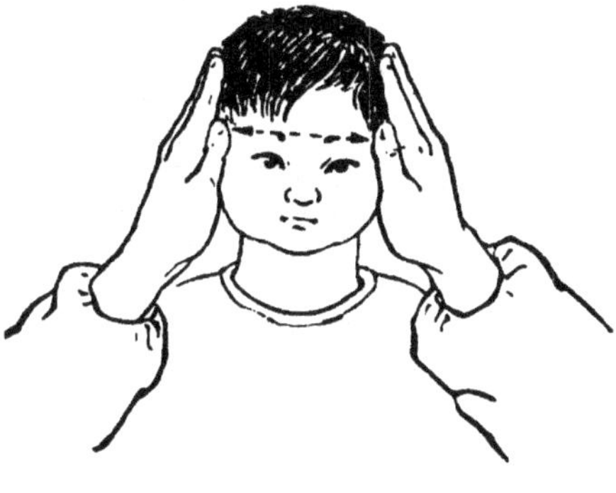

Figure 207 Pushing *Kǎn Gōng*, also known as disjoining *Yīn Yáng*

tàiyáng (EX-HN 5, 太阳): an acupoint that involves both a point and a line

Location In the depression posterior to the eyebrows of both sides.

Operations

1. *Pushing tài yang* Use the radial side of both thumbs to directly push the point in an anteroposterior direction.
2. *Kneading tài yáng or revolving tài yang* Use the tip of the middle finger to perform kneading or revolving on *tài yáng* (see Figure 208).

Number of times 30 to 50 times.

Indications Headache, fever, red and painful eyes.

Clinical Applications

1. It is a common maneuver in pediatric tui na for both exterior pattern with external contraction and interior damage.
2. For painful red eyes, pricking blood can be added to enhance the effect.

rén zhōng (also known as *shuĭ gōu*, DU 26, 人中, 水沟)

Location At the junction of the superior 1/3 and inferior 2/3 of the philtrum.

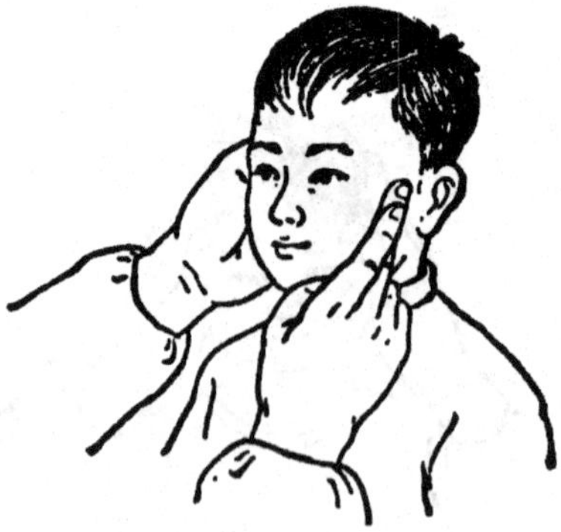

Figure 208 Kneading *Tài Yáng* (revolving *Tài Yáng*)

Operations Use the thumb nail to press it, known as nailing the *rén zhōng*.

Number of times 3 to 5 times or until the person is conscious.

Indications Convulsions, fainting, muscle jerking.

Clinical applications Mainly used in combination with nailing *shí xuān* (EX-UE 11) and *lǎo lóng* as first aid measures in conditions such as loss of consciousness, convulsion, and seizures.

yíng xiāng (LI 20, 迎香)

Location In the nasolabial groove, 0.5 cun from the border of the ala nasi.

Operations Kneading with the index and middle fingers, called kneading *yíng xiāng*.

Number of times 20 to 30 times.

Indications Nasal congestion, runny nose.

Clinical applications Mainly used for stuffed nose owing to externally contracted pathogens or chronic rhinitis. It may be combined with clearing *fèi jīng* and grasping *fēng chí* (GB 20).

bǎi huì (DU 20, 百会)

Location In the intersection of the anteroposterior mid-line and the line connecting the apexes of the ears.

Operations Use the thumb to perform pressing or kneading on *bǎihuì* (see Figure 209).

Number of times Apply pressing 30 to 50 times; apply kneading 100 to 200 times.

Indications Headache, convulsions, irritability, rectal prolapse, urinary incontinence.

Clinical Applications

1. *For convulsions and irritability* Combine with clearing *gān jīng*, clearing *xīn jīng*, nail-kneading *xiǎotiān xīn*.
2. *For enuresis and rectal prolapse* Combine with supplementing *pí jīng* and *shènjīng*, pushing *sān guān* and kneading *dān tián*.

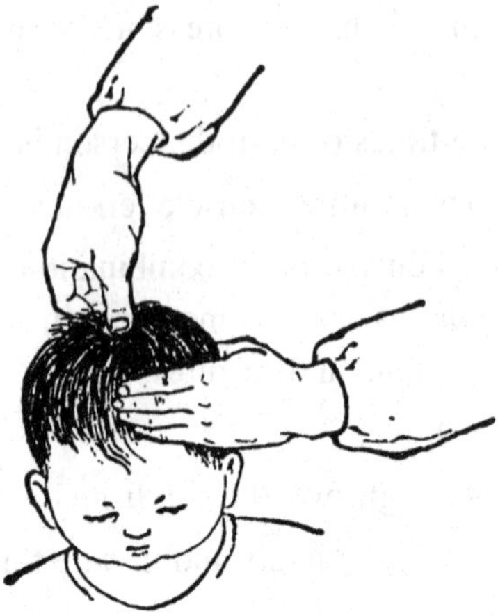

Figure 209 Pressing or kneading *Bǎi Huì*

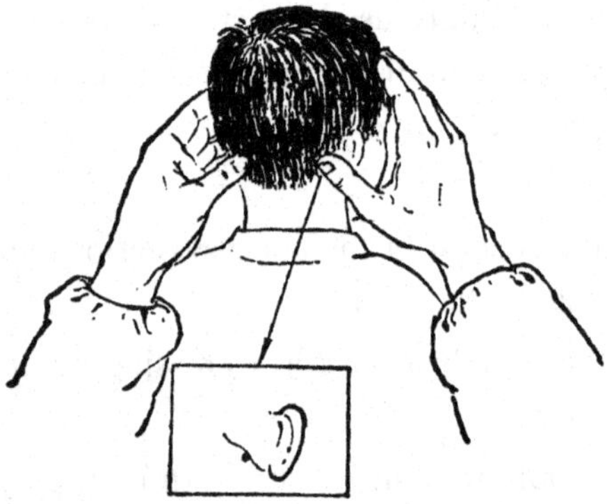

Figure 210 Kneading *Ěr Hòu Gāo Gǔ*

ěr hòu gāo gǔ (耳后高骨), bony prominence posterior to the ears

Location The depression right below the bony prominence posterior to the ear, level with the posterior hairline and equivalent to *wángǔ* (GB 12, 完骨).

Operations Use the thumbs or middle fingers to knead both sides of the points; this is called kneading *ěr hòu gāo gǔ* (see Figure 210).

Number of times 30 to 50 times.
Indications Headache, convulsions, irritability, restlessness.

Clinical Applications

1. *Headache of exogenous pattern* Commonly combined with clearing *fèijīng*.
2. *Convulsions, irritability and restlessness* Used in conjunction with kneading *bǎihuì* and clearing *xīnjīng*.

fēng chí (GB 20, 风池)

Location Below the occipital bone and between the sternocleidomastoid and trapezius.

Operations Grasping *fēng chí*.

Number of times Five to ten times.

Indications Colds, headaches, neck pain.

Clinical Applications

1. *Cold and headache* Commonly used in combination with clearing *fèijīng*.
2. *Stiff and painful neck* Combine with kneading on *liè quē* (LU 7) and neck muscles.

tiān zhùgǔ (天柱骨): a line-shaped pediatric tui na acupoint

Location The straight line between the posterior hairline and *dà zhuī* (DU 14).

Operations Use a thumb or the index finger to push the point in an up-down direction; this is called pushing *tiān zhù*.

Number of times Five to ten times.

Indications Fever, vomiting, stiff neck, convulsions.

Clinical Applications

1. *Fever of exogenous pattern and stiff neck* Combine with grasping *fēng chí*.
2. *Vomiting* Combine with kneading *bǎn mén* and *zhōngwǎn* (RN 12).

Summary of Commonly Used Acupoints and Techniques on the Head and Face

1. *Releasing the exterior* Pushing *cuán zhú, kăngong,* and *tiānzhù*; kneading *tài yang*; grasping *fēng chí*.
2. *Calming fright and opening orifices* Pressure kneading *băihuì*, and kneading *yíng xiāng*.
3. *Lifting yang from sinking* Pressure kneading *băihuì*.

Everyday Exercises

1. What are the characteristics of pediatric tui na?
2. What are the commonly used maneuvers on the head and face in pediatric tui na?
3. What is the general order of pediatric tui na operations?

Day 2

THORACIC AND ABDOMINAL ACUPOINTS

tiāntū (RN 22, 天突)

Location In the center of the suprasternal fossa.

Operations Use the tip of the middle finger to press or knead the point, namely pressing *tiān tū* or kneading *tiān tū* (see Figure 211).

Number of times Ten to 15 times.

Indications Coughs, asthma, fullness of the chest, phlegm accumulation, shortness of breath, nausea, vomiting.

Clinical Applications

1. *Coughs, asthma, and phlegm accumulation* Combine with pushing kneading *dànzhōng* and revolving *nèi bā guà*.
2. *Nausea and vomiting* Used in conjunction with kneading *zhōngwǎn* (RN 12) and pushing the spleen earth (*pí jīng*).

dànzhōng (RN 17, 膻中): an acupoint that involves both a point and a line

Location In the anterior midline of the body, between the nipples.

Operations Kneading with the tip of the middle finger is called kneading on *dànzhōng*; disjoining pushing on *dànzhōng* is the operation that begins from

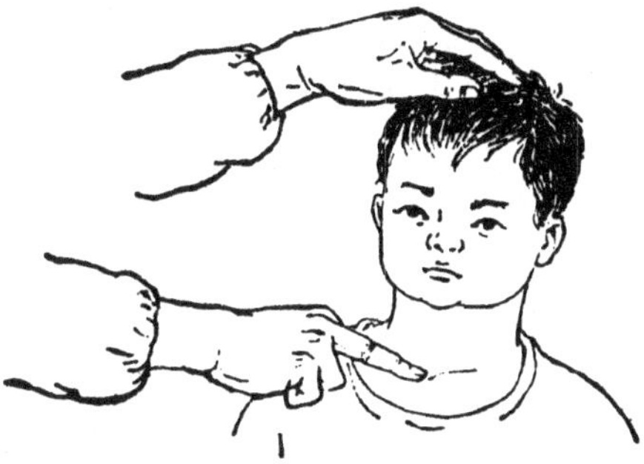

Figure 211 Kneading *Tiān Tū*

the middle of the point to where it is near both nipples using the thumbs; pushing *dànzhōng* uses the index and middle finger together, pushing from the sternal notch down to the xiphoid process. (See Figure 212.)

Number of times Pushing or kneading 50 to 100 times.

Indications Chest distension, coughs, labored breathing, wheezing due to phlegm accumulation, vomiting.

Clinical Applications

1. *Chest distension* Disjoining pushing *dànzhōng*.
2. *Coughs, labored breathing, and gurgling due to phlegm* Kneading *dànzhōng* and combine pushing *fèijīng* and kneading *fèishū* (BL 13).
3. *Vomiting* Pushing *dànzhōng*, combined with kneading *tiān tū* and pressure kneading *fēng lóng* (ST 40).

rŭ páng (乳旁), *rŭgēn* (乳根): point-shaped tui na acupoints that are often used together

Location Rŭ páng is 0.2 cun lateral to the nipple and *rŭgēn* is 0.2 cun inferior to it.

Operations Kneading with the index and middle finger combined, namely kneading *rŭ páng* and kneading *rŭgēn* maneuvers respectively.

Number of times 20 to 50 times.

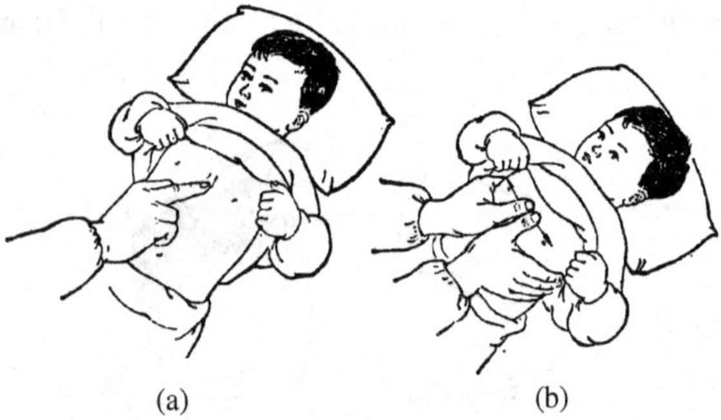

(a) 揉膻中	- Kneading *Dàn Zhōng*
(b) 分推膻中	- Disjoining Pushing *Dàn Zhōng*

Figure 212 Operational method on *Dàn Zhōng*

Indications Coughs, labored breathing, chest distension.

Clinical applications For coughs, labored breathing, and distended chest, combine the maneuver with kneading *dànzhōng* and *fèi shū*.

xiélèi (胁肋): as a surface-shaped acupoint, *xiélèi* literally means lateral thorax

Location Between the rib below the axillary and *tiān shū* (ST 25) on both sides.

Operations Foulage rubbing both sides of the ribs starting from the axillaries and gradually moving to *tiān shū*, namely foulage rubbing *xiélèi* (see Figure 213).

Number of times 50 to 100 times.

Indications Rib pain, chest distension, labored breathing triggered by phlegm, shortness of breath, infantile malnutrition with accumulation.

Clinical Applications

1. *Rib pain, chest distension, labored breathing due to phlegm* Combine with kneading or pushing *dànzhōng*.
2. *Infantile malnutrition with accumulation* Perform more foulage rubbing on *xiélèi*, and add spinal pinching.

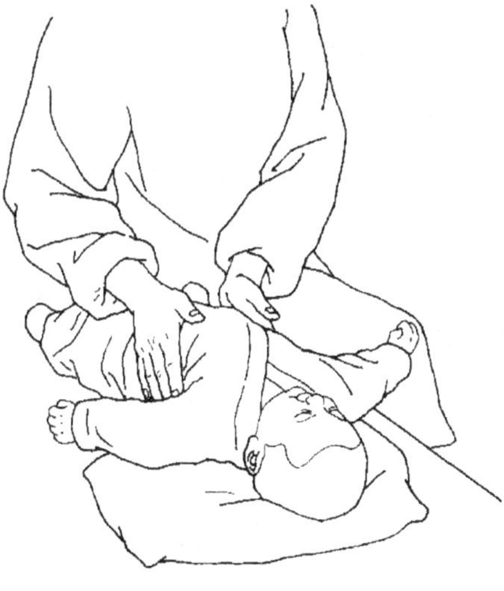

Figure 213 Foulage rubbing *Xié Lèi*

zhōngwǎn (RN 12, 中脘): an acupoint that combines a point, a line, and a surface

Location On the anterior midline, 4 cun above the umbilicus.

Operations

1. *Kneading* zhōngwǎn Use the pulp of the finger or the palm-heel to knead or pressure knead the acupoint (see Figure 214a).
2. *Rubbing* zhōngwǎn Use the center of the palm or four fingers to rub the acupoint.
3. *Pushing* zhōngwǎn Push from *tiān tū* along the anterior midline all the way to *zhōngwǎn* (see Figure 214b).

Number of times Kneading or pushing 100 to 300 times; rubbing for five minutes.

Indications Abdominal distension, eructation, food retention, poor appetite, vomiting, diarrhea.

Clinical Applications

1. For abdominal distension, eructation, food retention, poor appetite, vomiting and diarrhea, combine this maneuver with pushing *pí jīng* and pressure kneading *zú sān lǐ* (ST 36).
2. For rebellious stomach qi going upwards, eructation and vomiting, combine the maneuver with pushing *bǎn mén* and *tiān zhù*.

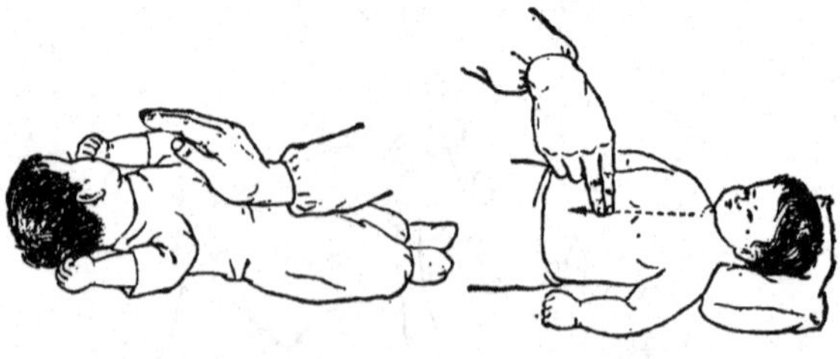

(a) (b)

(a) 揉中脘 - Kneading *Zhōng Wǎn*
(b) 推中脘 - Pushing *Zhōng Wǎn*

Figure 214 Operational methods of *Zhōng Wǎn*

fù (腹): an acupoint that combines a surface and a line

Location abdominal area, mainly the mid-abdomen.

Operations

1. *Disjoining pushing* fù Also known as pushing *fù yīn yáng*, use both hands to push along the edge of the xiphoid angles (see Figure 215a).
2. *Rubbing* fù Use a palm or pulps of the four fingers to perform the operation (see Figure 215b).

Number of times Disjoining pushing for 100 to 200 times; rubbing for five minutes.

Indications Indigestion, abdominal pain and distension, nausea, vomiting.

Clinical Applications

1. *Digestive disorders* Combine with kneading *zhōngwǎn* and pushing *pí jīng*.
2. *Preventative pediatric care* Often combined with spinal pinching and pressure kneading *zú sān lǐ*.
3. *Infantile diarrhea* Effective while combined with kneading *qí* (the navel) and *guī wěi*, and pushing upwards along *qī jié*.

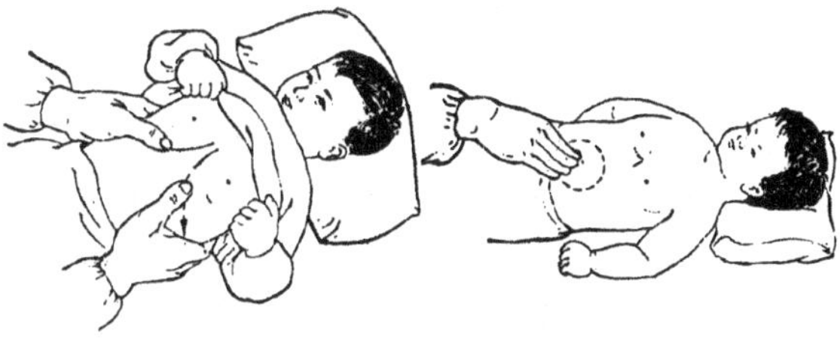

(a) (b)

(a)	分推腹阴阳	-	Disjoining Pushing the *Fù Yīn Yáng*
(b)	摩腹	-	Rubbing *Fù*

Figure 215 Operational methods on the abdomen

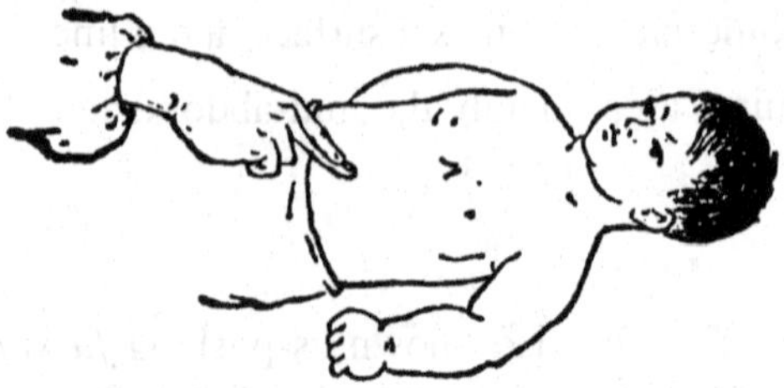

Figure 216 Kneading *Qí*

qí (脐): an acupoint that combines a point and a surface

Location The umbilicus.

Operations Use the tip of the middle finger or the palm-heel to apply kneading on *qí* (see Figure 216).

Number of times 100 to 300 times.

Indications Diarrhea, constipation, abdominal pain and distension, infantile malnutrition with accumulation.

Clinical Applications

1. *Diarrhea and constipation* Combine with rubbing *fù*, kneading *guī wěi,* and pushing *qī jié.*
2. *Infantile malnutrition with accumulation* Combine with spinal pinching, and kneading *zhōngwǎn* and *zú sān lǐ.*

tiān shū (ST 25, 天枢)

Location Bilateral points, 2 cun lateral to the navel.

Operations Place the index and middle fingers on the left and right side of *tiān shū* respectively, to perform kneading *tiān shū* (see Figure 217).

Number of times 50 to 100 times.

Indications Diarrhea, abdominal pain and distension, constipation, digestive disorders.

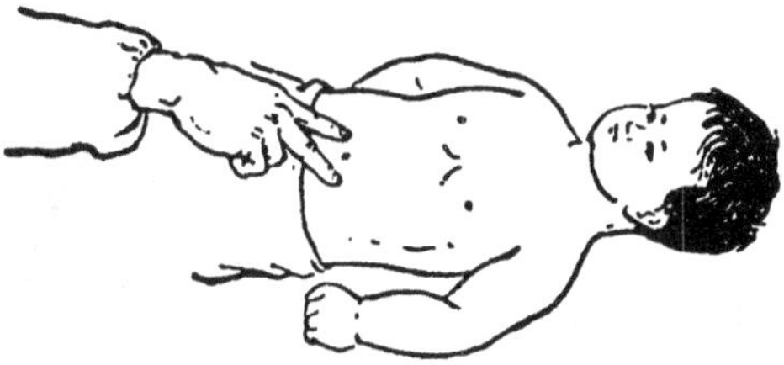

Figure 217 Kneading *Tiān Shū*

Clinical Applications

1. Combine with kneading *qí*, pushing *pí jīng,* and pressure kneading *zú sān lǐ* in treating acute or chronic gastroenteritis, and digestive disorders.
2. Clinically, *qí* and *tiān shū* can be manipulated concurrently by placing the middle finger on *qí* while the index and ring fingers knead on each side of *tiān shū* respectively.

dān tián (丹田): an acupoint that combines a point and a surface

Location In the lower abdomen, between the space of two to three cun below the umbilicus.

Operations Rubbing or kneading.

Number of times Kneading 50 to 100 times; rubbing for five minutes.

Indications Abdominal pain, enuresis, rectal prolapse, hernia, and urine retention.

Clinical Applications

1. *Hernia, enuresis or rectal prolapse* May combine with supplementing *shèn jīng*, pushing *sān guan,* and kneading *wài láo gōng* (EX-UE 8).
2. *Urine retention* Combine pressing *dān tián* with pushing *jī mén.*

dù jiǎo *(*肚角*)*

Location Two cun lateral from the bilateral points that are two cun below the umbilicus

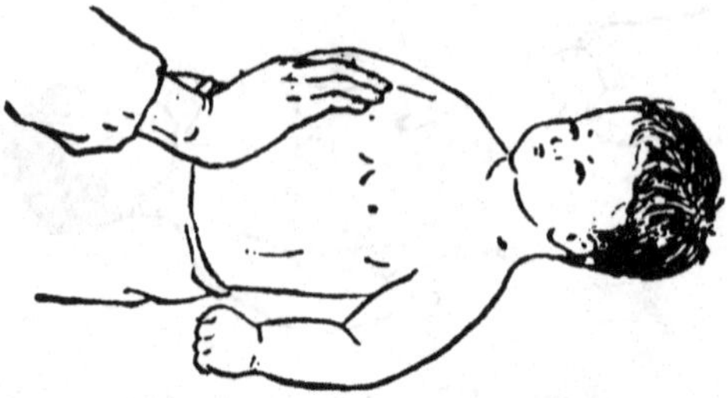

Figure 218 Kneading *Dān Tián*

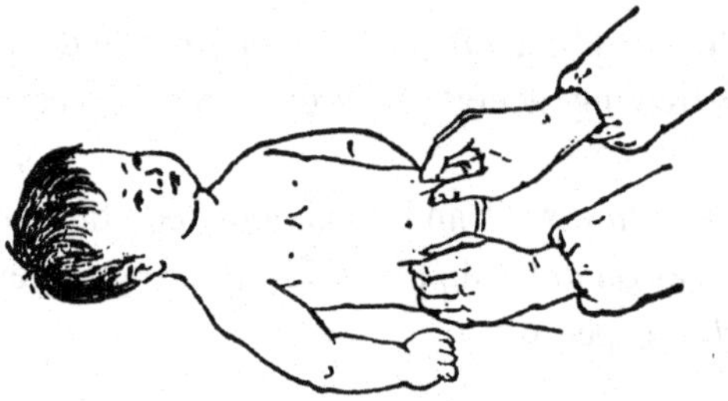

Finger 219 Grasping *Dù Jiăo*

Operations

1. *Grasping* dù jiăo Use the thumb, index finger, and middle finger to apply three-finger grasping to *dù jiăo*.
2. *Pressing* dù jiăo Use the middle finger to press *dù jiăo*.

Number of times Three to five times.
Indications Abdominal pain, diarrhea.
Clinical applications Combine with kneading *pí jīng*, rubbing *fù*, and kneading *dān tián*.

Summary of Commonly Used Acupoints and Techniques on the Chest and Abdomen

1. Acupoints of the chest are mainly used to treat respiratory disorders such as coughing, labored breathing, gurgling due to phlegm, and chest fullness.

2. Acupoints of the upper and middle abdomen are mainly used to treat digestive dysfunctions including indigestion, abdominal distension, diarrhea, and constipation.
3. Lower abdominal acupoints are mostly used to warm the lower *jiao*, fortify the kidney, and secure the life essence, treating diseases of the urinary system such as enuresis.

Everyday Exercises

1. Try to memorize the operations and clinical applications of *dànzhōng* and *zhōngwǎn*.
2. What are the effective acupoint combinations that are used to treat diarrhea?

Day 3

ACUPOINTS OF THE BACK

jiānjǐng (GB 21, 肩井): an acupoint that combines a point and a surface

Location At the midpoint between the line connecting *dà zhuī* (DU 14) and the acromion.

Operations

1. *Pressing* jiān jǐng Use a finger to press the *jiān jǐng* point.
2. *Grasping* jiān jǐng Grasp *jiān jǐng* between the thumb and the index and middle fingers (see Figure 220).

Number of times Pressing 30 to 50 times; grasping three to five times.

Indications Cold, convulsion, fainting, motion disorder of the arms.

Clinical Applications

1. *Common cold* Combine with the grasping *fēng chí* and commonly used pediatric tui na procedures.
2. *Pain of bì pattern* Combine with the corresponding local treatment maneuvers for pain of *bì* pattern in adults.
3. Use as the ending procedure in pediatric tui na.

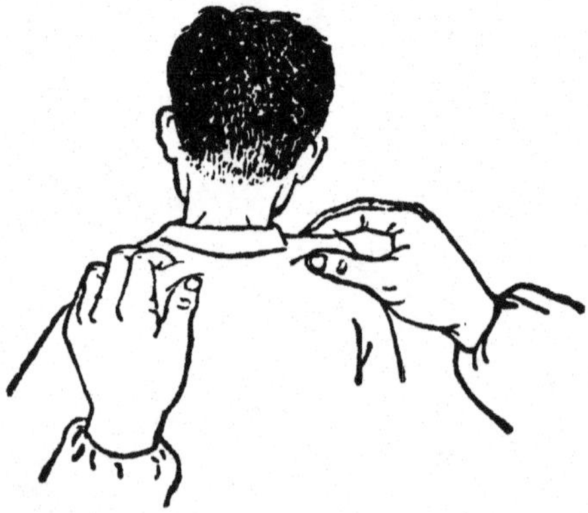

Figure 220 Grasping *jiān jǐng*

dà zhuī (DU 14, 大椎)

Location The interspinal space below the 7th cervical vertebra.

Operations Kneading *dà zhuī* with the middle finger.

Number of times 20 to 30 times.

Indications Stiff neck, fever, and coughing.

Clinical Applications

1. *Cold, fever, and stiff neck* Combine with commonly used pediatric tui na maneuvers and pushing *tiān zhù*.
2. *Coughs* Combine with kneading *rǔ páng* and *rǔgēn*.

fēngmén (BL 12, 风门)

Location 1.5 cun lateral from the posterior midline, between the 2nd and 3rd thoracic spinal process.

Operations Place the index and middle fingers on each side of the acupoint to apply kneading on *fēng mén*.

Number of times 20 to 30 times.

Indications Cold, cough, and labored breathing.

Clinical Applications

This acupoint is mainly used to treat exterior pattern of externally contracted wind-cold and can be combined with grasping *fēng chí* (GB 20), clearing *fèi jīng*, kneading *fèi shū,* and pushing *dànzhōng* (RN 17).

fèishū (BL 13, 肺俞)

Location 1.5 cun lateral from the posterior midline, between the 3rd and the 4th thoracic spinal process.

Operations

1. Place the index and middle fingers on each side of the acupoint to apply kneading on *fèi shū* (see Figure 221a).
2. Use both thumbs to push the medial edges of the scapular bones from the top to bottom; this is pushing *fèi shū* or disjoining pushing the scapulae (see Figure 221b).

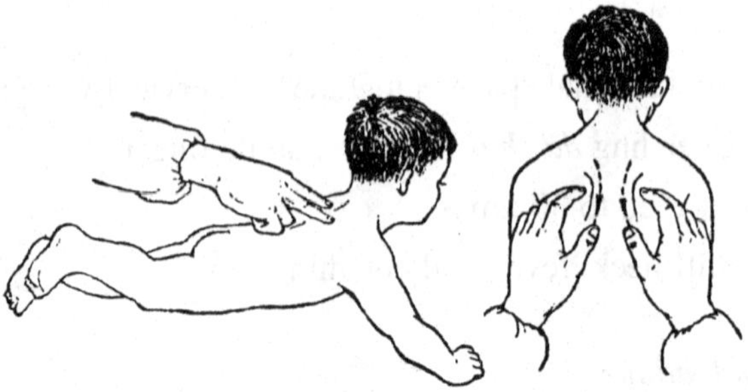

(a) 揉肺俞	-	Kneading *Fèi Shū*
(b) 推肺俞(分推肩胛骨)	-	Pushing *Fèi Shū* or Disjoining Pushing the Scapulae

Figure 221 Operating on *Fèi Shū*

Number of times Kneading 50 to 100 times; pushing 100 to 300 times.

Indications Labored breathing, cough, gurgling due to phlegm, chest pain or distension.

Clinical Applications

1. It is mostly used to treat respiratory diseases and can be combined with pushing or kneading *dànzhōng*, clearing *fèi jīng,* and kneading *fēng lóng* (ST 40).
2. For patients with chronic and refractory cough, a little granulated table salt can be used while performing the maneuver.

pí shū (BL 20, 脾俞)

Location 1.5 cun lateral from the posterior midline, between the 11th and 12th thoracic spinal process.

Operations Kneading *pí shū* by placing the index and middle fingers on each side of the acupoint.

Number of times 50 to 100 times.

Indications Diarrhea, indigestion, poor appetite, infantile malnutrition with accumulation, weakness of the four limbs.

Clinical applications The acupoint is mainly used to treat diseases of the digestive system. It can be used in conjunction with kneading *zhōngwǎn* (RN 12), pushing *pí jīng*, pressure kneading *zú sān lǐ* (ST 36), and spinal pinching.

shèn shū (BL 23, 肾俞)

Location 1.5 cun lateral from the posterior midline, between the 2nd and 3rd lumbospinal process.

Operations Kneading *shèn shū* with the index and middle fingers placed on each side of *shèn shū*.

Number of times 50 to 100 times.

Indications Diarrhea, constipation, lower abdominal pain, *wěi* pattern weakness of the lower extremeties.

Clinical Applications

1. For children with diarrhea or constipation owing to kidney deficiency, the maneuver can be used in conjunction with supplementing *pí jīng* and *shèn jīng*, and kneading *shàng mǎ*.
2. For *wěi* pattern weakness of the lower extremities, it can be used in combination with spinal pinching and tui na maneuvers of the lower limbs.

yāo shū (腰俞)

Location 3.5 cun lateral from the posterior midline, between the 3rd and 4th lumbospinal process.

Operations Kneading *yāo shū* is performed by either placing the index and middle fingers or thumbs on each side of the point.

Number of times 50 to 100 times.

Indications Lumbago, paralysis of the lower limbs.

Clinical applications It can be combined with tui na maneuvers of the trunk and lower limbs.

jí zhù (*jí*, 脊柱): a line-shaped acupoint

Location The straight line between *dà zhuī* (DU 14) and *cháng qiáng* (DU 1). It is the longest line-shaped acupoint in children.

Operations

1. *Pushing* jí Use the pulp of the index and middle fingers to push straight down from the top (see Figure. 222).
2. *Grand pushing* jí Start from *tiān zhùgŭ* while pushing *jí* is performed. This maneuver has a stronger action of clearing heat.
3. *Spinal* (jí) *pinching* If pinching is performed along *jí zhù*, it is called pinching *jí* or spinal pinching. Refer to page XX for details.

Number of times Pushing 300 to 500 or more times; pinching three to five times.

Indications Fever, convulsions, infantile malnutrition with accumulation, diarrhea, and constipation.

Clinical Applications

1. *Clearing heat* By using a small amount of water or alcohol while pushing *jí*, this becomes a great physical cooling method, often combined with pushing *liùfŭ* downwards, clearing *tiān hé shuĭ,* and pushing *yŏng quán* (KI 1).
2. *Maintaining the well being of children* Pinching *jí* (spinal pinching) regulates yin and yang, rectifies qi and blood, harmonizes *zang-fu* organs, unblocks meridians and collaterals, cultivates the original qi, and improves physical strength. It is often combined with supplementing *pí jīng* and *shènjīng*, pushing the upper three *guan*, rubbing *fù,* and pressure kneading *zú sān lĭ* (ST 36) in treating chronic diseases due to natal or postnatal deficiencies.

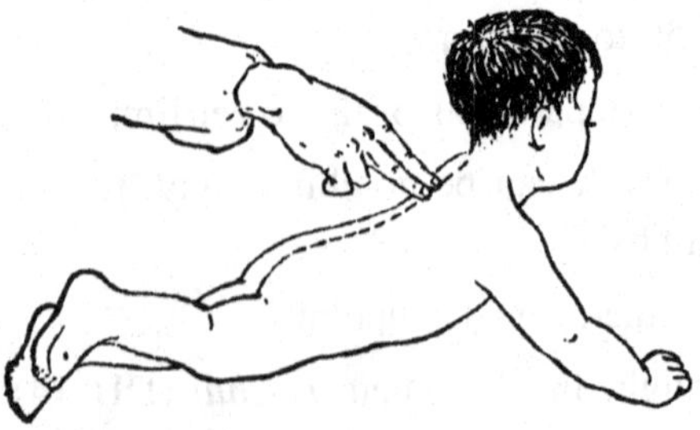

Figure 222 Pushing *Jí*

qī jié gŭ (*qī jié*, 七节骨, 七节): a line-shaped acupoint

Location The straight line between the depression under the 4th lumbospinal process and the tip of the tail bone where *cháng qiáng* is located.

Operations

1. *Pushing upwards along qī jié* Use the radial aspect of the thumb or the pulps of the index and middle fingers to push straight up from the lower end of *qī jiégŭ* till its upper end.
2. *Pushing downwards along* qī jié The maneuver is the same as the above, except in the opposite direction.

Number of times 100 to 300 times.

Indications Diarrhea, constipation, and rectal prolapse.

Clinical Applications

1. *Pushing upwards along qī jié* For diarrhea, combine it with kneading *guī wĕi*, rubbing *fù,* and kneading *dān tián*; for rectal prolapse and enuresis due to deficient sinking qi, add pressure kneading *băi huì* (DU 20) and kneading *dān tián.*
2. *Pushing downwards along qī jié* For constipation, combine pushing downwards along *qī jié* with kneading *bó yáng chí.*

guī wĕi (龟尾)

Location At the tip of the tail bone, which is equivalent to *cháng qiáng* (DU 1).

Operations Use the tip of the thumb or middle finger to perform kneading on *guī wĕi.*

Number of times 100 to 300 times.

Indications Diarrhea, constipation, rectal prolapse, enuresis.

Clinical applications With the ability to smooth out qi flow in *dumai*, the acupoint has a two-way regulatory function in the large intestines.

1. *Diarrhea and constipation* Combine with pushing *qī jié*, rubbing *fù,* and kneading *qí.*
2. *Rectal prolapse and enuresis* Add kneading *dān tián* and pressure kneading *băihuì.*

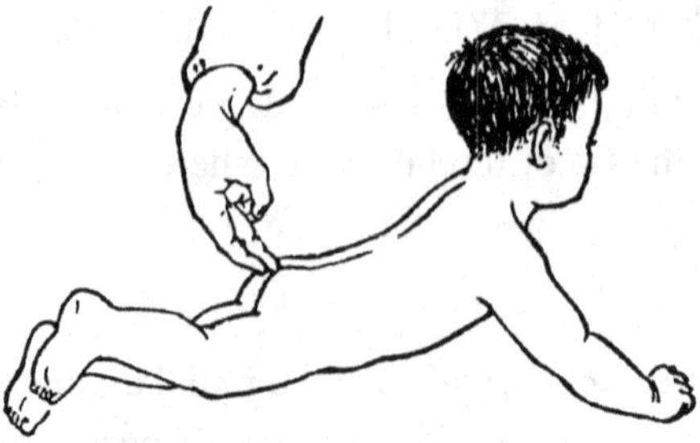

Figure 223 Kneading on *Guī Wěi*

Summary of Commonly Used Acupoints and Techniques on the Back

1. *Supplementing and draining* With pressure kneading *fèi shū*, *pí shū*, and *shèn shū*, it regulates and treats diseases of or related to the corresponding *zang* organs of the lung, spleen and kidney respectively, supplements their deficiencies, or drains its excess.
2. *Clearing heat, releasing the exterior, and calming panting* pushing *jí*, and kneading *dà zhuī* (DU 14) or *fēng mén* (BL 12) can clear the heat. Among these maneuvers, pushing *jí* has a stronger effect in clearing the heat while the other two are more effective in releasing the exterior and calming labored breathing.
3. *Regulating the function of the large intestines* The combination of *guī wěi* and *qī jié* has a two-way regulatory function on the large intestines.

Everyday Exercises

1. Master the locations, operations, and clinical applications of *fèi shū*, *pí shū*, and *shèn shū*.
2. How would you operate on the acupoint of *jí zhù* and what are the clinical applications?
3. What are the operating methods on *qī jié gǔ*? What are the correct clinical usage of pushing upwards and downwards along *qī jié*?

Day 4

ACUPOINTS OF THE UPPER EXTREMITIES, PART I

pí jīng (the acupoint for the spleen meridian, 脾经): an acupoint combining a line and a surface

Location The pulp of the thumb.

Operations (see Figure 224)

1. *Supplementing* pí jīng Flex the child's thumb and push straight from the distal edge to the palm-heel along the radial side; or, perform circling pushing on the pulp of the thumb.
2. *Clearing pí jīng* Extend the child's thumb, push straight from the tip of the thumb, and pass over the pulp toward the root of the finger.
3. *Pushing pí jīng* This is the common name for the combination of supplementing and clearing *pí jīng*.

Number of times 100 to 500 times.

Indications Diarrhea, constipation, poor appetite, indigestion.

Clinical Applications

1. *Supplementing pí jīng* The maneuver fortifies the spleen and the stomach while supplementing qi and blood concurrently. It can be used in patients with poor appetite and indigestion if it is combined with kneading *zhōngwǎn* (RN 12), *pí shū* (BL 20), and *zú sān lǐ* (ST 36).
2. *Clearing pí jīng* The maneuver clears damp-heat and can be combined with clearing *tiān hé shuǐ* and *dà cháng*. The spleen and stomach of small children are delicate. Therefore, it is not appropriate to overly use purging methods. In general, the supplementing method should be used on *pí jīng*. On the other hand, the clearing method should be used in children with stronger constitution, or supplementing it should be added afterwards.

gān jīng (the liver meridian, 肝经): an acupoint combining a line and a surface

Location The pulp of the index finger.

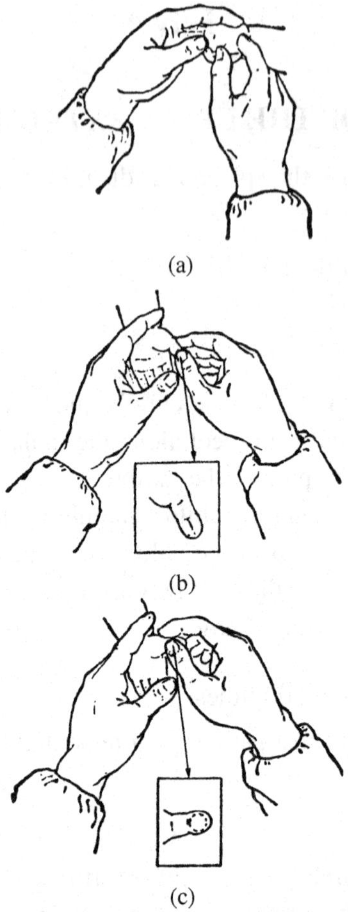

(a) 屈指直推脾经(补脾经)	-	Pushing *Pí Jīng* with Thumb Flexed (Supplementing *Pí Jīng*)
(b) 直推脾经(清脾经)	-	Pushing *Pí Jīng* with Thumb Extended (Clearing *Pí Jīng*)
(c) 旋推脾经(补脾经)	-	Circling Pushing *Pí Jīng* (Supplementing *Pí Jīng*)

Figure 224 Operation on *Pí Jīng*

***Operations* (see Figure 225)**

1. *Clearing* gān jīng Extend the child's index finger and push from the tip toward the root over the finger pulp.
2. *Supplementing* gān jīng Circling push over the pulp of the index finger.
3. *Pushing* gān jīng This is the common name for both of the above maneuvers.

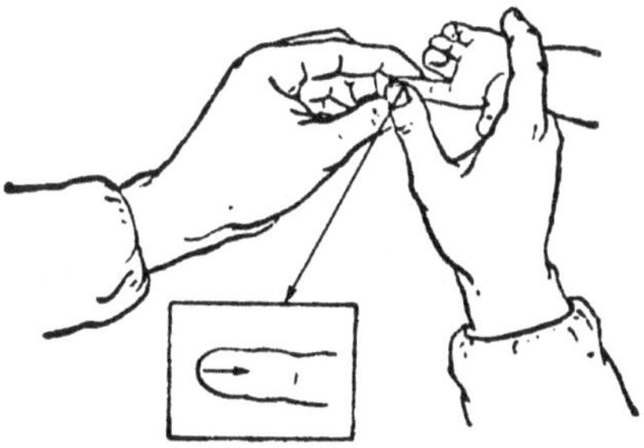

Figure 225 Pushing (clearing) G*ān Jīng*

Number of times 100 to 500 times.
Indications Irritability, restlessness, convulsion, five-center vexing heat, red eyes, bitter mouth, dry throat.

Clinical Applications

1. *Clearing gān jīng* With the effects of calming the liver, draining the fire, extinguishing the wind, suppressing fright, resolving constraint and dissolving vexation, it may be combined with clearing *tiān hé shuǐ* and pushing *yǒng quán* (KI 1).
2. *Supplementing gān jīng* Most times, it is appropriate to clear *gān jīng* rather than supplement it. Therefore, when there is a liver deficiency that needs to be supplemented, the clearing method should be added after supplementing it. Another way is to supplement *shèn jīng* instead, which is the method of nourishing the kidney to cultivate the liver, or nourishing water to cultivate wood.

xīn jīng (the heart meridian, 心经): an acupoint combining a line and a surface shape
Location The pulp of the middle finger.

Operations (see Figure 226)

1. *Clearing xīn jīng* Extend the child's middle finger and push from the tip toward the root over the finger pulp.

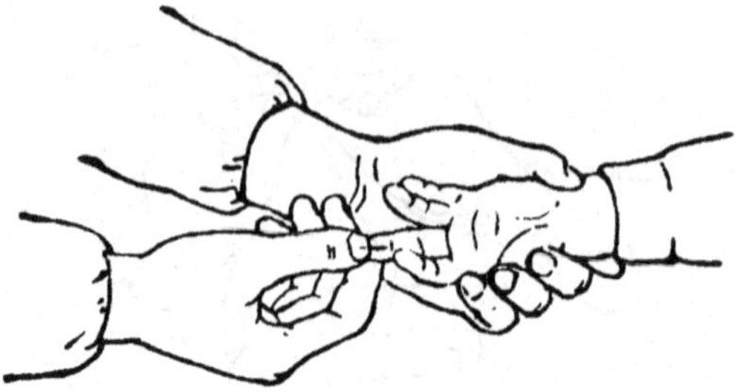

Figure 226 Pushing *Xīn Jīng*

2. *Supplementing xīn jīng* Circling push over the pulp of the middle finger.
3. *Pushing xīn jīng* This is the common name for both of the above maneuvers.

Number of times 100 to 500 times.
Indications High fever with loss of consciousness, five-center vexing heat, mouth ulcer, tongue boil, dark and difficult urination, deficient heart-blood, fright, restlessness.

Clinical Applications

1. *Clearing xīn jīng* It clears heat and resolves heart fire, and is often used in combination with clearing *tiān hé shuǐ* and *xiǎocháng*.
2. *Supplementing xīn jīng* It is usually appropriate to clear *xīnjīng* rather than supplement it. When there is a deficiency showing vexation, restlessness, and unable to fully close eyes while sleeping, clearing should be performed after supplementing it. A substitute supplementing method is to supplement *shèn jīng*.

fèijīng (the lung meridian, 肺经): a point combining a line and a surface
Location The pulp of the ring finger.

***Operations* (see Figure 227)**

1. *Supplementing fèi jīng* Circling push the pulp of the ring finger.
2. *Clearing fèi jīng* Push the pulp straight, with the direction going from the finger tip to the root.

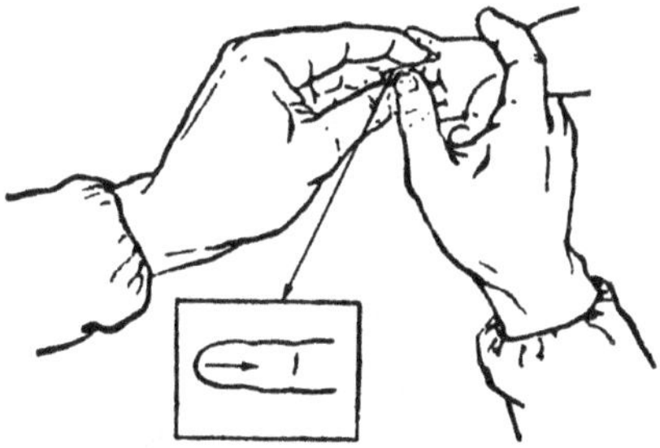

Figure 227 Pushing *Fèi Jīng*

3. *Pushing fèi jīng* This is the common name for both of the above maneuvers.

Number of times 100 to 500 times.

Indications Common cold, fever, cough, fullness of the chest, labored breathing, debilitating sweat, rectal prolapse.

Clinical Applications

1. *Boosting lung qi* Apply supplementing *fèi jīng*; this may be combined with kneading *fèi shū* (BL 13).
2. *Clearing fèi jīng* It can diffuse lung qi, clear lung heat, disperse wind, release the exterior, transform phlegm, and relieve cough; it may be combined with pushing *dànzhōng* (RN 17) and kneading *fēng mén* (BL 12).

shènjīng (the kidney meridian, 肾经): an acupoint combining a line and a surface
Location The pulp of the little finger.

Operations **(see Figure 228)**

1. *Supplementing shèn jīng* Circling push the pulp of the little finger.
2. *Clearing shèn jīng* Push the pulp straight, with the direction going from the finger tip to the root.
3. *Pushing shèn jīng* This is the common name for both of the above maneuvers.

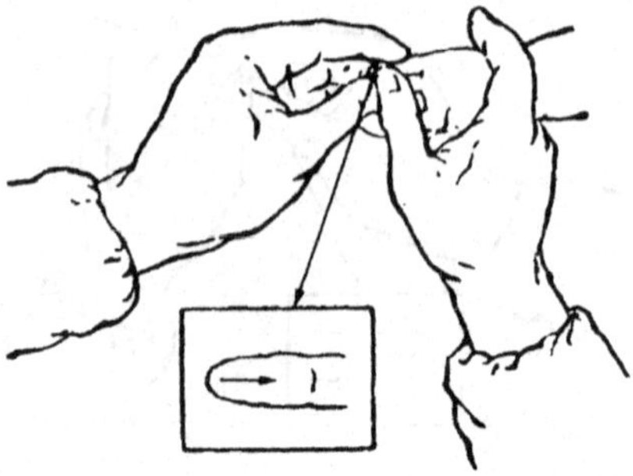

Figure 228 Pushing *Shèn Jīng* (using the clearing method)

Number of times 100 to 500 times.

Indications Natal deficiency, debility owing to chronic diseases, debilitating panting, diarrhea and bed-wetting due to kidney deficiency, heat accumulation in the bladder, painful and dripping urination.

Clinical Applications

1. *Supplementing shèn jīng* It can fortify the kidney, benefit the marrow, warm the original qi of the lower *jiao* when it is combined with kneading *shèn shū* (BL 23) and *dān tián*.
2. *Clearing shèn jīng* It can clear damp-heat of the lower *jiao* and may be substituted by clearing *xiǎo cháng*.

dà cháng (large intestines, 大肠): a line-shaped acupoint

Location A straight line along the radial side of the index finger from the tip to the web.

Operations (see Figure 229)

1. *Supplementing dà cháng* Push straight from the tip of the index finger to the web.
2. *Clearing dà cháng* Push to the opposite position of supplementing *dà cháng*.
3. *Pushing dà cháng* This is the common name for both of the above maneuvers.

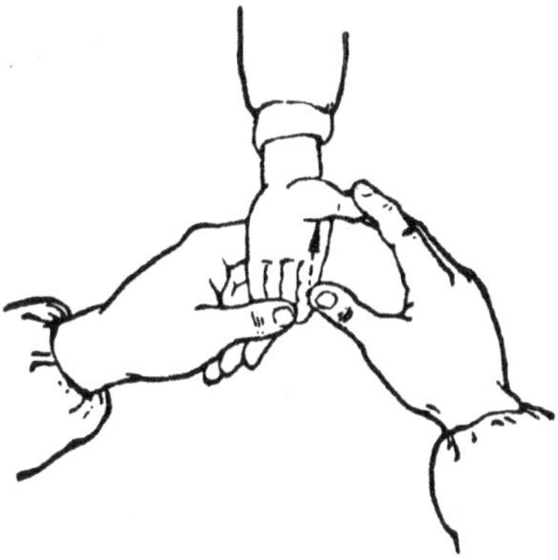

Figure 229 Pushing *Dà Cháng*, supplementing method

Number of times 100 to 500 times.

Indications Diarrhea, rectal prolapse, constipation.

Clinical Applications

1. *Supplementing* dà cháng It can be used in combination with kneading *dān tián* and *wài láo gōng* (EX-UE 8), and pushing *sān guān* to astringe the intestines, rescue it from desertion, and warm the center to arrest diarrhea.
2. *Clearing* dà cháng It can be used in combination with pushing *liùfǔ* and rubbing *fù* to clear intestines, benefit the bowels, resolve damp-heat, and dissolve food retention.
3. *Finger venule diagnosis* Another name for *dà cháng* acupoint is *sānguān* of the finger. See details in "Observing Infantile Finger Venules" in Week 11.

xiǎo cháng (small intestines, 小肠): a line-shaped acupoint

Location The straight line from the tip to the root along the ulnar side of the little finger.

***Operations* (see Figure 230)**

1. *Clearing xiǎo cháng* Push straight from the root of the little finger to the tip.

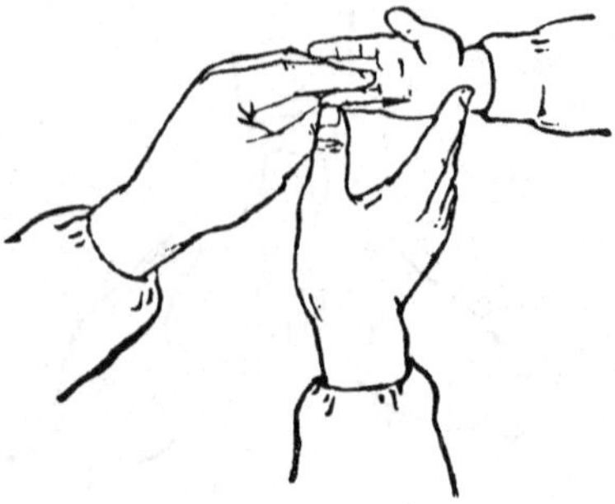

Figure 230 Pushing *Xiǎo Cháng*, supplementing method

2. *Supplementing xiǎo cháng* Push to the opposite position of clearing *xiǎo cháng*.
3. *Pushing xiǎo cháng* This is the common name for both of the above maneuvers.

Number of times 100 to 500 times.

Indications Dark and difficult urination, anuria, enuresis.

Clinical Applications

1. *Clearing xiǎo cháng* It may be used in conjunction with clearing *tiān hé shuǐ* to remove damp-heat of the lower *jiao* and separate the clear from the turbid.
2. *Supplementing xiǎo cháng* It can treat enuresis and urorrhagia while being used in conjunction with kneading *dān tián* and *shèn shū* (BL 23).

sì héng wén (*sì fèng*, EX-UE10, 四横纹, 四缝): a short line-shaped acupoint

Location In the midpoint of the palmar side of the transverse creases of the proximal interphalangeal joints of the index, middle, ring, and little fingers.

Operations

1. *Pushing sì héng wén* Have the four fingers close together, and push from the palmar side of transverse crease of the index finger to that of the little finger.

2. *Nailing sì héng wén* Use the nail to press the transverse creases of the proximal interphalangeal joints of all four fingers.

Number of times Push 100 to 300 times; nail five times.

Indications Abdominal distension, infantile malnutrition with accumulation, indigestion.

Clinical applications Sì héng wén can be used to treat indigestion and infantile malnutrition with accumulation. Pushing *sì héng wén* can be performed together with supplementing *pí jīng* and kneading *zhōngwǎn* (RN 12). The same result can be achieved by nailing *sì héng wén* or pricking them to draw some blood or yellowish fluid.

bǎn mén (板门): a surface-shaped acupoint

Location The surface of the palmar aspect of the thenar.

Operations

1. *Kneading* bǎn mén Use a finger to apply kneading on *bǎn mén* (see Figure 231a).
2. *Pushing* bǎn mén Push from the root of the thumb or *bǎn mén* to the transverse creases (see Figure 231b).

Number of times 100 to 300 times.

Indications Food accumulation, abdominal distension, poor appetite, vomiting, diarrhea, belching.

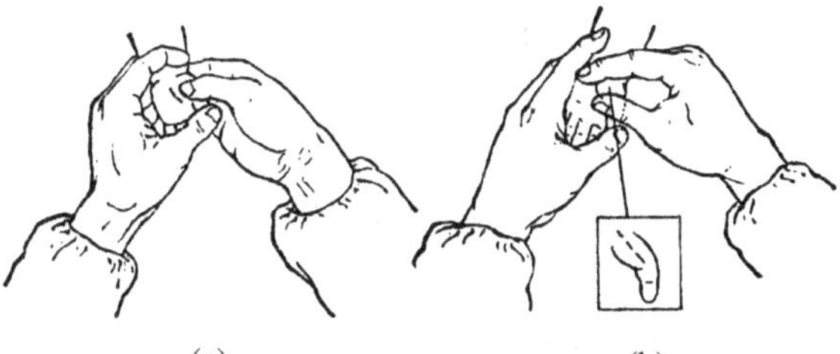

(a) (b)

(a) 揉板门 - Kneading *Bǎn Mén*
(b) 推板门 - Pushing *Bǎn Mén*

Figure 231 Operational method on *Bǎn Mén*

Clinical Applications

1. *Fortify the spleen and harmonize the stomach* Kneading *bǎn mén* combined with supplementing *pí jīng*, anc kneading *zhōng wǎn* and *pí shū* (BL 20).
2. *Arrest diarrhea* Pushing from *bǎn mén* to the transverse crease of the wrist.
3. *Stop vomiting* Pushing from the transverse crease of the wrist to *bǎn mén*.

nèiláo gōng (*láo gōng*, PC 8, 内劳宫, 劳宫)

Location In the center of the palm, between the 2nd and 3rd metacarpal bones, closer to the 3rd metacarpal bone.

Operations Finger kneading *nèi láo gōng*.

Number of times 100 to 300 times.

Indications Fever, irritability, thirst, mouth ulcer, gum erosion, deficient vexation with internal heat.

Clinical applications Kneading *nèi láo gōng* clears heat and resolves vexation, and can be used in conjunction with clearing *xīn jīng* and *tiān hé shuǐ*.

nèibā guà (内八卦)

Location The surface by taking 2/3 of the distance between the center of the palm and the transverse crease of the root of the middle finger as the radius to draw a circle (Fig. 204).

Operations The common manuever used is evolving *nèi bā guà*.

Number of times 100 to 300 times.

Indications Cough with phlegm, labored breathing, fullness of the chest, poor appetite, abdominal distension, vomiting.

Clinical applications Revolving *nèi bā guà* can comfort the chest, benefit the diaphragm, rectify qi, transform phlegm, remove stagnant food, and resolve food accumulation. It can be used in combination with pushing *pí jīng* and *fèi jīng*, kneading *zhōngwǎn* (RN 12), and pressure kneading *zú sān lǐ* (ST 36).

Everyday Exercises

1. Memorize the locations, operations, and clinical applications of the five *jīng* acupoints of *gān*, *xīn*, *pí*, *fèi*, and *shèn*.
2. Master the operational methods and clinical applications of *sì héng wén* acupoint.

Day 5

ACUPOINTS OF THE UPPER EXTREMITIES, PART II

xiǎotiān xīn (minor heavenly center, 小天心, a.k.a. *yú jì jiāo*, 鱼际交)

Location On the root of the palm, in the depression where the thenar and hypothenar intersect.

Operations

1. Kneading *xiǎotiānxīn* with the middle finger (see Figure 232).
2. Nailing *xiǎotiān xīn*.
3. Pounding *xiǎotiān xīn* with the middle finger.

Number of times kneading 100 to 300 times; nailing or pounding five to 20 times.

Indications Convulsions, spasms, vexation, night crying, dark and difficult urination, red and painful eyes, and incomplete eruption of rashes and poxes.

Clinical Applications

1. *Kneading xiǎo tiān xīn* When it is used in combination with clearing *xīn jīng*, *xiǎo cháng,* and *tiān hé shuǐ*, it clears heat, promotes urination, and benefits the eyes.

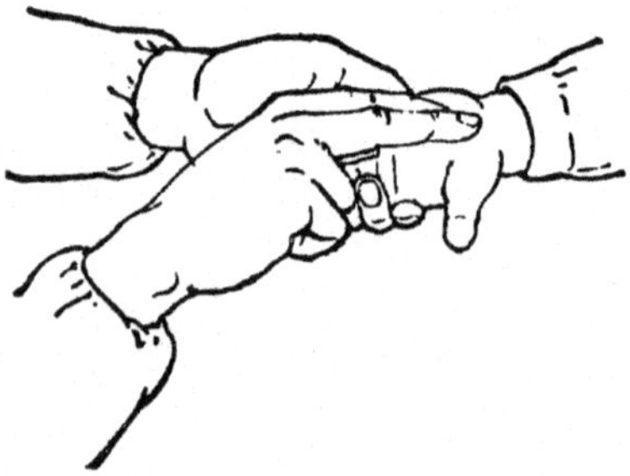

Figure 232 Kneading *Xiǎo Tiān Xīn*

2. *Nailing and pounding* xiǎo tiān xīn Combine with clearing *gān jīng*, pressure kneading *bǎi huì* (DU 20), nailing *rén zhōng* (DU 26) and *lǎo lóng* to ease fright and calm the mind.

Transporting water to earth and *transporting soil to water* (运水入土, 运土入水)

Location At the palmar side — an arc line along the edge of the palm from the root of the thumb to the little finger.

Operations

1. *Transporting water to earth* Start from the root of the thumb along the edge of the palm, pass *xiǎotiān xīn,* and push until the root of the little finger.
2. *Transporting earth to water* Same maneuver, but in the opposite direction to *transporting water to earth.*

Number of times 100 to 300 times.

Indications Dark and difficult urination, abdominal distension, diarrhea, poor appetite, constipation.

Clinical Applications

1. *Transporting water to earth* Used in combination with pushing *sānguān* (*dáchàng*) upwards to fortify the spleen and assist its transporting ability, moisten dryness and promote defecation.
2. *Transporting earth to water* Used in conjunction with pushing *liù fǔ* downwards to clear damp-heat of the spleen and stomach, promote urination, and arrest diarrhea.

zǒng jīn (总筋)

Location In the midpoint of transverse crease on the palmar side.

Operations Kneading (see Figure 233) or nailing *zǒng jīn*.

Number of times Kneading 100 to 300 times; nailing three to five times.

Indications Convulsions with spasms, mouth ulcer, tongue boil, night crying, hot flashes.

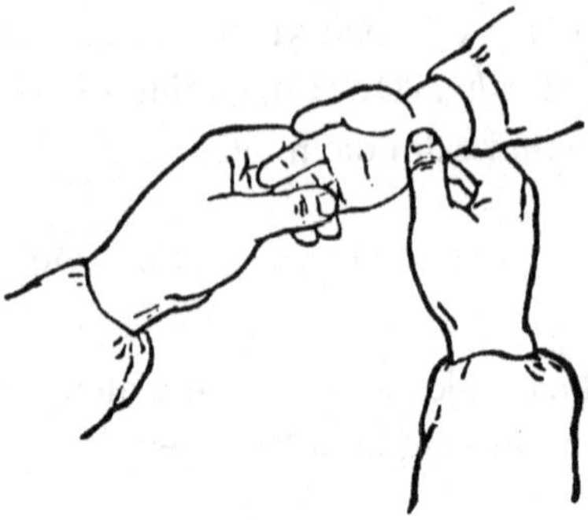

Figure 233 Kneading *Zǒng Jīn*

Clinical Applications

1. *Kneading zǒng jīn* It clears the heat of *xīn jīng*, dissipates masses, relieves pain, unblocks and rectifies the overall qi mechanism when combined with clearing *xīn jīng* and *tiān hé shuǐ.*
2. *Nailing zǒng jīn* It treats convulsions and spasms when combined with pounding *xiǎo tiān xīn*.

dàhéng wén (hand yin yang, 大横纹, 手阴阳): line-shaped acupoint

Location Palmar side of the transverse crease of the wrist. The radial end is called *yáng chí* (阳池) while the ulnar end is called *yīn chí* (阴池).

Operations

1. *Disjoining pushing dà héng wén* Use both thumbs to push simultaneously from the center of the palmar side of the transverse crease of the wrist to both sides; this maneuver is also known as disjoining hand yin yang (see Figure 234).
2. *Joining yin yang* Push from *yáng chí* and *yīn chí* at the same time toward *zōng jīn* in the center of the wrist.

Number of times 30 to 50 times.

Indications Alternating chills and fever, abdominal distension, diarrhea, vomiting, food accumulation, irritability, and restlessness.

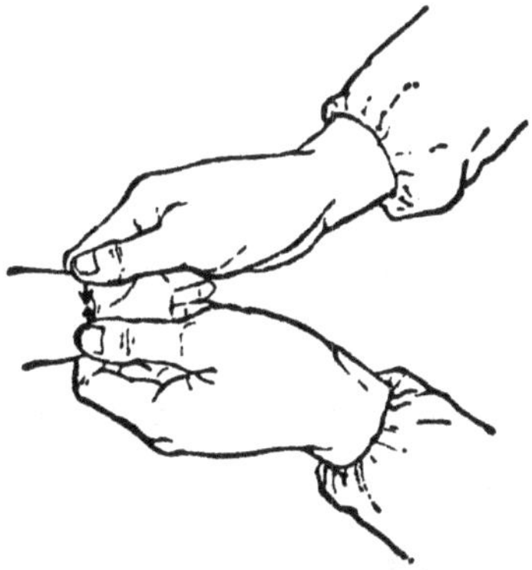

Figure 234 Disjoining pushing *Dà Héng Wén*, also known as disjoining hand Yin Yang

Clinical Applications

1. *Disjoining hand yin yang* It balances yin and yang, regulates and harmonizes qi and blood, moves stagnant food, and resolves food accumulation. It can be combined with rubbing *fù* and pushing *pí jīng*. If the child is showing excess heat pattern, allocate more strength to disjoining *yīn chí*. If the child suffers deficient cold pattern, there should be more emphasize on disjoining *yáng chí*.
2. *Joining yin yang* It removes phlegm and dissipates masses. It can be used in conjunction with clearing *tiān hé shuǐ*.
3. *Disjoining hand yin yang and kneading zǒngjīn* These serve as regular hand maneuvers in pediatric tui na.

shí xuān (EX-UE 11, 十宣)

Location The tips of all ten fingers adjacent to the nails on the white skin.

Operations Nailing *shí xuān*.

Number of times Five times on each finger tip, or until the patient resumes consciousness.

Indications Coma with high fever.

Clinical applications Nailing *shí xuān* is mostly used in first aid emergency situations with the function of clearing heat and opening orifices. It can be combined with nailing *lǎo lóng* and rén *zhōng* (DU 26) and grand pushing *jí* (the spine).

lǎo lóng (老龙)

Location 0.1 cun posterior to the center of the nail base of the middle finger.

Operations Nailing *lǎolong* (see Figure 235).

Number of times Five times or until the child resumes consciousness.

Indications Acute infantile convulsions.

Clinical applications Nailing *lǎo lóng*, with functions of reviving consciousness and opening orifices, is mainly used in first aid emergency situations. If the patient responds by making sounds to the painful nailing maneuver, it is relatively easier to treat. On the other hand, if neither does he or she feel the pain nor respond to the stimulation of nailing, it generally indicates that the condition is difficult to treat.

èr shàn mén (double-paneled door, 二扇门)

Location On the dorsal aspect of the hand, in the depressions on both sides of the metacarpophalangeal joint of the middle finger.

Operations

1. *Kneading èr shàn mén* Use both the index and middle fingers to apply pressure knead on the bilateral point (see Figure 236a).
2. *Nailing èr shàn mén* Use the thumb nail to perform nailing on the acupoint (see Figure 236ba).

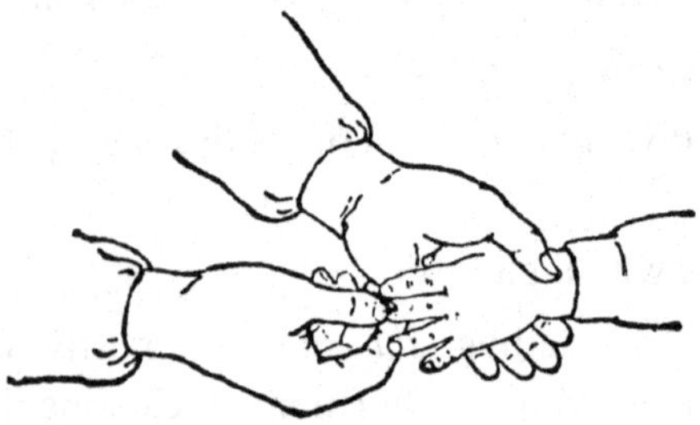

Figure 235 Nailing *Lǎo Lóng*

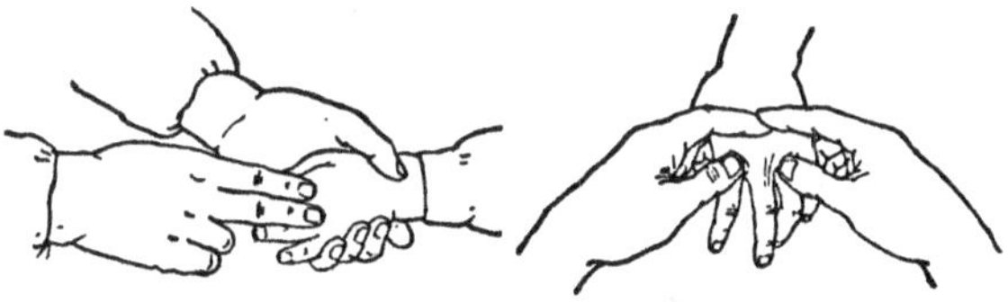

(a) (b)

(a) 揉二扇门 - Kneading *Èr Shàn Mén*
(b) 掐二扇门 - Nailing *Èr Shàn Mén*

Figure 236 Operational Methods on *Èr Shàn Mén*

Number of times Kneading 100 to 300 times; nailing three to five times.

Indications Fever without sweat.

Clinical Applications

1. As an empirical sweat-inducing acupoint, *èr shàn mén* induces sweat, vents the exterior, dissolves fever, and calms labored breathing while kneading or nailing is performed.
2. If the child has high fever without perspiration, sweating can be induced after pressure kneading is performed for one or two minutes.
3. If the child is of weak constitution, and is prone to contracting exterior pathogens, exterior securing methods such as supplementing *pí jīng* and *shènjīng* can be performed prior to applying kneading or nailing on *èr shàn mén* to induce sweat.

shàng mǎ (上马)

Location On the dorsum of the hand, between the metacarpophalangeal joints of the ring and little finger.

Operations

1. *Kneading shàng mǎ* Use the tip of the thumb to perform kneading on the acupoint.
2. *Nailing shàng mǎ* Use the nail of the thumb to apply nailing on the acupoint.

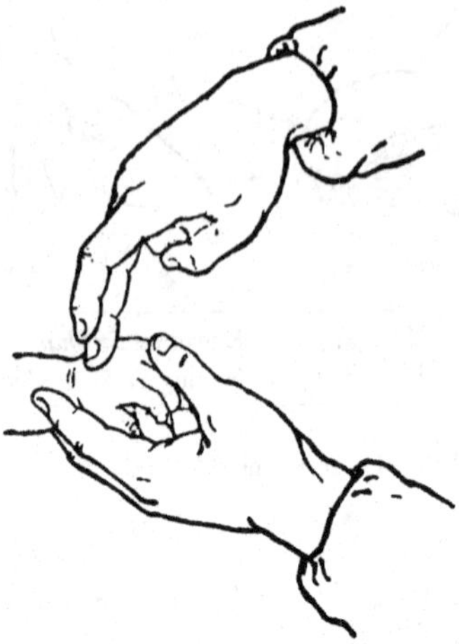

Figure 237 Kneading *Wài Láo Gōng*

Number of times Kneading 100 to 500 times; nailing three to five times.

Indications Labored breathing and coughing due to yin deficiency heat; dark, dripping, and difficult urination.

Clinical Applications

1. *Nourishing kidney yin* This is an important acupoint to nourish kidney yin and can be combined with kneading *fèi shū* (BL 13) and supplementing *shèn jīng*.
2. *Clearing the lung* For those suffering lung infection with persistent dry rales, combine the operation of *shàng mǎ* with pushing *xiǎo héng wén*, consisting of transverse crease of the on the palmar side

wàiláo gōng (also known as *lào zhěn xué*, EX-UE 8, 外劳宫, 落枕穴)

Location On the dorsum of the hand, opposite to where *nèiláo gōng* is located.

Operations Kneading or nailing *wài láo gong* (see Figure 237).

Number of times Kneading 100 to 300 times; nailing three to five times.

Indications Common cold owing to wind-cold contraction, abdominal distension, diarrhea, rectal prolapse, enuresis.

Clinical Applications

With its warming nature, the acupoint is great to warm yang, dissipate cold, raise yang, and lift the sunken. In addition, it induces sweating and releases the exterior. When it is applied to treat rectal prolapse and enuresis, it can be combined with supplementing *pí jīng* and *shèn jīng*, pushing *sān guān*, and kneading *dān tián*.

sān guān (三关): line-shaped acupoint.

Location The straight line from *yáng chí* (SJ 4) to *qǔ chí* (LI 11) on the radial side of the forearm.

Operations (see Figure 238)

1. *Pushing sān guan* Use the radial side of the thumb or the pulps of the index and middle fingers to push from the wrist to the elbow; this is also known as pushing *sān guān* upwards.
2. *Grant pushing sān guan* Have the child's thumb flexed, and perform pushing from the radial side of the thumb all the way to the elbow.

Number of times 100 to 300 times.

Indications Qi and blood deficiency, debilitation after being sick, cold limbs owing to yang deficiency, abdominal pain, diarrhea, incomplete eruption of rashes, common cold of wind-cold contraction, and all conditions that are owing to deficient cold.

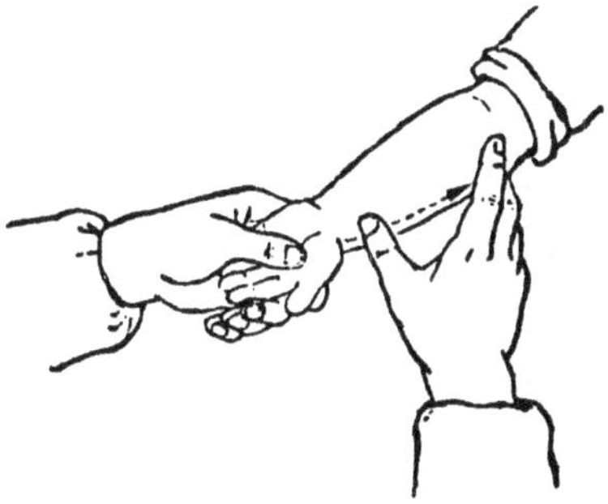

Figure 238 Pushing *Sān Guān*

Clinical Applications

1. *Diseases of deficient cold pattern* With its warming nature, pushing *sān guān* can boost qi, invigorate the blood, warm yang, dissipate cold, induce sweat, and release the exterior. It can be combined with supplementing *pí jīng* and *shèn jīng*, kneading *dān tián*, rubbing *fù*, and spinal pinching.
2. For the common cold due to wind-cold contraction, aversion to cold without sweating, or incomplete eruption of rashes, the maneuver can be used in combination with clearing *fèi jīng*, and nailing and kneading *èr shàn mén*.

liù fŭ (six bowels, 六腑): line-shaped acupoint

Location The straight line between *yīn chí* and *shào hăi* (HT 3) on the ulnar side of the forearm.

Operations Using the thumb or the pulps of the index and middle fingers, pushing *liù fŭ* downwards from the elbow to the wrist.

Number of times 100 to 300 times.

Indications High fever, irritability, thirst, convulsion, sore throat, numbness of the tongue, mumps, and constipation.

Clinical Applications

1. *Excess heat pattern* The nature of pushing *liù fŭ* is cool and cold; therefore, it is applicable to all diseases of excess heat pattern. It can

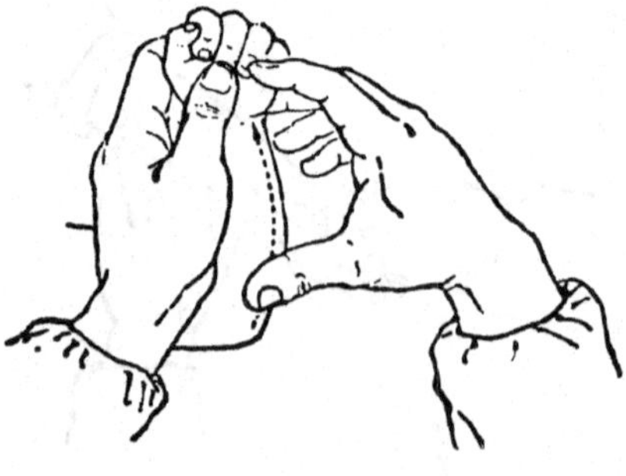

Figure 239 Pushing *Liù Fŭ* downwards

be used in conjunction with clearing *fèijīng*, *xīn jīng*, and *gān jīn,* and pushing *jí*.

2. *Using pushing liù fŭ downwards alone or combining it with sān guān*
   a. Because of the great cooling nature of pushing *liù fŭ* downwards, it can be used to treat high fever, irritability, and thirst in children, while pushing *sān guān* can be applied in aversion to cold for its great heating nature for children with qi deficiency and weak constitution.
   b. With the combination of the two acupoints, they can balance yin and yang to prevent excessive cold or heat from damaging the healthy qi. If the pattern is cold-heat complex with heat being dominant, the ratio of pushing *liù fŭ* downwards and pushing *sān guān* should be 3:1. On the other hand, it should be 1:3 when the disease pattern is the same with cold being dominant.

tiān hé shuĭ (heavenly river water, 天河水): line-shaped acupoint

Location The straight line between *zŏngjīn* and *hóng chí*, i.e., *qŭ zé* (PC 3) in the midline of the forearm.

Operations

1. *Pushing* tiān hé shuĭ Use the pulps of the index and middle fingers to push from the wrist to the elbow; this maneuver is also known as clearing *tiān hé shuĭ* (see Figure 240).

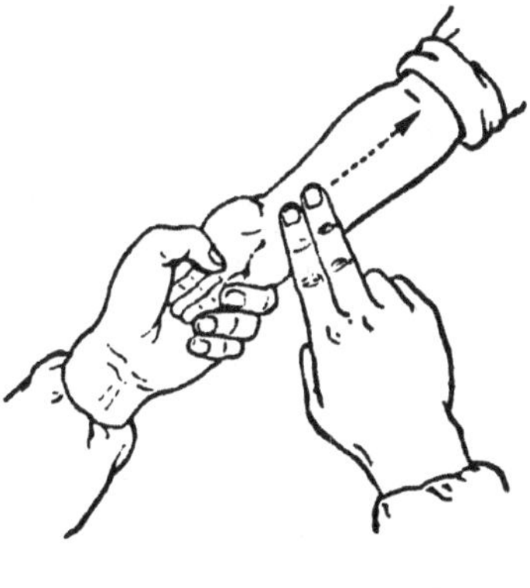

Figure 240 Clearing *Tiān Hé Shuĭ*

2. *Spurring the horse to cross* tiān hé Dip the index and middle fingers into water, flick up and down starting from *zǒngjīn* all the way to *hóng chí* and blow air to where it is being stricken.

Number of times 100 to 300 times.

Indications Diseases showing excessive heat pattern including fever due to external contraction, tidal fever, and internal heat.

Clinical Applications

1. *Clearing heat, releasing the exterior, draining fire, and resolving irritability* With the mild cooling and gentle nature of clearing *tiān hé shuǐ*, it can be used to counter heat patterns. It may be combined with clearing *fèi jīng*, pushing *cuán zhú* (BL 2) and *kǎn gōng*, and kneading *tài yáng* to treat heat owing to external contraction. On the other hand, it can be used to treat internal heat patterns when combined with clearing *xīn jīng* and *gān jīng*, and kneading *yǒng quán* (KI 1).
2. *For excessive heat and high fever* Usually, spurring the horse to cross *tiān hé* is more appropriate since its clearing heat effect is greater than clearing *tiān hé shuǐ*.

Summary of Commonly Used Acupoints and Techniques on the Upper Limbs

1. *Treating diseases of designated zang-fu organs* Acupoints such as *pí jīng*, *gān jīng*, *xīn jīng*, *fèi jīng*, *shèn jīng*, *wèi jīng*, *dà cháng,* and *xiǎo cháng* are mainly used in treating diseases of their designated *zang-fu* organs. A supplementing maneuver can supplement the deficiency while a clearing maneuver drains the excess. Among these, the appropriate method of using *gān jīng* and *xīn jīng* is meant to clear but not supplement, while *pí jīng* and *shèn jīng* should be used to supplement but not clear.
2. *Heat clearing acupoints and maneuvers*
   a. *Fever owing to external contraction* Use clearing heat maneuvers such as nail-kneading *èr shàn mén*, clearing *tiān hé shuǐ,* and pushing *sān guan*.

b. *Clearing ying blood level heat* Clearing *tiān hé shuǐ*, spurring the horse to cross *tiān hé*, pushing *liù fǔ* downwards, and kneading *xiǎotiān xīn*.
c. *Clearing deficient and vexing internal heat* Kneading *nèi láo gōng* (PC 8) and *shàng mǎ*.
d. *Clearing the heat of the heart meridian* Kneading *nèi láo gōng* (PC 8) and *xiǎo tiānxīn*.
e. *Alternating cold and heat* disjoining hand yin yang can be used owing to its ability of regulating qi and blood.

3. *Spleen-fortifying acupoints* Maneuvers such as pushing and kneading *bǎn mén*, and pushing *sì héng wén* and *xiǎohéng wén* can fortify the spleen, harmonize the center, assist transporting, and resolve food retention.

Everyday Exercises

1. Memorize the locations, operations, indications, and clinical applications of *pí jīng*, *gān jīng*, *xīn jīng*, *fèi jīng*, *shèn jīng*, *wèi jīng*, *dà cháng*, and *xiǎo cháng*.
2. Memorize the locations, operations, indications and clinical applications of *sān guān*, *liù fǔ*, and *tiān hé shuǐ*.

Day 6

ACUPOINTS OF THE LOWER EXTREMITIES

jī mén (箕门): line-shaped acupoint

Location A straight line between the upper corner of the patella and the midpoint of the groin on the medial side of the thigh.

Operations Pushing *jī mén*, which uses both the index and middle fingers to push straight from the medial aspect of the upper corner of the patella to the groin.

Number of times 100 to 300 times.

Indications Dark urine and difficult urination, anuresis and watery diarrhea.

Clinical applications Pushing *Jī mén* is fairly effective in promoting urination with its gentle and harmonizing nature.

1. *Urine retention* It may be combined with kneading *dān tián* and pressure kneading *sān yīn jiāo* (SP 6).
2. *Dark urine and difficult urination* It may be combined with clearing *xiăo cháng*.

băi chóng (百虫)

Location On the medial side above the knee where the muscle bulges out.

Operations Pressing or grasping *băi chóng* (see Figure 241).

Number of times Five to ten times.

Indications Twitching of the four limbs, *wěi* and *bì* patterns of the lower limbs.

Clinical applications Pressing and grasping *băi chóng* can unblock the meridians and collaterals and relieve twitching. It is often used in treating *wěi* and *bì* patterns and paralysis of the lower limbs when combined with grasping *wěi zhōng* (BL 40), pressure kneading *zú sān lǐ* (ST 36) and kneading *jiě xī* (ST 41). If the maneuver is used to treat convulsion and twitching, it should be applied with greater stimulation.

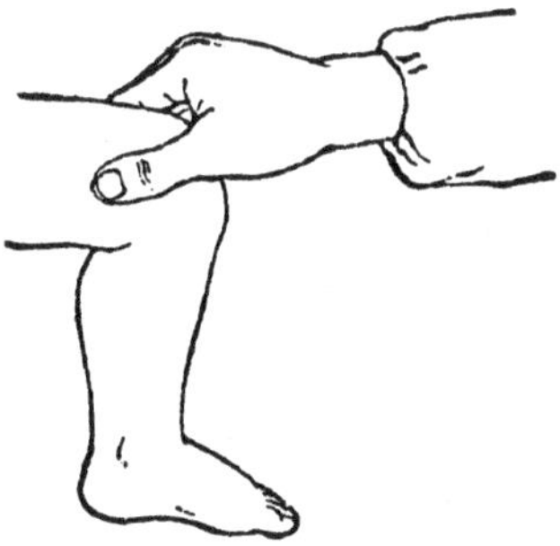

Figure 241 Grasping *Bǎi Chóng*

zú sān lǐ (ST 36, 足三里)

Location Three cun below the lateral space of the knee, one middle-finger width lateral to the anterior crest of the tibia.

Operations Pressure kneading using the tip of the finger.

Number of times 50 to 100 times.

Indications Pain and distention of the abdomen, diarrhea, vomiting, *wěi* and *bì* patterns of the lower extremities.

Clinical applications As the *He*-Sea point of the foot *yangming* stomach meridian and a main point treating digestive disorders, *zúsān lǐ* fortifies the spleen, harmonizes the stomach, regulates the center, rectifies qi, resolves stagnation, and unblocks the collaterals.

1. *Abdominal pain and distention* Combine with rubbing *fǔ* and kneading *pí shū* (BL 20).
2. *Vomiting* Combine with pushing *tiān zhùgǔ* and disjoining *fǔ* yin yang.
3. *Diarrhea owing to spleen deficiency* Combine with pushing *qī jié* upwards and supplementing *dà cháng*.
4. *General pediatric wellness* Combine with spinal pinching, i.e., pinching *jí* and rubbing *fǔ*.
5. *Wěi and bì of the lower limbs* Supplement with maneuvers seen in tui na for adults introduced in previous chapters.

qiánchéng shān (前承山)

Location Anterior-lateral of the tibia, opposite of *hòu chéng shān.*

Operations Nailing or kneading *qián chéng shān.*

Number of times Nailing five times; kneading 30 times.

Indications Twitching of the lower limbs.

Clinical applications It is often combined with grasping *wěi zhōng* (BL 40), pressing *bǎi chóng* and nailing *jiě xī* (ST 41) to treat opisthotonus and twitching of the lower extremities.

fēng lóng (ST 40, 丰隆)

Location Eight cun above the lateral malleolus, 1.5 cun lateral to the anterior border of the tibia between the tibia and the fibula.

Operations Kneading *fēng lóng* with the thumb or the middle finger.

Number of times 50 to 100 times.

Indications Cough, gurgling due to phlegm, labored breathing.

Clinical applications Kneading *fēng lóng* can regulate stomach qi and transform phlegm and dampness. It is mainly used to treat excessive phlegm, cough, and labored breathing, and may be combined with kneading *dànzhōng* (RN 17), *fèi shū* (BL 13), and revolving *nèi bā guà.*

sān yīn jiāo (SP 6, 三阴交)

Location Three cun above the medial malleolus, at the posterior border of the tibia.

Operations Pressure kneading *sān yīn jiāo* using the thumb or the index finger (see Figure 242).

Number of times 100 to 300 times.

Indications Bed-wetting; painful, difficult and frequent urination; *wěi* and *bì* of the lower extremities.

Clinical Applications

1. *Enuresis, anuresis and difficult urination* *Sān yīn jiāo* is a major acupoint in treating diseases of the urinary system. Pressure kneading this point not only unblocks blood vessels, invigorates meridians and collaterals, dredges the lower *jiao*, resolves damp-heat, and frees and

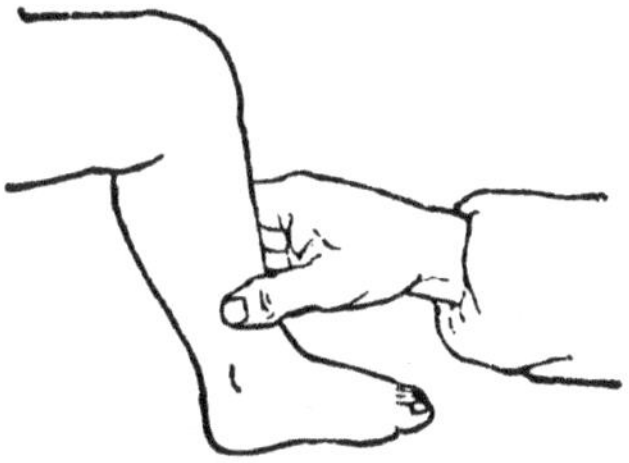

Figure 242 Pressure kneading *Sān Yīn Jiāo*

adjusts the waterway, but it also fortifies the spleen and stomach and assists transporting and transforming nutrients. It can be combined with kneading *dān tián*, and pushing *jī mén* and *shèn jīng*.

2. *Bì pattern pain of the lower limbs* This refers to the relevant content in the tui na for adults sections of this book.
3. *Fortifying the spleen and stomach, and assisting in transporting and transforming* It can be combined with kneading *zhōngwǎn* (RN 12) and pushing *pí jīng*.

jiě xī (ST 41, 解溪)

Location In the midpoint of the anterior transverse crease of the ankle, between the tendons of muscle extensor hallucis longus and digitorum longus.

Operations Nailing and kneading *jiě xī*.

Number of times Nailing three to five times; kneading 50 to 100 times.

Indications Convulsions, incontinent vomiting and diarrhea, restricted flexion and extension of the ankle joint.

Clinical Applications

1. *Convulsions, vomiting, and diarrhea* Nailing *jiě xī* may be combined with pressing *bǎi chóng* and pressure kneading *zú sān lǐ* (ST 36).
2. *Restricted flexion and extension of the ankle* Use the kneading maneuver and supplement it with related adult tui na maneuvers in the previous sections.

wěizhōng (BL 40, 委中)

Location In the middle of the popliteal space, between the two major tendons.

Operations Grasping *wěi zhōng* (see Figure 243) is the maneuver that uses the tip of the index finger to lift, grasp, hook, and pluck the soft tissue of the popliteal space.

Number of times Three to five times.

Indications Convulsions, twitching, and *wěi* pattern weakness of the lower limbs.

Clinical Applications

1. *Convulsions and twitching* Combine it with pressing *bǎi chóng* and nailing *lǎo lóng*.
2. *Wěi pattern weakness of the lower limbs* Pressure kneading *zú sān lǐ*, quadriceps femoris, and anterior tibial muscle.

hòu chéng shān (also known as *chéng shān*, BL 57, 后承山, 承山)

Location The depression of the belly of the gastrocnemius.

Operations Grasping *hòu chéng shān*.

Number of times Three to five times.

Indications Pain and twitching of the legs, and *wěi* pattern weakness of the lower limbs.

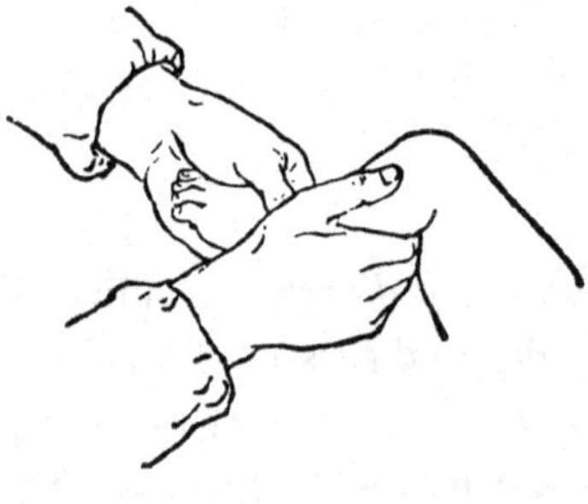

Figure 243 Grasping *Wěi Zhōng*

Clinical applications Grasping *chéng shān* can relieve convulsions, and unblock the related meridians and collaterals. It may be combined with grasping *wěi*zhōng, pressure kneading *zú sān lǐ*, and grasping the gastrocnemius to treat muscle spasms and *wěi* pattern weakness of the lower limbs.

pú cān (BL 61, 仆参)

Location The depression inferior to the lateral malleolus.

Operations Grasping or nailing *pú cān* (see Figure 244).

Number of times Three to five times.

Indications Fainting and convulsions.

Clinical applications It is mainly used to treat fainting and may be combined with nailing *rén zhōng* (DU 26) and *lǎo lóng*.

yǒng quán (KI 1, 涌泉): an acupoint combining a point and a line

Location In the depression at the anterior 1/3 to the center of the sole while the foot is flexed.

Operations

1. Pushing *yǒng quán* straight from the acupoint toward the direction of the toes using the thumb (see Figure 245a).
2. Kneading *yǒng quán* using the tip of the finger (see Figure 245b).

Number of times 50 to 100 times.

Indications Fever, vexing heat of the five centers, vomiting, diarrhea.

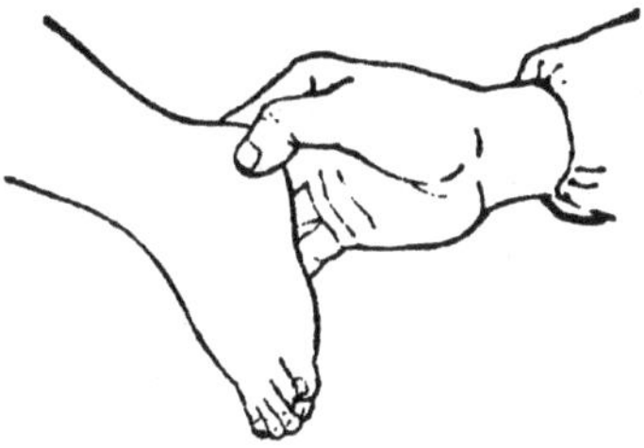

Figure 244 Nailing *Pú Cān*

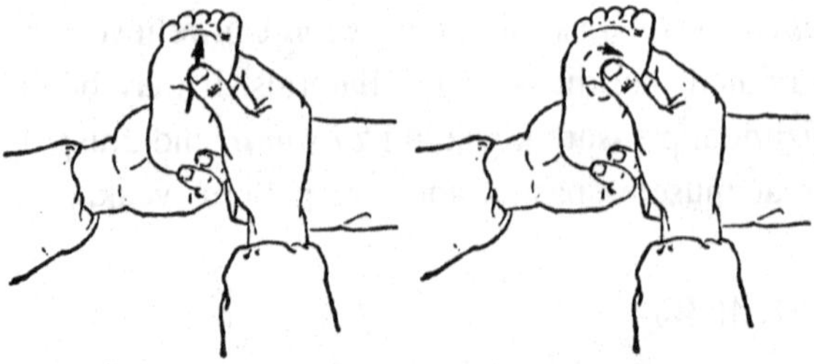

(a) 推涌泉	-	Pushing *Yǒng Quán*
(b) 揉涌泉	-	Kneading *Yǒng Quán*

Figure 245 Operational methods of *Yǒng Quán*

Clinical Applications

1. *Guide the fire down to its origin and resolve deficient-heat* Pushing *yǒng quán* can treat vexing heat of the five centers, irritability, and restlessness. It may be combined with kneading *shàng mǎ* and revolving *nèi láo gōng* (PC 8).
2. *Remove excessive heat* Pushing *yǒng quán* can be used in conjunction with pushing *jí*, pushing *liù fǔ* downwards, and clearing *tiān hé shuǐ.*
3. *Vomiting and diarrhea* In men, kneading the right *yǒng quán* counter-clockwise stops vomiting and diarrhea while kneading it clockwise. In women, the operation should be applied to the left foot in the opposite direction.

Summary of Commonly Used Acupoints and Techniques on the Lower Limbs

1. *Bǎi chóng*, *chéng shān*, *qiánchéng shān*, *jiě xī*, *wěi zhōng,* and *pú cān* can be used to treat convulsions, spasms, twitching, and *wěi* and *bì* patterns of the lower limbs.
2. *Jī mén* and *sān yīn jiāo* are able to treat diseases of the urinary systems such as anuresis and difficult urination.
3. *Zú sān lǐ*, a unique acupoint, is also the primary point in treating digestive disorders, while *fēng lóng* is capable of transforming phlegm and

dampness, relieving cough, and calming labored breathing. Last but not least, pushing *yǒng quán* pertains to the treatment method of removing firewood under a boiling cauldron that can not only resolve excess but also deficient heat.

Everyday Exercises

1. Memorize the locations, operations, indications, and clinical applications of *zú sān lǐ, fēng lóng, sān yīn jiāo, and yǒng quán.*
2. Memorize three to five acupoints that treat convulsions, spasms, and twitching.

WEEK 13

Day 1

Subject 4 — Tui Na for Common Pediatric Diseases

Infantile Diarrhea

Infantile diarrhea, also known as infantile indigestion, is a gastrointestinal disorder with diarrhea as the main symptom. It is a common condition in infants below two years of age, with half the incidents occurring in infants below one. The condition is a great threat to the health of small children. Causes of diarrhea can be divided into non-infectious and infectious causes. The former may include an under-developed digestive system, low activity of digestive enzymes, poor regulatory function of the nervous system to the gastrointestinal tract, an immature immune system, improper feeding, or climatic factors. The latter includes internal and extrogenous intestinal infections.

The condition can occur in all four seasons but it occurs more commonly in the summer and autumn. If it is untreated or poorly treated, it may become protracted and impact the nutrition, growth, and development of the child in mild cases. In more serious situations, it can cause severe dehydration, metabolic acidosis, or even life-threatening conditions. Therefore, physicians should take it very seriously in clinical practice.

Clinical Manifestations

In mild cases of diarrhea, symptoms include mild simple dyspepsia with the increased frequency of defecation, with thin or watery stools that may be mixed with undigested food residue and a small amount of mucus. In more serious cases, symptoms include severe toxic indigestion, with the child passing motion more than ten times a day, accompanied by fever, vomiting, poor appetite, dry skin, and listlessness. There would be large amounts of water and mucus in the stool. If a serious cases of diarrhea is not treated in time, the child may suffer dehydration and metabolic acidosis; therefore, changes of the condition must be carefully observed.

According to TCM pattern differentiation rules, infantile diarrhea can be classified as damp-cold, damp-heat, food damage, and spleen deficiency diarrhea.

1. *Damp-cold diarrhea* Signs and symptoms may include thin, frothy, pale, and odorless stool; abdominal pain; bowel noises; pale complexion; no thirst; lengthy urination and clear urine; greasy tongue coating; soggy pulse; and red finger venule.
2. *Damp-heat diarrhea* Signs and symptoms may include abdominal pain followed by diarrhea with urgent burst; dark, yellowish, hot, and smelly stool; low grade fever; thirst; oliguria with dark yellow color; yellow and greasy tongue coating; slippery and rapid pulse; and purple finger venule.
3. *Food damage diarrhea* Signs and symptoms may include abdominal distention; crying and irritability prior to diarrhea; relieved pain after the diarrhea; large amount of stool with spoiled smell containing undigested food; a lot of gas; vomiting of acrid and spoiled food; bad breath; poor appetite; no desire for milk; thick or greasy tongue coating; and slippery pulse.
4. *Spleen deficiency diarrhea* Signs and symptoms may include chronic and often recurrent diarrhea; yellowish facial complexion; loss of appetite; loose stool mixed with tiny milk chunks or food residue; diarrhea right after meals; thin tongue coating; and soggy pulse. If the diarrhea is protracted, it can further damage the kidney yang, so that there will be incontinence diarrhea with undigested food, cold limbs, listlessness, pale tongue, and soft and feeble pulse.

Diagnosis and Differentiation

Diagnosis It is not difficult to diagnose the disease based on the clinical manifestations.

Differential Diagnosis

1. *Physiological diarrhea* This is more common in infants less than six months old, and is caused by a developmental defect of the digestive system. The infant usually has a puffy appearance, often accompanied with eczema. The only symptom is increased frequency of defecation.
2. *Bacillary dysentery* The main symptoms include abdominal pain, diarrhea, and tenesmus with sepsis. The child generally has a history of dysentery contact, and a stool bacterial culture can detect Shigella bacteria.

Treatment

1. *Treatment principles* These are based on the type of diarrhea after pattern differentiation.
   a. *Damp-cold diarrhea* Warming the center to dissipate cold, and transforming dampness to stop diarrhea.
   b. *Damp-heat diarrhea* Clearing heat and resolving dampness, and regulating the center to stop diarrhea.
   c. *Diarrhea due to food damage* Promoting digestion to guide out food stagnation, harmonizing the stomach to stop the diarrhea.
   d. *Diarrhea due to spleen deficiency* Fortifying the spleen to boost its qi, warming yang to stop diarrhea.
   e. *Spleen and kidney yang deficiency* Warming and supplementing the spleen and kidney, and consolidating the essence to stop diarrhea.
2. *Commonly used maneuvers* rubbing, kneading, pushing, pressing, scrubbing, and pinching *jí* (spine).
3. *Commonly used acupoints* *fù* (abdomen), *qí* (navel), *qījiégǔ*, *guīwěi*, *píjīng*, *dàcháng*, *zúsānlǐ* (ST 36).
4. *Operational methods*
   a. *Basic operations*

Have the child in a supine position, with the parent holding the child. The practitioner sits to the right of the child. Use one palm to apply palmar-rubbing on the whole abdomen of the child with mild force following a certain direction such as clockwise from beginning to end. The maneuver should cover all three areas of the upper, lower and the entire abdomen and last for eight to ten minutes. Place the index, middle, and ring fingers on the left *tiānshū*, *qí,* and right *tiānshū,* respectively, and apply triple-finger kneading for one to two minutes. Work on the acupoints on the hand, including supplementing *píjīng* and pushing *dàcháng*, each for 100 times. Apply pressure kneading to the bilateral *zúsānlǐ* for about a minutes or two. Lastly, perform kneading on *guīwěi* 300 times followed by pushing *qījié* upwards 300 times.

b. *Modifications based on pattern differentiation*

- *Damp-cold diarrhea* Add kneading *wàiláogōng* (EX-UE 8) 100 times, pushing *sānguān* upwards 300 times, and supplementing *píjīng*100 times.
- *Damp-heat diarrhea* Add clearing *píjīng*, *dàcháng,* and *xiǎocháng*, each for 200 times; clearing *tiānhéshuǐ* and pushing *liùfǔ* downwards, each for 300 times.
- *Diarrhea due to food damage* Add supplementing *píjīng* 300 times, supplementing *dàcháng* 200 times, and pushing *sānguān* 300 times. Then, add pressure kneading on both sides of *píshū* (BL 20) and *wèishū* (BL 21) for one minute each.
- *Diarrhea of spleen and kidney yang deficiency* Add supplementing *píjīng* and *shènjīng* for 300 times each, supplementing *dàcháng* 200 times, pressure kneading on *shènshū* (BL 23) for a minute, and scrubbing *bāliào* (BL 31 to 34) horizontally until frictional heat is felt.

Precautions

1. Although tui na can be used to treat infantile diarrhea, it is limited to treating children suffering diarrhea caused by digestive disorders of the gastrointestinal tract or simple diarrhea resulting from rotavirus, without significant dehydration and acidosis.
2. A child suffering from bacillary dysentery should first be given antibiotics.

3. The sick child should be on a proper diet. Use warm water to clean the anus thoroughly after each bowel movement. Change diapers frequently to keep the skin clean and dry.
4. Feed the child appropriately by following a regular schedule as much as possible with reasonable quantity while breast-feeding or giving supplementary baby food. Please note that supplementary food should not be given too early and too much in variety. Be cautious about climate change and dress the child accordingly. Pay attention to food hygiene to prevent intestinal diseases.

Everyday Exercises

1. What is infantile diarrhea?
2. How would you differentiate infantile diarrhea from bacterial dysentery?
3. What kind of diarrheas is tui na be able to treat? What are the basic operations?

Day 2

FEVER

Fever is the pathological increase in body temperature, a systemic response of the human pathogenic factor. It is an accompanying symptom of many diseases. Due to faster metabolism and a still-developing thermoregulatory center, the body temperature of a small child is slightly higher than that of an adult. A child's normal rectal temperature is between 36.9°C (98.4°F) and 37.5°C (99.5°F), about 0.5°C (32.9°F) higher than the oral temperature, while the axillary temperature is 0.5°C lower than the oral temperature. In general, it is more convenient to measure the rectal temperature of a child. In addition, normal body temperature fluctuates slightly in 24 hours; it is lower in the morning and higher in the afternoon, with the difference no more than 1°C (33.8°F). It is considered normal if a child's body temperature increases temporarily while eating, crying, moving around, or wearing too much clothes; or if the external room temperature is high.

There are many diseases that may cause fever. Diseases can be divided into two major categories: infectious and non-infectious. We will only describe those of acute and functional type, results of upper respiratory tract infections.

Clinical Manifestations

An abnormal rise in body temperature with a rectal temperature above 37.5°C (99.5°F) is the main characteristic of fever. The child may have other signs and symptoms including irritability, shortness of breath, flapping of nose ala, startling seizures, listlessness, coma, delirium, fatigue, weakness, and lack of appetite.

According to TCM pattern differentiation, the patterns of fever generally include exogenous contraction, excess heat of the lung and stomach, and internal heat due to yin deficiency.

1. *Exogenous contraction*

   a. *Externally contracted wind-cold* Fever, aversion to cold, headache, absence of sweat, nasal congestion, runny nose, no thirst, coughs, watery sputum, thin and white tongue coating, floating pulse, red finger venule.

b. *Externally contracted wind-heat* Fever, slight sweating, headache, nasal congestion, turbid nasal discharge, coughs, thick yellow sputum, sore throat, dry mouth, red tongue, thin yellow tongue coating, floating pulse, and reddish purple finger venule.

2. *Excess heat of the lung and stomach* Relatively high fever, vermilion face and lips, dry mouth and nose, strong thirst, rapid and labored breathing, no appetite, constipation, scanty dark urine, red tongue with dry and yellow coating, rapid pulse, and deep purple finger venule.
3. *Internal heat due to yin deficiency* Hot flashes or low grade fever in the afternoon is the main symptom accompanied by slim and frail figure, spontaneous and night sweating, vexing heat of five centers, dry mouth and lips, decreased appetite, red tongue and peeled coating, rapid pulse, and lilac finger venule.

Diagnosis and Differentiation

Key diagnostic criteria

1. Rectal temperature above 37.5°C associated with upper respiratory catarrhal symptoms and throat congestion.
2. Auscultation detects thickening breath sounds of the lungs, and dry or moist rales.
3. Laboratory tests show an increase in the total number of WBCs and neutrophils.
4. Chest X-rays show thickened texture of lung tissue or inflammatory changes.

Differential Diagnosis

The differential diagnosis of fever is quite complex. It is based on the medical history of the child, signs, symptoms, and laboratory tests. This section only describes fever due to the common cold.

Treatment

1. *Treatment principles*

   a. *Fever due to exogenous contraction* clearing heat, releasing the exterior and dispersing external pathogen.
   b. *Fever of excess heat of the lung and stomach* diffusing the lung qi, clearing heat, promoting digestion, and rectifying qi.
   c. *Internal heat due to yin deficiency* nourishing yin, clearing vexing heat, supplementing the lung and the kidney.

2. *Commonly used maneuvers* pushing, kneading, smearing, rubbing, pressing.
3. *Commonly used acupoints* *sānguān*, *liùfŭ*, *tiānhéshuĭ*, *fèijīng*, *fèishū* (BL 13) and *fēngchí* (GB 20).
4. *Operational methods*

   a. *Fever of exogenous contraction pattern* Opening *tiānmén*, disjoining head yin-yang, and kneading *tàiyáng* (EX-HN 5) 30 times for each maneuver; clearing *fèijīng* and *tiānhéshuĭ* 300 times for each acupoint.

      - *Wind-cold pattern* Add pushing *sānguān* upwards and kneading *èrshànmén* 300 times per acupoint, and grasping *fēngchí* three to five times.
      - *Wind-heat pattern* Add pushing *jí* (spine) 300 times.
      - *Complicated by coughing and gurgling due to phlegm* Add push-kneading *dànzhōng* (RN 17) 50 times, kneading *fèishū* 100 times, and kneading *fēnglóng* (ST 40) 50 times.

   b. *Excess heat in the lung and stomach* Clearing *fèijīng* and *wèijīng* 300 times each, clearing *dàcháng*, kneading *bănmén,* and revolving *nèibāguà* 200 times each, clearing *tiānhéshuĭ* and pushing *liùfŭ* downwards 300 times each, kneading *zhōngwăn* (RN 12) 150 times and *tiānshū* 100 times.
   c. *Internal heat due to yin deficiency* Supplementing *píjīng*, *fèijīng,* and *shènjīng* 300 times each, clearing *gānjīng* 200 times, kneading *shàngmă* and clearing *tiānhéshuĭ* 300 times each, pushing *yŏngquán* (KI 1) 50 times, and pressure kneading *zúsānlĭ* (ST 36) 100 times.

Precautions

1. Prior to treating a child with fever, the tui na practitioner must examine the child carefully to identify the reasons, confirm the diagnosis, and rule out acute contagious and infectious diseases in order to avoid misdiagnosis and wrong treatment. If there is high fever, even that of external contraction pattern, the child should treated with a comprehensive method such as intravenous fluids.
2. During the period of fever, encourage the child to drink sufficient boiled water and have nutritious, easy-to-digest food.
3. Encourage the child to exercise on a regular basis to enhance the physical constitution.

Everyday Exercises

1. How should we differentiate the patterns of fever in traditional Chinese medicine? What are the patterns?
2. How would you apply tui na in treating various types of fever?

Day 3

BRONCHIAL ASTHMA

Bronchial asthma (*xiàochuăn*, 哮喘) is a very common condition — the result of bronchial obstruction due to bronchospasms, mucosal edema, and increased secretions. Some of its symptoms include paroxysmal dyspnea, asthma, coughs, and expectoration. It is reversible, with the symptoms disappearing completely after the asthma attack is treated.

Typical cases of asthma are more common in children over the age of four or five, occurring in more boys than girls. It also occurs in children who are prone to allergies. About 50% of children who suffer from asthma have a history of infantile eczema and the other 50% have a family history of allergies with a genetic predisposition. Asthma can occur throughout the year, but a child is more susceptible to it in spring and autumn, during sudden weather changes, and when the child succumbs to respiratory infections, especially viral infections.

In Chinese medical practice, it is believed that the occurrence of asthma is due to "congested qi internally, non-epidemic contraction externally, and gelatinous phrenic phlegm. With the three combined, the airway is blocked, [forcing] qi to dash against [the air tract], causing *xiàochuăn* (内有壅塞之气，外有非时之感，膈有胶固之痰三者相合，闭拒气道，搏击后，发为哮喘)." Its symptoms are wheezing (*xiào*) and labored breathing (*chuăn*). Clinically, both symptoms co-exist and are closely related. Therefore, the common name is *xiàochuăn* (asthma).

Clinical Manifestations

There are usually prodromes prior to a typical bronchial asthma attack, such as coughs, chest tightness, continuous sneezing, or nasal itching. If left untreated, labored breathing will soon follow. Children suffering an acute attack of asthma have symptoms including shortness of breath, wheezing, panting, coughing, and expelling a large amount of sputum. As the bronchial lumen narrows, breathing becomes particularly difficult, resulting in shortness of breath. Patients are typically found in a forced sitting position, hands extended to the front, shoulders shrugged, mouth open, cold sweat on their foreheads. Each attack could last for several hours or even several days in a continuous attack, before it gradually eases. The physical examination shows expanded chest, excessive voiceless sounds, and wheezing. In serious cases, cyanosis can occur on lips and fingers.

In TCM, asthma generally can have three patterns: excess cold, excess heat, and deficiency patterns.

1. *Excess cold pattern* Coughs, labored breathing, gurgling phlegm in the throat, clear and thin sputum with a lot of foam, pale face, cold limbs, absence of thirst, clear urine, and lengthy urination. The color of the tongue is pale with thin white coating, and the pulse is floating and tight or floating and slippery.
2. *Excess heat pattern* Coughs, heavy and labored breathing, loud gurgling phlegm in the throat, thick yellow sputum, red face, very warm body, fullness of the chest and hypochondria, irritability, restlessness, strong desire for cold drinks, constipation, scanty dark urine, and red tongue with thin or thick yellow coating. The pulse is rapid floating or wiry and slippery.
3. *Deficiency pattern* Shortness of breath with even mild physical activity, cyanotic face and lips, sweaty head, panting while sitting up, cold limbs, and feeble waist and legs. Other symptoms are listlessness, fatigue, lack of appetite, greenish watery stool, clear urine, and lengthy urination. The tongue is pale with white coating and the pulse is thready and weak.

Diagnosis and Differentiation

Key diagnostic criteria

1. The patient has the clinical manifestations of asthma.
2. Laboratory tests show an increase in blood eosinophils.
3. Chest X-rays show that there is increased brightness of both lungs accompanied by a lowered diaphragm. For those who have a repetitive occurrence of asthma, there is thickened texture of the tissues and emphysema.

Differential Diagnosis

1. *Cardiac asthma* Frequent coughing with pink, bloody, and foamy phlegm; difficulty breathing; auscultation can detect rales on the bottom of both lungs with signs of heart disease.
2. *Chronic bronchitis* Relatively longer course of the disease with gradually aggravated shortness of breath and typical emphysema signs. Bronchial spasmolytic medications have a demonstrable effect.

Treatment

1. *Treatment principles* directing qi downwards, transforming phlegm, relieving coughs, and calming labored breathing.
2. *Commonly used maneuvers* pushing, kneading, rubbing, foulage, grasping, and scrubbing.
3. *Commonly used acupoints fèijīng, nèibāguà, bǎnmén, dànzhōng* (RN 17), *dìngchuǎn* (EX-B 1), *fèishū* (BL 13) and *xiélèi.*
4. *Operational methods*
   Basic operations
   a. Face the child. Apply regular head maneuvers first, with pushing *cuánzhú* (opening *tiānmén*) and *kǎngōng* (disjoining head yin-yang), and kneading *tài yáng* (EX-HN 5) 30 times each. Apply pressure kneading on *dànzhōng*, *rǔpang,* and *rǔgēn* (the pediatric one), each for one to two minutes. These manipulations comfort the chest and diffuse lung qi. Next, work on acupoints on the hands. Perform supplementing *píjīng* 500 times, revolving *nèibāguà* 400 times, nailing *sìhéngwén* with each *héngwén* for three to five times, and kneading *bǎnmén* 500 times. In particular, kneading *bǎnmén* can direct rebellious qi downwards when combined with foulage and scrubbing *xiélèi* for 100 times.
   b. Now work on the back of the child. First, place the middle finger on *dàzhuī* (DU 14) with the index and ring fingers on the left and right *dìngchuǎn* (EX-B 1), respectively. Apply triple-finger kneading on the three acupoints for 100 times. Then, apply double-finger kneading on *fèishū* (BL 13) and disjoining pushing the scapulas for 100 times each. Next, perform scrubbing on *fèishū* left and right until the heat from the friction is felt. End the treatment with grasping *jiānjǐng* (GB 21).

Modifications Based on Pattern Differentiation

a. *Cold pattern* Add pushing *sānguān* upwards 300 times, pressure kneading *fēngchí* (GB 20) ten to 20 times, and scrubbing the spine and both sides of the bladder meridians until the heat is felt.
b. *Heat pattern* Add clearing *fèijīng* 300 times, clearing *dàchángjīng* 200 times, pushing *liùfǔ* downwards 300 times, pushing *jí* 300 times, and kneading *fēnglóng* (ST 40) 100 times.
c. *Deficient pattern* Add supplementing *fèijīng* 300 times, *shènjīng* 500 times, kneading *dāntián* for three to five minutes, and pressure kneading on *zúsānlǐ* (ST 36) 20 times. Then, apply double-finger kneading on *fèishū* (BL 13), *píshū* (BL 20), and *shènshū* (BL 23), one minute for each acupoint.

Precautions

1. Increase physical and outdoor activities to strengthen the child's physical constitution and reduce the number of attacks.
2. Have children who suffer from repeated attacks receive asthma vaccine.
3. Identify allergens, receive desensitization therapy, and avoid contact with allergens.
4. Keep warm and prevent respiratory tract infections.
5. If tui na therapy is not effective, the child should be immediately given comprehensive treatment including fluids, oxygen, and infection control.
6. Based on the view in Chinese medical practice of "a disease that often attacks in winter needs to be treated in summer," treating asthma with tui na during hot summer days is more effective. In addition, during the remission period after the onset, tui na can have a preventive effect and reduce the severity if there is an onset.

Everyday Exercises

1. What is bronchial asthma and what are the TCM patterns?
2. How should bronchial asthma be treated using tui na therapy?

Day 4

COUGHS

Coughing is the most common respiratory symptom of many diseases, including influenza and pneumonia. As a defensive reflex activity of our body, coughing removes excessive secretions and foreign objects in the trachea and bronchi with an explosive expiratory movement. Coughing in children is usually the result of acute or chronic respiratory infection, because the respiratory tract in children is rich in blood vessels while the mucosa of trachea and bronchia are yet delicate and more prone to inflammatory degeneration. Coughs can occur throughout the year, but are most common in the winter and spring.

In Chinese medical practice, it is believed that the lungs, in charge of respiration and located on top of other organs, are fairly delicate. When external pathogens attack the body, they first invade the lungs. Thus, the exterior of the body is fettered and the lungs fail to diffuse, vent, and descend qi, leading to rebellious qi going upwards and bursting forth as coughs. People in ancient times named a bursting sound without phlegm "*ké*", which is different from the name given to phlegm without sound, which is "*sòu.*" The two sounds combined give the so-called *késòu* (cough).

Clinical Manifestations

In TCM, coughs are divided into two common types: those of exterior patterns and those of interior damage patterns.

1. *Coughs of exterior patterns*

   a. *Exterior wind-cold* The main symptom is coughing. Other symptoms may include coughing up clear and thin sputum, nasal congestion with clear discharge, headache, body pain, aversion to cold, absence of fever or mild fever, absence of sweat, and no thirst. The tongue coating is thin and white, and the pulse is floating and tight.

b. *Exterior wind-heat* The main symptom is coughing. Others symptoms may include thick yellow sputum that is difficult to spit out; fever; aversion to wind; sweating; turbid nasal discharge; sore, dry, or itching throat; thirst; constipation; and dark yellow urine. The tongue is quite red with thin yellow coating, and the pulse is floating and rapid.

2. *Coughs of internal damage patterns* The main symptom is protracting unhealed coughs. There can be a large amount of phlegm, dry coughs without phlegm, or thick phlegm that is difficult to expectorate. Other symptoms may include pallor, cold limbs, shortness of breath, sweating, chest tightness, poor appetite, emaciation, listlessness, and fatigue. The tongue coating is white and greasy and the pulse is thready, or thready and rapid.

Diagnosis and Differentiation

Diagnosis of coughs in children should not be difficult based on the symptoms. In addition to coughs, lung auscultation can detect audible rough breathy sounds, and dry or moist rales. Laboratory tests show increased blood leukocytes and neutrophils. Chest X-ray show a slightly thickened texture of tissues or shadows owing to lung inflammation.

Treatment

1. *Treatment principles*

   a. *Coughs due to exogenous contraction of wind-cold* The appropriate treatment is to dissipate cold, release the exterior, diffuse the lung, and relieve coughs.

   b. *Coughs due to exogenous contraction of wind-heat* The proper treatment is to clear the heat, release the exterior, purify lung qi, and relieve coughs.

   c. *Coughs due to internal damages* The correct treatment is to fortify the spleen, nourish the lung, relieve coughs, and transform the phlegm.

2. *Commonly used maneuvers* pushing, kneading, pressure kneading, nailing, and grasping.

3. *Commonly used acupoints* *fèijīng*, *nèibāguà*, *rǔpáng*,*rǔgēn* (pediatric), *dànzhōng* (RN 17), *fèishū* (BL 13), *píshū* (BL 20), and *zúsānlǐ* (ST 36).
4. *Operational methods*
   Basic operations
   a. Face the child. Apply regular facial and head maneuvers, i.e., opening *tiānmén*, disjoining head yin-yang, and kneading *tàiyáng* (EX-HN 5) 30 times each. Apply disjoining pushing *dànzhōng* 100 times, and kneading *rǔpáng* and *rǔgēn* 30 times each. Next, work on hand acupoints — revolving *nèibāguà* 200 times, clearing *fèijīng* 300 times, and supplementing it 500 times. Then, apply kneading on *fēnglóng* (ST 40) and *zúsānlǐ* (ST 36) bilaterally, one minute for each acupoint.
   b. Upon completion of the above maneuvers, let the child lie prone or have the practitioner facing the child's back with the child sitting. Apply pressure kneading on *fēngmén* (BL 12) and *fèishū* (BL 13), each for a minute. Then, apply disjoining pushing the scapulas 100 times followed by scrubbing the child' sback-*shu* points until the frictional heat is felt.

Modifications Based on Pattern Differentiation

a. *Externally contracted wind-cold* Add kneading *wàiláogōng* (EX-UE 8) 30 times, pushing *sānguān* 300 times, grasping *hégǔ* (LI 4) five to ten times and *fēngchí* (GB 20) ten times.
b. *Externally contracted wind-heat* Add clearing *fèijīng* and pushing *liùfǔ* downwards 500 times each and pushing *tiānzhùgǔ* 100 times.
c. *Internal damages* Add supplementing *píjīng* 500 times and *shènjīng* 300 times, kneading *zhōngwǎn* (RN 12) 200 times and kneading *dāntián* for two minutes. Then, apply pressure kneading on *píshū* (BL 20), *wèishū* (BL 21), and *shènshū* (BL 23) for one minute each.

Precautions

1. Coughing is just a symptom. Therefore, it is necessary to find out the cause of it in a timely manner in order to treat it accordingly as early as possible.

2. While the child is ill, make sure he or she rests appropriately, eats light and easy-to-digest food, and avoids salty and spicy food.
3. Keep the chest and abdomen warm, and especially watch out for weather changes.

Everyday Exercises

1. What is the definition of coughs and what are the types according to the TCM pattern differentiation?
2. Memorize the basic tui na operations in treating coughs.

Day 5

INFANTILE MALNUTRITION WITH ACCUMULATION

Infantile malnutrition with accumulation (*gānjī*, 疳积) is the collective name for infantile malnutrition (*gānzhèng*, 疳证) and food accumulation (*jīzhì*, 积滞), with the two having different levels of severity. Food accumulation refers to the condition in children as a result of improper feeding of milk or food, causing damage to the spleen and stomach, so that these organs fail to transport and transform the food, leading to food stagnation. Infantile malnutrition refers to the depletion of qi and body fluids, leading to emaciation and weakness, which is the result of further development of food accumulation. Therefore, an ancient saying says, "no accumulation, no infantile malnutrition (无积不成疳)."Another cause of malnutrition in children is parasite infection.

Modern Western medicine regards infantile malnutrition as a chronic nutritional deficiency. The main causes of infantile malnutrition are inadequate intake of food, improper feeding, the child's fastidiousness to food, and poor digestion and absorption. Besides, the condition can be secondary to a variety of chronic diseases, causing lack of, or increased consumption of, protein and calories, which leads to the abnormal metabolism of the body and the consumption of its own tissue. As a result, there will be weight loss and reduction of subcutaneous fat that gradually leads to edema and stagnant growth. In severe situations, there may be dysfunction of multiple organs.

Clinical Manifestations

The main symptoms of this disease are listlessness, fatigue, poor facial luster, emaciation, growth retardation, obviously reduced subcutaneous fat, and muscular atrophy. According to TCM pattern differentiation, infantile malnutrition falls into two categories.

1. *Milk or food stagnation* Symptoms include abdominal distention, poor appetite, nocturnal restlessness, lassitude, and irregular defecation accompanied by bad smell or constipation. There may also be vexing

heat in the center of the palms and soles. The tongue coating is thick, greasy, light yellow, and lack fluids; the pulse is weak or weak and rapid; and the finger venule is purple.

2. *Qi and blood deficiency* Symptoms include pale white or dark yellowish complexion; shriveled facial appearance like in an elderly person; sparse hair that falls out easily; extremely skinny, dry and scurfy skin; listlessness; low and deep crying; drowsiness and weakness; and profuse sweating with minimal activities. The limbs are cold, and may be accompanied by edema; the condition being more common in the lower extremities. Other symptoms are no desire or an abnormally strong desire for food, developmental disorders, depressed abdomen, and loose stool. The tongue is pale with a thin coating, and the finger venule is pale.

Diagnosis and Differentiation

Key diagnostic criteria

It should not be difficult to diagnose the disease based on the physical appearance of the child and various clinical manifestations. At the same time, it is necessary to further identify predisposing factors and complications to properly estimate the severity of the disease and facilitate the treatment. The following list can serve as a reference:

1. The extent of weight loss.
2. The extent of swelling.
3. Whether the concentration of the plasma protein is normal or obviously decreased, the basal metabolic rate, and excretion of creatine and creatinine.

Differential Diagnosis

1. *Primary tuberculosis* In addition to a weight loss and poor appetite, main symptoms also include long-term fever, coughs, hemoptysis, hot flashes, and night sweats. A chest X-ray can confirm the diagnosis.
2. *Parasitic diseases* In addition to weight loss, the child can often have abdominal pain and anal itching, and a stool examination will show eggs of intestinal parasites.

Treatment

1. *Treatment principles* For milk and food stagnation, it is appropriate to disperse accumulation by guiding it out, fortifying the spleen, and harmonizing the stomach. For those that are of qi and blood deficiency pattern, it is proper to warm the center, fortify the spleen, and replenish qi and blood.
2. *Commonly used maneuvers* pushing, kneading, rubbing, pinching, nailing, pressure kneading.
3. *Commonly used acupoints píjīng, bănmén, sìfèng (sìhéngwén), nèibāguà, fù*, qí, *zúsānlĭ* (ST 36), the spine.
4. *Operational methods*
   Basic operations

   a. Have the child in a supine position. Start by pushing *píjīng* 500 times, *bănmén* 300 times, and *sìhéngwén* 200 times, and revolving *nèibāguà* 200 times. Next, combine rubbing *fù* and kneading *qí* for a total of five minutes to make the abdomen warm. Then, apply pressure kneading on both sides of *zúsānlĭ* (ST 36) for one minute.
   b. Have the child in a prone position. Use the index and middle fingers to perform double-finger kneading on both sides of *píshū* (BL 20), *wèishū* (BL 21) and *sānjiāoshū* (BL 22), each for a minute. Then, apply spinal pinching starting from *guīwěi* and all the way up to *dàzhuī* (DU 14) for three to five times. For an enhanced stimulation, add lifting pinching on *píshū*, *wèishū,* and *sānjiāoshū.*

Modifications Based on Pattern Differentiation

a. *Milk and food accumulation* Add clearing *píjīng* 500 times, supplementing *píjīng* 300 times, clearing *dàcháng* 300 times and *shènjīng* 100 times, and kneading *zhōngwăn* (RN 12) for five minutes.
b. *Qi and blood deficiency* Add supplementing *píjīng* 500 times, pushing *sānguān* upwards 300 times, knead-rubbing *zhōngwăn* for five minutes, rubbing *dāntián* for two minutes, kneading *xuèhăi* (SP 10)

30 times, finger-kneading *shènshū* (BL 23) and *mìngmén* (DU 4) for one minute peracupoint.

Precautions

1. Feed small children appropriately, and breast-feed whenever it is possible. Add supplementing food at the right time, and ensure a normal nutritional diet high in protein or calories. The food needs to be soft, and be given in smaller portioned, multiple meals.
2. Correct bad eating habits such as being choosy about food.
3. Arrange proper outdoor activities and physical exercises for the child to increase his or her appetite and improve digestion.
4. Ensure that the child sleeps adequately.
5. Pay attention to food hygiene to prevent the child from catching intestinal infectious and parasitic diseases.

Everyday Exercises

1. What is infantile malnutrition with accumulation?
2. What are the two patterns of infantile malnutrition with accumulation in clinical Chinese medicine, and what are the treatment principles and basic tui na treatment for these?

Day 6

CONSTIPATION

Constipation is characterized by a reduction in the number of bowel movements, dry feces, and difficult defecation. Under normal circumstances, it takes 24 to 48 hours for food to pass through the gastrointestinal tract, and be digested and absorbed, with the residue then being excreted. If the defecation intervalis over 48 hours, constipation would be said to have occurred. However, there are also healthy individuals who have bowel movements every other day or once every three days. As long as the bowel movements follow a regular schedule, the individual may not necessarily have constipation.

There are many causes of constipation, such as insufficient food intake and poor eating habits like including too little fiber in the diet. Dietary fiber adds bulk to your stool and makes it easier to pass. Also, the food residue in the colon may advance too slowly and cause constipation if the person lacks defecating power, or related muscles (like the diaphragm, abdomen, anal levator, and intestinal smooth muscles) are too weak as the result of malnutrition and cachexia. Some other causes of constipation include intestinal malformation, perianal inflammation, extra intestinal tumor oppression, and abuse of strong laxatives.

In TCM, it is believed that constipation is the result of several causes. Firstly, dry and accumulated feces is difficult to be eliminated owing to accumulated heat in the stomach and intestines, or depletion of body fluids after suffering diseases of the heat pattern. Secondly, some cases are due to the large intestines not being moistened because of deficiency of body fluids in people of weak constitution.

Clinical Manifestations

According to TCM pattern differentiation, constipation is of two types: excess and deficiency constipation.

1. *Excess constipation* Symptoms include dry stools, scanty dark urine, red face, warmer than normal body, bad breath, red lips, dry mouth

with a desire to drink, belching, sour regurgitation, reduced food intake, and abdominal fullness. The tongue coating is dry and yellow or thick and greasy, the pulse is wiry and rapid, and the finger venule is purple.

2. *Deficiency constipation* The stool may not be very dry, however, it is difficult to be eliminated. Other symptoms may include clear urine, pallor, lassitude, low in vital energy, cold limbs, in favor of warmth and aversion to cold. The tongue is pale with thin and white coating, the pulse is thready and weak, and the finger venule is pale.

Diagnosis and Differentiation

The condition is easy to diagnose because of its clear clinical manifestations. For a detailed differential diagnosis, refer to the section on constipation in adultson page.

Treatment

1. *Treatment principles* The proper treatment for excess pattern is to rectify qi, guide stagnation, clear heat, and unblock the feces, while for deficient pattern, it is appropriate to boost qi, nourish blood, moisten dryness, and unblock the feces.
2. *Commonly used maneuvers* pushing, rubbing, kneading and pressure kneading.
3. *Commonly used acupoints zhōngwǎn* (RN 12), *fù*, *tiānshū* (ST 25), *dàhéng* (SP 15), *dàchángshū* (BL 25), *bóyángchí*, *qījiégǔ*, *guīwěi*, and *zúsānlǐ* (ST 36). *Bóyángchí* is on the dorsal aspect of the forearm, threecun above the transverse crease of the wrist, which is equivalent to *zhīgōu* (SJ 6) in adults.
4. *Operational methods*
   Basic operations

   a. The child is supine, with the practitioner facing the child. Apply finger-kneading on *zhōngwǎn* for two minutes. Apply rubbing *fù* clockwise for two to three minutes. Put more focus on the left side of *tiānshū* and *dàhéng,* and apply double-finger kneading for three to five minutes. Apply pressure kneading to both sides of *bóyángchí* and *zúsānlǐ*, one minute for each acupoint.

b. Have the child in a prone position. Perform double-finger kneading on *dàchángshū* for one to two minutes. Then, push *qījiégǔ* straight, top-down 300 times. Complete the basic operations with finger-kneading *guīwěi* 300 times.

Modifications Based on Pattern Differentiation

a. *Excess constipation* Add clearing *tiānhéshuǐ* 300 times, pushing *liùfǔ* downwards 300 times, clearing *dàcháng* 300 times, clearing *píjīng* 200 times, and pushing *bǎnmén* 200 times.
b. *Deficiency constipation* Add pushing *sānguān* upwards 300 times, fortifying *píjīng* 500 times, clearing *dàcháng* 200 times, supplementing *shènjīng* 300 times, and double-finger kneading *shènshū* (BL 23) for a minute.

Precautions

1. Eat more vegetables and fruits rich in fiber.
2. Develop a regular schedule for defecation.
3. For constipation due toother reasons, find out the cause for appropriate treatment.

Rectal Prolapse

Rectal prolapse is a condition in which the rectum becomes stretched out and protrudes out of the anus. This is a common condition in children under the age of three. As the sacral curvature in children is not fully formed, the rectum is in a vertical position. In addition, the supporting tissues of the rectum are relatively weak. When there is increased intra-abdominal pressure, the rectum may not have enough support from the sacrum and surrounding tissues, causing it to slide down easily, resulting in a rectal prolapse.

In TCM, it is believed that the occurrence of this condition in children is due to several causes including congenital deficiency, frailty after sickness, and chronic diarrhea. All of these would deplete healthy qi, leading to the sinking of qi and powerlessness of the qi to lift and hold, resulting in a rectal prolapse.

Clinical Manifestations

According to TCM pattern differentiation, rectal prolapse can be divided into deficient and excess patterns, with most cases of the deficient pattern type.

1. *Rectal prolapse of deficient pattern* The prolapsed rectum is light red, not easy to retract on its own, and without much swelling and pain. The child's facial complexion is pale or sallow. Other symptoms may include emaciation, listlessness, fatigue, cold limbs, and spontaneous sweating. The color of the tongue is pale with a thin white coating, the pulse is thready and weak, and the finger venule is pale.
2. *Rectal prolapse of excess pattern* The prolapsed rectum is bright red, with a small amount of bright red exudates. It is often associated with perianal swelling, a hot sensation, pain, and itching. There can be dry stool and scanty dark urine. The sick child often cries with anxiety and restlessness. The tongue is red with a yellow greasy coating, the pulse is rapid, and the finger venule is purple.

Diagnosis and Differentiation

The diagnosis of the disease is not difficult based on its clinical manifestations. It is also easily differentiated from perianal abscess.

Treatment

1. *Treatment principles* For patients of deficient pattern, boosting qi, lifting up the prolapsed rectum, and rescuing it from slipping out. For those of excess pattern, clearing heat, lifting up the prolapsed rectum, and rescuing it from slipping out.
2. *Commonly used maneuvers* pushing, kneading, pressure kneading.
3. *Commonly used acupoints bǎihuì* (DU 20), *dāntián*, *dàcháng*, *guīwěi*, *qījiégǔ*, etc.

4. *Operational methods*
   Basic operations
   a. The child is supine, with the practitioner facing the child. Apply pressure kneading on *bǎihuì* for two minutes. Apply kneading to *dāntián* at the lower abdomen for about five minutes.
   b. Next, have the child in prone position. Apply straight pushing on *qījiégǔ* bottom-up followed by finger-kneadingon *guīwěi*, each for 300 times. For those of frail constitution, add spinal pinching bottom-up for three to five times.

Modifications Based On Pattern Differentiation

A. *Deficient pattern* Add supplementing *píjīng* 500 times and *dàcháng* 300 times, pushing *sānguān* upwards 300 times, and supplementing *shènjīng* 500 times.
b. *Excess pattern* Add clearing *dàcháng* and *xiǎocháng* 300 times each, kneading *qǔchí* (LI 11) 30 times, and pushing *liùfǔ* downwards 200 times.

Precautions

1. Pay attention to the personal hygiene and care of the anal area. Wash the anus with warm water after each bowel movement. Apply lifting and kneading maneuvers to the prolapsed rectum to make it retract in a timely manner.
2. Do not allow the child to sit on the toilet for a long time upon bowel movement.
3. Improve nutritional and food hygiene, and prevent diarrhea or constipation.
4. Encourage the child to do levatorani exercises.

Everyday Exercises

1. Master the basic tui na treatment methods for children with constipation.
2. What is rectal prolapse?
3. Master the tui na operational methods in treating rectal prolapse.

WEEK 14

Day 1

NOCTURIA

Nocturia is the need to wake up in the night to urinate. Nocturia is more common in boys, with the male to female ratio at approximately 6 to 2. Occurrence is more in the first half of the night, usually two to three hours after bedtime. Nocturia, which is a type of sleep disorder, is different from urinary incontinence, which is an organic disorder. The latter can occur at any time while nocturia occurs only during sleep. When the patient is unable to wake up, but urinates during sleep, the condition is known as nocturnal enuresis (commonly called bedwetting). This is particularly common in infants, whose central nervous systems regulating urination are not yet fully developed. When a child reaches three to four years of age, urination will become conscious and voluntary once the bladder is filled.

Pediatric nocturnal enuresis is mostly a functional change, triggered by factors such as change of environment, impact of mood, over-excitement during the day, tiredness, and psychological stimulation. It is necessary to treat the condition as early as possible, since an extended period of bedwetting can affect a child's physical and mental health and his or her normal development.

In Chinese medical practice, it is believed that the condition is mostly related to congenital kidney qi deficiency, causing deficient cold of the kidney. The kidney governs hiding and storing with its orifices as the anterior yin (external genitalia) and posterior yin (anus). It also controls both urination and bowel movements and forms the interior-exterior pair with the bladder. When the qi of both the kidney and bladder is deficient, they fail to restrict the waterway, causing nocturia.

Clinical Manifestations

Nocturia occurs easily when the child is over-excited or has had an exhausting day. In mild cases, the child will have one occurrence every few nights. In more severe cases, it may happen once, twice or even more times every night. When the child suffers nocturia for a long time, symptoms can include sallow facial complexion, mental retardation, dizziness, fatigue, weakness and soreness of the waist and knees, and cold limbs. Older children suffering from nocturnal enuresis may also appear to be shy, suffer from mental stress, or have an inferiority complex.

Diagnosis and Differentiation

Nocturia can be confirmed after obtaining a detailed medical history and ruling out organic enuresis through a neurological physical examination.

Treatment

1. *Treatment principles* supplementing and warming the spleen and the kidney, and consolidating and astringing the lower origin (kidney essence).
2. *Commonly used maneuvers* pushing, kneading, pressure kneading, scrubbing, and pinching.
3. *Commonly used acupoints bǎihuì* (DU 20), *píjīng, shènjīng, sānguān, dāntián, shènshū* (BL 23), *mìngmén* (DU 4), and *sānyīnjiāo* (SP 6).
4. *Operational methods*

   Basic operations

   a. Have the child in a supine position, with the practitioner facing the child. First, apply pressure kneading *bǎihuì* for two minutes, supplementing *píjīng* and *shènjīng* for 500 times each, and pushing *sānguān* 300 times. Then, perform kneading to *dāntián* for three to five minutes and pressure kneading on *sānyīnjiāo* for 30 to 50 times.

b. Have the child change to a prone position. Place the middle finger on *mìngmén*, the index finger on the left *shènshū*, and the ring finger on the right *shènshū*. Apply three-finger kneading on the three points for two minutes and scrubbing them horizontally until the heat can be felt. Finally, apply spinal pinching bottom-up for three to five times.

Modifications Based on Pattern Differentiation

a. *Kidney qi deficiency* Add supplementing *shènjīng* 100 times, pushing *sānguān* 100 times, and pressure kneading *yǒngquán* (KI 1) 50 times.
b. *Lung qi deficiency* Add supplementing *fèijīng* 300 times, kneading *wàiláogōng* (EX-UE 8) 50 times and pushing *sānguān* 100 times.
c. *Damp-heat of the liver meridian* Add clearing *gānjīng* 100 times and *xiǎocháng* 100 times, pushing *liùfǔ* downwards 100 times, and foulage on *xiélèi* 50 times.

Precautions

1. Correctly guide the child suffering from nocturia and nocturnal enuresis to build up self-confidence and avoid fearful feelings and stress, so as to prevent the conditions from affecting his or her physical and mental health.
2. Help the child to cultivate the good habit of going to the bathroom on a regular schedule. Avoid drinking water and liquid food two hours before bed. Wake up the child on a certain schedule to go to the bathroom.

Urinary Retention

Urinary retention is the condition where the patient finds it difficult to empty his or her bladder completely, or at all, despite an urge to urinate. Urination is a complex reflection. The functions of the bladder are storing urine and urination. When the bladder is filled with urine, it produces the desire to urinate and results in urination. The completion of the function depends on the performance of nerves and muscles under the regulation of the cerebral cortex. When there is a dysfunction of the nerves and muscles due to causes such as encephalitis coma, spinal or epidural anesthesia, postural changes such as bed rest or adverse effect of certain drugs, it causes the inability of the bladder to discharge urine, resulting in urinary retention.

In Chinese medical practice, it is believed that the condition is due to unsmooth bladder qi transformation as the result of closure and blockage of the waterway, or insufficient kidney yang and depleted life-gate fire.

Clinical Manifestations

Symptoms include lower abdomen pain and fullness, a strong desire to urinate but unable to micturate, and an obviously full bladder with the bottom below the belly button.

Treatment

1. *Treatment principles* opening up the occlusion.
2. *Commonly used maneuvers* pushing, kneading, rubbing, pressure kneading, intense pressing.
3. *Commonly used acupoints dāntián, jīmén* (SP 11), *sānyīnjiāo* (SP 6).
4. *Operational methods*
   Have the child in a supine position. Select distal points and apply pressure kneading on *sānyīnjiāo* with relatively stronger stimulation for 50 to 100 times. Use the index and middle fingers to perform straight pushing from the upper edge of the medial side of the knee to the groin, namely pushing *jīmén,* for 300 times. Then, apply agile rubbing on the lower abdomen from one to two minutes followed by pressure kneading on *dāntián* for three to five minutes. Overlap the thumbs, place them on top of *dāntián,* and apply pressing on the acupoint with gradually increasing strength, following the rhythm of abdominal breathing until the child urinates. When 100–200 ml of urine is discharged, apply the palm-pressing maneuver using the root of the palm to press where the bladder bottom is located, following the rhythm of the abdominal breathing to raise and press the area, until the urine is completely drained.

Precautions

1. The key to treating urinary retention is to use appropriate force while applying intense pressing. The level of the force depends upon individual tolerance. Brute force should be avoided.
2. If tui na treatment is not effective, catheterization is an option; this can relieve the condition instantly.

Everyday Exercises

1. What is nocturia?
2. Master the treatment of nocturia using tui na therapy.
3. Master the method of using tui na to treat urinary retention and its precautions.

Day 2

INFANTILE MUSCULAR TORTICOLLIS

Infantile muscular torticollis is a condition in which an infant has his or her head tilted or twisted to one side. This is due in most cases to the unilateral contracture (or shortening) of the sternocleidomastoid muscle, which is the muscle that extends down the side of the neck. Besides congenital malformations, many scholars believe that the shortening is the result of ischemia of the sternocleidomastoid muscle, causing muscle fibrosis. Ischemia can be the result of various factors. For example, the head of the fetus could have been tilted to one side for a long time. Another factor is the temporary stagnation of blood flow, causing insufficient blood supply of the muscle during the delivery process. As a result, fusiform scar tissues or fiber cords replace the muscle, causing contracture.

Clinical Manifestations

1. A prism-shaped swelling can be found on one side of the neck after the birth of the child, which is consistent with the direction of the sternocleidomastoid muscle, and more confined to the middle and lower segments. Later on, the ipsilateral sternocleidomastoid develops contracture and tension that gives it a prominent and cord-like appearance. The muscle spasms and traction then lead to torticollis deformity.
2. Unique torticollis postures are observed, including head tilted to the affected side, leaning forward, or rotated to the contralateral side with the ipsilateral ear leaning downwards, close to the sternoclavicular joint. If the abnormality is not corrected in time, it would cause atrophy of the face on the ipsilateral side, making it look significantly smaller than the contralateral side. A small number of patients can have fixed scoliosis of the cervical or upper thoracic spine.
3. Activities of the neck are restricted, particularly in ipsilateral rotation and contralateral flexion.
4. Hard cord-like masses can be palpated in the ipsilateral sternocleidomastoid toward the middle to lower segments.

Diagnosis and Differentiation

Diagnosis The diagnosis of the disease is not difficult based on its clinical manifestations and can be confirmed after differentiation diagnosis ruling out other diseases.

Differential Diagnosis

1. *Congenital spinal deformity* Although there is also torticollis deformity, no swelling masses in the neck can be detected. Anteroposterior and lateral X-rays show congenital spinal deformities such as hemivertebra, wedge vertebra, or butterfly vertebra of the cervical spines.
2. *Diplopia with compensatory abnormal head position* Compensatory abnormal head position has a direct relationship with diplopia as the result of extraocular muscle paralysis. The left or right skew of the head are related to the superior rectus, inferior rectus, superior oblique and, inferior oblique.

Treatment

1. *Treatment principles* relaxing the sinews, invigorating blood, softening hardness, and dissipating masses.
2. *Commonly used maneuvers* push-kneading, grasping, plucking, and passive movement of the neck.
3. *Commonly used acupoints and areas ā shìxué*, ipsilateral sternocleidomastoid and lateral aspect of the neck.
4. *Operational methods*

   The child is supine, with the practitioner facing the child. Apply finger kneading on the sternocleidomastoid muscle up and down and back and forth for about two minutes with gentle force in order for the child to be able to adapt to the treatment. Then, apply grasping to the sternocleidomastoid up and down and back and forth for about one to two minutes with the focus on the swelling mass. Again, the stroke should be gentle and flexible; this maneuver reaches deeper tissues than the kneading maneuver does. Next, apply plucking up and down and back and forth on the sternocleidomastoid with the focus on the mass or swelling and supplement with kneading to relieve the pain response to the plucking. Use one hand to hold the child's ipsilateral shoulder and press down, while the other hand supports the ipsilateral temporal side of the head and slowly pushes it to the contralateral side to complete a lateral movement for three to five times, or more. This is called passive stretching of the sternocleidomastoid. Finally, let the sternocleidomastoid muscle relax for about one minute.

Precautions

1. During tui na treatment, apply talcum powder on the ipsilateral sternocleidomastoid muscle to prevent the delicate skin from being damaged. For child who sweats during the treatment, wipe the sweat off and make the skin dry before applying the powder.
2. Ask the parents to help their child daily with passive stretching exercises of the ipsilateral sternocleidomastoid muscle. While the child is sleeping, place a pillow on both sides of the head to stabilize its position.
3. Make the child turn his or her head and neck in the opposite direction of the deformity to help correct torticollis in day-to-day life. For example, feed the child from the desired direction, or position toys so that the child has to turn his or her head in the desired direction to see them.
4. The earlier the treatment, the better the efficacy in treating torticollis. If there is no significant improvement under conservative treatment for more than six months, orthopedic surgery should be considered to correct the problem.

Everyday Exercises

1. What is muscular torticollis? How do you differentiate it from congenital spinal deformity?
2. How would you use tui na to treat children with muscular torticollis?

Day 3

SCOLIOSIS

In a normal child, the spine runs straight down the middle of the back. In a child with scoliosis, the spine has a lateral curvature. In most cases, the cause of scoliosis unknown; it is then called primary scoliosis. Other types of scoliosis can be the result of congenital malformations, such as hemivertebrae, wedged vertebrae, hypoplasia of vertebral arches, nerve paralysis, lesion of the chest, spinal infection, and tumor. In addition, scoliosis can occur if a child has bad reading and writing postures, or carries single-strap school bags and heavy objects for an extended period of time. Usually, scoliosis occurs at the thoracolumbar or lumbosacral segment of the spine at an early age when there is rapid development. Usually, by the age of three to four years, the child can show an obvious deformity. However, the majority of the cases are discovered at age ten. Incidences of scoliosis are higher in girls than in boys.

Clinical Manifestations

Mild scoliosis does not cause any symptoms. They are usually discovered by chance when a parent is giving the child a bath or changing his or her underwear. In children with more obvious symptoms, it can be seen that the scapulae (shoulder blades) are not level or not in the same plane. In more severe cases of scoliosis, the deformities can cause visceral dysfunctions, such as heart and lung hypoplasia and low vital capacity. The patient often senses shortness of breath, palpitations, and chest tightness while performing physical activities. The gastrointestinal system can also be affected, with the child having indigestion and loss of appetite. In the nervous system, there may be symptoms owing to compression of the spinal cord or nerve root. Patients with severe scoliosis may have systemic dysplasia, thin and short bodies, numbness of the limbs, and physical fragility as a result of major visceral dysfunctions. Local pain or compression pain between the ribs and the iliac wings can occur once the patient reaches middle age or above.

A physical examination can detect S-shaped scoliosis with a localized arch on one side of the back. In addition, it is very important during a physical examination to determine whether the child with the disease has compensatory ability for scoliosis. First of all, observe if the inferior angles of both scapulae and the iliac wings are in the same plane. If they are, there is compensatory ability; i.e., scoliosis is considered to be compensatory when the pelvis is tilted laterally. Curving the lumbar spine to an angle equal to the pelvic tilt helps to hold the trunk vertically. Usually, the spine itself is not abnormal, and the scoliosis disappears when the pelvic tilt is corrected. If this does not happen, the scoliosis is said to show decompensation. (Decompensation refers to the loss of spinal balance when the thoracic cage is not centered over the pelvis.) Secondly, ask the child to pull a horizontal bar using both hands. If the body naturally hangs with disappearance of the original curvature of the spine, then the child has compensatory scoliosis. However, if the original curvature of the spine does not change, there is decompensation.

X-rays show an S-shaped spine. The middle part with the biggest curvature is called primary scoliosis. On the upper or lower part of it, compensatory scoliosis can be seen with relatively smaller reverse curvatures. The left and right gaps of the affected vertebra in primary scoliosis are unequal in width while the vertebral body is tilted to the concave side and shifted to the convex side. Moreover, there are different degrees of rotation of spines; and in the advanced stages of the disease, osteoarthritis changes are observed.

Diagnosis and Differentiation

Diagnosis Diagnosis is based on clinical symptoms and spinal X-rays. While performing scoliosis checks on a child, a special optical grating can be used for back Moiré inspection to help identify the disease at the early stage and in mild cases.

Differential diagnosis A differential diagnosis must done to rule out scoliosis caused by other factors including spinal infections and tumor. The physician needs to obtain a detailed medical history of the patient, perform physical examinations, and offer laboratory tests, X-rays and CT scans.

Treatment

Tui na therapy is only applicable in children suffering from compensatory scoliosis.

1. *Treatment principles* relaxing sinews, unblocking the collaterals, and correcting deformities.
2. *Commonly used maneuvers* grasping, pressing, intense pressing, pressure-kneading, and passive movements of the spinal stretching and rotation.
3. *Commonly used acupoints and areas fēngchí* (GB 20), *tiānzōng* (SI 11), *ā shìxué*, the neck, the thoracic and lumbar segments of the spine, and bilateral sacrospinalis muscles.
4. *Operational methods*
   a. Have the child in a prone position, with the practitioner on one side. Start from applying on *fēngchí* on both sides of the neck, manipulate along both sides of the paraspinal muscles, past the thoracic area and reaching the lumbosacral segment with the kneading maneuver up and down and back and forth for about two to three minutes. Apply grasping on *fēngchí* and the sacrospinal muscles with the focus on the thoracic and lumbar segments, especially the arched portion of the spine. If the force of the maneuver is superficial, it will not be effective; thus, the force must reach the deeper level of the muscles, the range of the kneading stroke should be small, and the top-down transition needs to be slow. This step should last for about five minutes. Apply plucking on the same muscles. Lastly, use the pressing maneuver to work on the spine from the thoracic section to the lumbar segment with thumbs overlapped.
   b. Next, with the help of X-ray films of the spine to guide you, perform the scoliosis reduction maneuver. Place a thumb on the curved spinous process to get ready for the push to the opposite side, then support the anterior shoulder and stretch it in a posterior direction with the other hand. Make sure to apply the forces at the same time to complete the maneuver. The manipulation is similar to unilateral vertebral stretching with chest outin treating ankylosing spondylitis in Day 2 of Week 9. This correction should put more emphasis on

the spot of the primary scoliosis. Finally, apply scrubbing on the erector sacrospinous muscles to end this part of the operation.

c. Now, have the child change to a sitting position. Stand to the back of the child. First, apply grasping on *fēngchí*, *jiānjǐng* (GB 21), and the sacralspinous muscle top down for one to two minutes. Then, use both hands to lift up the child's elbows to perform passive chest expansion with back stretching, and ask the child to take slow deep breaths coordinating with the passive movement.
d. Use a knee to support the spine with the primary protrusion, and using both hands, pull back the child's elbows; this is the passive chest expansion movement. Lastly, apply grasping on *jiānjǐng* and patting on the back, starting from the thoracic segment to the lumbar, back and forth two to three times to end the treatment.

Precautions

1. It is necessary to detect and treat the condition as early as possible.
2. Have the child sleep on a hard-board bed in supine position.
3. Do horizontal bar pulling and sitting-up exercises every day.
4. Whenever the condition allows, combine with traction treatment, and make the child wear plastic or steel vests to slow down the abnormal development.
5. For patients with severe deformity and ineffective conservative medical treatment, surgical correction may be considered.

Everyday Exercises

1. What is scoliosis? What are the main clinical manifestations?
2. How do you distinguish compensatory from decompensated scoliosis?

Day 4

SEQUELA OF POLIOMYELITIS

Poliomyelitis is an acute infectious disease caused by a neurotropic virus. The disease symptoms are fever, sore throat, and body pains. Since it is more common in children, and since the disease can give rise to flaccid paralysis, i.e., lower motor neuron paralysis, it is also known as infantile paralysis. Epidemically, the disease is a disseminated one (i.e., it can spread from its initial point of origin to other regions in the body), with the highest incidence among children between the age of one to five years, and with the highest outbreaks in summer and fall. The polio virus has the characteristic of neurotropic toxicity with less damage to other tissues. Although the virus can spread to the entire central nervous system, it mainly causes damage to the spinal cord and the brain stem, with the motor neurons being the most affected. Therefore, it is common to see flaccid paralysis of the limbs and the body clinically. There is a rapid recovery period from paralysis in varying degrees, mostly within the first four to six months, after which the recovery slows down. Failure of timely treatment will cause muscle atrophy in the paralyzed limbs. In this case, the blood supply is poor and the bone development is retarded, leading to deformity sequela. The paralysis tends to occur on the lower limbs, with less chance of the upper limbs being affected.

In Chinese medical practice, it is believed that the disease pertains to the scope of *wěi* (atrophy, 痿) pattern. One source has recorded that "lung heat toasts the lobes (肺热叶焦), causing *wěipǐ* (则生痿躄)." *Wěi* means withered, signifying atrophy and weakness.

Clinical Manifestations

1. *Prodromal stage* At this stage the symptoms are low-grade to moderate fever, with sore throat, fatigue, coughs, and other respiratory symptoms. Gastrointestinal symptoms may include poor appetite, nausea, vomiting, and diarrhea. This is because the virus first attacks the respiratory and gastrointestinal tracts. Three to four days later, in the

majority of patients, the body temperature decreases, then returns to normal, namely the formefruste type, while a proportion of patients enter the pre-paralysis stage.

2. *Pre-paralysis stage* When the temperature drops and then rises again, in addition to fever, upper respiratory tract and gastro-intestinal symptoms, neurological symptoms appear. These include headache and generalized muscle pain. The child shows an unwillingness to be held, and cry when touched.
3. *Paralysis stage* There are reduced or disappeared tendon reflexes after the fever, followed by progressive paralysis in different parts of the body characterized by flaccid to normal sensation. The distribution is uneven and asymmetrical with decreased muscle tensility.
4. *Sequela stage* The sequela stage is about one to two weeks after the acute paralysis phase, with paralyzed limbs gradually being restored to their range of motion and muscle strength starting from the distal ends. At the same time, tendon reflexes gradually return to normal. If the disease is not treated on time, the nerves will lose their autonomous recovery function, resulting in the occurrence of various polio deformities, such as clubfoot, high foot arches, and genu recurvatum.

Within one week from the onset of the disease, the poliomyelitis virus can be isolated from the pharynx and feces, and a positive fecal result can be sustained for two to three weeks. There is greater clinical significance in separating the virus from the blood and cerebrospinal fluid in the early stage.

Diagnosis and Differentiation

Diagnosis It is relatively difficult to diagnose polio in mild cases and in the pre-paralysis stage. On the other hand, diagnostic accuracy can be improved with a good understanding of the child's medical history, epidemic trend, physical examination, and virus isolation.

Differential Diagnosis

1. *Infectious polyneuritis* Usually there is no fever but inflammation of the upper respiratory tract. Flaccid paralysis that is symmetrical and

ascending gradually appears. In severe cases, there will be paralysis of respiratory muscles that is life-threatening. It is often accompanied by sensory disturbances and general paralysis, but the patient recovers fairly quickly and completely with very few sequelae.

2. *Cerebralpalsy* There is rapid onset, and associated with disturbance of consciousness and spastic paralysis commonly on one side of the limbs, i.e., hemiplegia. Virus isolation is helpful in differential diagnosis.

Treatment

This disease should be treated as early as possible. In general, when the fever is gone, the patient should be isolated while tui na is carried out. Or, wait for four to six weeks until the infectious period has elapsed before performing tui na.

1. *Treatment principles* warming the meridians, unblocking the collaterals, nourishing sinews, fortifying muscles, and correcting deformities. We will use the lower limbs as an example to explain the treatment.
2. *Commonly used maneuvers* finger kneading, palm-heel pressure kneading, grasping, scrubbing, and passive joint movements.
3. *Commonly used acupoints and areas jiájǐ* (EX-B 2), *huántiào* (GB 30), *wěizhōng* (BL 40), *bìguān* (ST 31), *fútù* (ST 32), *xuèhǎi* (SP 10), *zúsānlǐ* (ST 36), *yánglíngquán* (GB 34), *chéngshān* (BL 57), *kūnlún* (BL 60), *jiěxī* (ST 41), and the entire limb.
4. *Operational methods*
   a. Have the child in a prone position, with the practitioner standing at the affected side. Apply finger-kneading for about two minutes on *jiájǐ* points of the ipsilateral lumbar, preferably obtaining the soreness *de*-qi sensation. Apply palm-heel pressure kneading top down and back and forth in this order: the waist, hip, posterior part of the thigh, calf, and the Achilles tendon. Supplement these maneuvers by stronger stimulation such as point-pressing and intense pressing on points such as *huántiào*, *chéngfú* (BL 36), *wěizhōng*, *chéngshān,* and *kūnlún* for five to eight minutes.

If there is clubfoot deformity, the Achilles tendon is the focus of the treatment. In addition to applying pressure kneading on the Achilles tendon, which is the focus of the treatment, coordinate the treatment with passive ankle hyperextension. Finally, apply scrubbing to the Achilles tendon until the hot frictional sensation is felt.

b. Have the child change to a supine position, with the practitioner standing on the ipsilateral side. Focus the operations on the antero-lateral leg muscles. According to the TCM belief that "in treating *wěi*, choose *yangming* exclusively (治痿独取阳明)," *yangming* meridians should be used as the main channel while treating this ailment. First of all, use the palm-heel pressure kneading maneuver on the quadriceps and anterior tibialis muscles, top down and back and forth. At the same time, coordinate the operations with finger-kneading on *bìguān*, *fútù*, *xuèhǎi*, zúsānlǐ, *yánglíngquán*, *xuánzhōng* (GB 39), and *jiěxī,* preferably until obtaining the sense of *de*-qi. Then, apply passive flexion and extension on the ipsilateral limb, and passive rotation of the hips and ankles. Next, apply grasping on the anterior tibialis muscle to enhance the stimulation. Lastly, apply scrubbing on the anterior tibialis muscle and the dorsal side of the feet until the frictional heat is sensed. The entire treatment should total up to about ten minutes.

Precautions

1. Keep in mind that prevention comes first and actively promote live polio vaccination pill in order to improve the level of population immunity.
2. The child should be put under the respiratory and gastrointestinal tracts isolation for at least 40 days from the onset of the disease.
3. Avoid bringing small children to public places in the polio epidemic season.
4. Treat sequelae of polio as early as possible to prevent the occurrence of deformities.
5. Keep the ipsilateral limb warm all the time. Encourage and guide the child to perform function exercises and restore muscle strength.

Everyday Exercises

1. What is sequela of poliomyelitis? What kind of paralysis can it give rise to?
2. What are the clinical stages of polio and what are the main symptoms at each stage ?
3. Be aware of the precautions for polio.

Day 5

CEREBRAL PALSY

Cerebral palsy is a neurological disorder that appears in infancy or early childhood and affects body movement and muscle coordination. The course of the disease is generally non-progressive and there is a tendency to gradual improvement. The most common cause is cerebral hypoxia as the result of various perinatal problems. Other causes may include gestosis, infection, radiation, dystocia, brain contusion, and choking. On the other hand, the pathologic cause cannot be confirmed among many patients. The main symptom of the disease is mobile dysfunction of voluntary muscles, causing spastic paralysis.

Clinical Manifestations

The symptoms of this disease vary in severity. In mild cases, the child's intelligence level is normal, with only mild rigidity and weakness of the lower extremities that gradually improve with the increase of age. However, in severe cases, the child often has mental hypoplasia, poor language skills, learning difficulties, impaired vision and hearing, and severe paralysis. Patients often die of concurrent infections during childhood.

Due to the involvement of the nervous system, including the pyramidal tract and the extra pyramidal system, a patient manifests a bilateral, symmetrical, and spastic paralysis, more in the lower limbs, forming a unique scissors-like gait. The gait is also known as the spastic paraplegic gait with the thighs close to each other, knees touching each other tightly, the thighs and calves semi-flexed with slight pronation, foot dropped with internal rotation and a certain degree of varus, toes close to each other and heels separated. When the child tries to extend his thighs and calves, the entire lower extremities or the trunk will move concurrently. When the child is standing, the toes touch the floor with foot virus, knees closed, making the legs cross-shaped (see Figure 246).

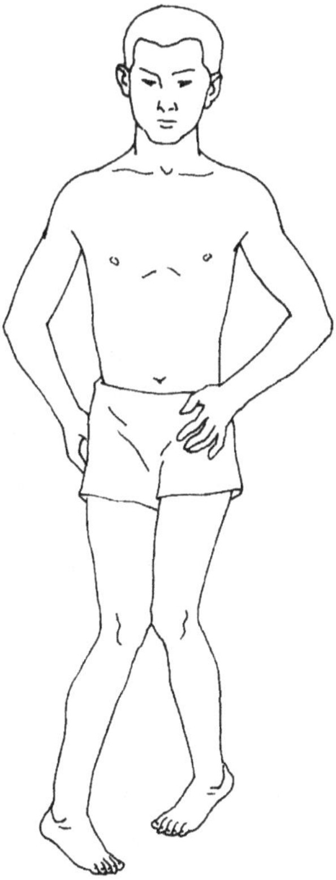

Figure 246 Spastic paraplegic gait

A physical examination reveals the following: mental retardation, slow response, behavioral disorders; internally rotated upper arm affixed to the chest, pronation of the forearm, flexed hands, wrists and fingers, and adduction of the thumbs. There is an obvious spastic paraplegic gait of the lower limbs. Other symptoms include tendon hyperreflexia, increased muscle tension; pyramidal tract damage with positive Hoffmann sign of the upper limbs, and positive Babinski sign of the lower extremities.

Diagnosis and Differentiation

The diagnosis is fairly straightforward, and is based on the clinical history of the child, clinical manifestations, and the spastic paraplegic gait. Intracranial progressive and space-occupying lesions can be ruled out through a detailed neurological examination, laboratory tests, skull X-rays, and CT and MRI scans.

Treatment

1. *Treatment principles* boosting qi, invigorating blood, benefiting joints, and restoring functions of the limbs.
2. *Commonly used maneuvers*: kneading, intense pressing, scattering sweeping, grasping, scrubbing, and passive joint movement.
3. *Commonly used acupoints and areas bǎihuì* (DU 20), *sìshéncōng* (EX-HN 1), *fēngchí* (GB 20), *dàzhuī* (DU 14), back-*shu* points, *zhìyáng* (DU 9), *jīnsuō* (DU 8), *mìngmén* (DU 4), *qìhǎi* (RN 6), *guānyuán* (RN 4), *qǔchí* (LI 11), *hégǔ* (LI 4), *huántiào* (GB 30), *chéngfú* (BL 36), *fēngshì* (GB 31), *wěizhōng* (BL 40), *yánglíngquán* (GB 34), *kūnlún* (BL 60), the head, and flexors of the four limbs.
4. *Operational methods*

   Basic operations

   a. Have the child sit, with the practitioner facing the child. Use one hand to perform pressure kneading on *bǎihuì* followed by double-handed pressure kneading on *sìshéncōng*, one minute each acupoint. Then, apply scattering sweeping on both temples 30 to 50 times, grasping on *fēngchí* and paraspinal cervical muscles top-down and back-and-forth, and finger-kneading on *dàzhuī* for about two minutes.
   b. Have the child in a prone position and apply palm-heel pressure kneading bilaterally along the sacrospinal muscles top-down and back-and-forth for one to two minutes. Then perform two-finger kneading to the back-*shu* points along the bilateral bladder meridian top-down, and back-and-forth many times, focusing more on *xīnshū* (BL 15), *géshū* (BL 17), *píshū* (BL 20), and *shènshū* (BL 23), one minute for each acupoint. Apply finger-kneading on *zhìyáng*, *jīnsuō*, and *mìngmén* along *dumai*, one minute on each acupoint. Apply scrubbing along *dumai* and the bilateral bladder meridian until frictional heat is felt.
   c. Have the child in asupine position, with the practitioner sitting to the right of the child. Apply rubbing on *fù* and finger-kneading on

qìhǎi (RN 6) and *guānyuán* (RN 4) for a total of five minutes. Lastly, use both thumbs to perform pressure kneading on the bilateral *zúsānlǐ* (ST 36) respectively for one minute.

Modifications Based on Pattern Differentiation

a. *Paralysis of the upper extremities* Apply palm-heel pressure kneading on the deltoid muscle, foulage on the shoulder joint, and intense pressing on *jiānsānxuè*, coordinating with passive circular shoulder rotation for about three minutes. Apply grasping on the triceps and forearm flexors with passive elbow and forearm supination for about two minutes. Apply finger-kneading on *wàiguān* (SJ 5) and *yángchí* (SJ 4) with passive movements including wrist dorsiflexion, metacarpophalangeal hyperextension, and thumb abduction for about three minutes.
b. *Lower limb paralysis* Have the patient in a prone position. Focus on intense pressing and pressure kneading on huántiào and chéngfú with passive external hip rotation and extension for about two minutes. Apply palm-heel kneading on the posterior thigh, calf, and the Achilles tendon with more focus on the Achilles tendon, and coordinate with the grasping, scrubbing and passive ankle dorsiflexion for about three minutes. Next, have the patient supine, and concentrate on the adductors with palm-heel kneading on the muscles, passive hip abduction, and grasping and plucking of the adductors for about another three minutes. Apply finger-kneading on *xuèhǎi* (SP 10), *yánglíngquán* and *jiěxī* (ST 41), followed by scrubbing on the anterior tibial muscles until the frictional heat is felt. This step should last for about three minutes. End the operation with flexing the knee and pressing the foot (see Figure 247).

Precautions

1. Help the child to maintain mental health, and encourage the child to take part in activities within the full extent of his or her physical ability. Try to prevent the child from assuming an unhealthy state of mind or having undesirable feelings like a low self-esteem and loneliness.

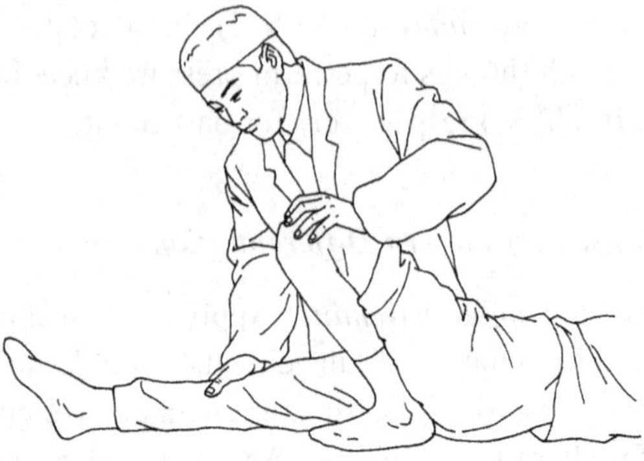

Figure 247 Flexing the knee and pressing the foot to make the ankle dorsiflex

2. In clinical practice, tui na should be pertinent to paralyzed muscles in order to speed up the restoration of the functions and reduce spasms.
3. Increase the care level for children with severe cerebral palsy, pay attention to their nutritional needs, and prevent complications such as pneumonia from occurring.

Everyday Exercises

1. What is cerebral palsy?
2. What are the characteristics of the scissors gait?

Day 6

ǑU TÙ (VOMITING)

Ǒutù is a common symptom among infants and has many causes. This chapter will focus on *ǒu tù* as the result of digestive tract lesions. Generally, it is associated with reverse peristalsis of the esophagus, stomach, or intestinal tracts, often accompanied by strong spasmodic contraction of the abdominal muscles, forcing the contents in the esophagus or stomach out from the mouth or nose. In severe *ǒu tù*, the infant can even have temporary apnea and choking. If improper care is given, or if the infant inhales the spew, it can lead to secondary respiratory infections. Furthermore, repeated *ǒu tù* tends to cause disorders of water and electrolyte metabolism, which can be life-threatening in severe cases. At the same time, long-term *ǒu tù* can affect the absorption of nutrients, resulting in malnutrition and stunted growth in children. On the other hand, if a baby is fed improperly, such as when the baby is given too much milk while in haling a lot of air, a small amount of milk may be throw up; this is known as milk spitting, which is a normal condition.

In Chinese medical practice, it is believed that *ǒu tù* is due to rebellious stomach qi going upwards. Vomiting actions that produce sounds while throwing up content are called *ǒu* (呕) while those that do not have a sound while throwing up content are named *tù* (吐). The third type, which produces sounds without spewing anything is called *gānǒu* (dry vomiting, retching, 干呕).

Clinical Manifestations

According to TCM pattern differentiation rules, *ǒu tù* can be divided into the following categories:

1. *Tù of cold pattern* Vomiting while eating occurs just slightly more than usual; it occurs and then stops. The content is usually clear, thin, and watery sputumor undigested milk and food with mild acrid odor. The infant has abdominal pain that eases with warmth. The limbs are cold

and the stool is loose and thin or with undigested food, and the urine is clear and copious. The tongue is pale with thin and white coating, the pulse is thready and weak, and the finger venule is red.

2. *Tùof heat pattern* The infant spits up right after eating. The content has a foul smell. The infant has fever, thirst, and a red face, is irritable, may be constipated, and passes foul-smelling stool and dark yellow urine. The tongue is red with yellow and greasy coating, the pulse is rapid, and the finger venule is purple.
3. *Ǒutù of food damage pattern* There is frequent vomiting. The content has a putrid and rancid smell and contains undigested food residue or milk tablets. There is bloating, abdominal distension, anorexia, foul flatus, and constipation or diarrhea with rancid smell. The tongue coating is thick and greasy and the pulse is slippery and rapid.

Diagnosis and Differentiation

Ǒutù (vomiting) is a symptom rather than a disease. The problem is that there are many causes of *ǒutù*, in particular, the central nervous system type needs to be differentiated. Increased intracranial pressure owing to any lesions of the central nervous system can induce *ǒutù*; it is often accompanied by a significant headache. Spurting *ǒutù* in this case often occurs when the headache becomes severe. Thus, based on the relationship between *ǒutù* and headaches, we can differentiate normal *ǒutù* from *ǒutù* caused by problems of the central nervous system, such as traumatic brain injury and meningitis.

Treatment

1. *Treatment principles*
    a. *Cold pattern* It is appropriate to warm the center, dissipate cold, harmonize the stomach and bear down rebellious qi.
    b. *Heat pattern* The proper treatment is to clear heat, harmonize the stomach, bear down rebellious qi, and relieve vomiting.
    c. *Food damage* The proper treatment promotes digestion by guiding out food stagnation, harmonizing the center, and bearing down rebellious qi.

2. *Commonly used maneuvers* pushing, kneading, rubbing, and pressing.
3. *Commonly used acupoints píjīng, bǎnmén, fùyīnyáng, zhōngwǎn* (RN 12), *píshū* (BL 20), *wèishū* (BL 21), *zúsānlǐ* (ST 36), etc.
4. *Operational methods*

   Basic operations

   a. The child is supine, with the practitioner sitting to the right of the child. Apply kneading on *tiāntū* (RN 22) 30 times followed by straight pushing on *dànzhōng* (RN 17) 500 times and kneading on *zhōngwǎn* for three minutes. Using both thumbs, start from *tiāntū*, maneuver down along the lower edge of the costal arch on both sides, and perform disjoining pushing, namely pushing *fùyīnyáng* for about 50 times. Rub *fù* (abdomen) for three minutes. Apply kneading on *bǎnmén* 300 times and use both thumbs to apply kneading on the bilateral *zúsānlǐ* for a minute.
   b. Change the child to a prone position. The practitioner should sit at the left side of the child. Use the thumb and forefinger to push *tiānzhùgǔ* from top to bottom 200 times. Then apply double-finger kneading on *píshū* and *wèishū*, each for one minute.

Modifications Based on Pattern Differentiation

a. *Tù of cold pattern* Add supplementing *píjīng* 300 times, kneading *wàiláogōng* (EX-UE 8) 30 times, and pushing *sānguān* up to 300 times.
b. *Tù of heat pattern* Add clearing *píjīng* 100 times and *dàcháng* 300 times, pushing *liùfǔ* downwards 200 times, and kneading *wàiláogōng* 30 times.
c. *Tù of food damage pattern* Add clearing the supplementing *píjīng* 300 times, clearing *dàcháng* 300 times, pushing *qījié* downwards 100 times, and foulage rubbing *xiélèi* 50 times.

Precautions

1. Control the amount of milk and supplemental food given to children suffering *ǒu tù*. For those with repeated *ǒu tù*, fasting may be necessary until the symptom is reduced; then gradually increase the amount of milk or food.

2. Turn the child's head to the side when *ǒu tù* occurs to avoid the spew from being inhaled into the trachea.
3. As repeated *ǒu tù* can result in a disruption in water and electrolyte metabolism, intravenous fluids should be given to the child

Pediatric Tui Na for Health Maintenance

You can apply pediatric health maintenance tui na to a child to regulate functions of the meridians and collaterals, raise the clear qi up, direct the turbid qi down, and adjust deficiency and excess. All these ensure that the *ying* and *wei* levels are in harmony, the qi and blood are flowing freely, and yin and yang are balanced. Cell metabolism is promoted, and so are physiologic growth and development, immunity, the physical constitution, and the health of the *zang-fu* organs. In addition, the tui na maneuvers calm the *shen*, open the orifices, fortify the brain, and enhance mental ability.

We now introduce a few maneuvers of health maintenance tui na.

Raising the Clear Qi up, Directing the Turbid Qi down, Calming the Shen, Opening the Orifices, and Enhancing Mental Ability

1. Rubbing *xìnmén* (fontanel) 50 to 100 times.
   In infants aged 18 months or younger, the *xìnmén* is not completed fused. Therefore, there are two alternative operational methods:
   a. Use the finger pulp to touch the center of xìnmén where it pulsates and rub it very gently.
   b. Use the finger to gently rub the area around xìnmén (see Figure 248).

2. Kneading *bǎihuì* (DU 20) 50 to 100 times.

Smoothening, Regulating All Vessels, and Fortifying Zang-Fu Organs

1. Pushing the five *jīng* 100 to 200 times.

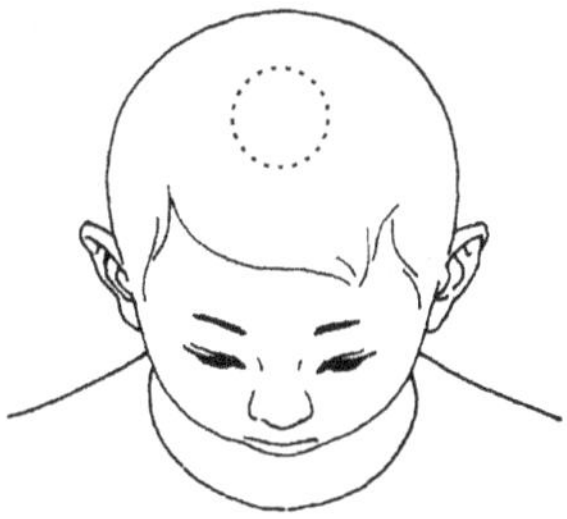

Figure 248

a. Location of the five *jīng*: at the tip of the five fingers, from the thumb to the little finger; the order is *píjīng*, *gānjīng*, *xīnjīng*, *fèijīng,* and *shènjīng* respectively.
b. *Operations* The child should have the palmar side down and fingers close to each other. Putting your thumb on the dorsum of the child's hand, with your other fingers closed and the palm of your hand facing the child's palm, apply pushing from the root of the finger toward the tip. In addition, you can put more focus on the three *jīng* of *pí*, *fèi,* and *shèn* with a finger-rotating maneuver, which is the concurrent supplementing method for both the innate and the post-natal basis.

2. Rubbing *fù* and kneading *dāntián* (see Figure 218) for a total of three to five minutes.
3. Pushing and kneading *yǒngquán* (KI 1) 50 to 100 times.

Improving Immunity and Enhancing Body Constitution

1. *Jí* (spine) pinching for three to five times (see Figure 203): as an important health maintenance maneuver for children, the method can pep up *du mai*, fortify the spleen, benefit the stomach, improve appetite, enhance immunity, and strengthen body constitution.
2. Kneading *zhōngwǎn* (RN 12) 100 to 200 times: this maneuver can fortify the spleen, harmonize the stomach, and regulate the function of the digestive tract.
3. Kneading *zúsānlǐ* (ST 36) 50 times.

Zúsānlǐ is a strengthening acupoint for the entire body and mainly used in treating diseases of the digestive system. As a commonly used method in pediatric health maintenance tui na, Kneading *zúsānlǐ* is often combined with pinching *jí* and kneading *zhōngwǎn*.

Preparation and Application of the Spring Onion and Ginger Juice Combo

1. *Preparation*
   a. Rinse the spring onion until it is clean. Use only the white stem and root.
   b. Rinse the ginger and use only the peel, slicing it into thin pieces.
   c. Put equal amounts of spring onion stem and ginger slices into a container, add 75% ethylalcohol until the solid material is completely immersed, and soak it for a week.
2. *Application* For every unit of the spring onion and ginger juice, add two units of clean water, and use the solution as a medium in pediatric tui na.

Precautions

1. The skin of children is particularly fragile and easily damaged. Tuina maneuvers in children must be gentle, soft, and slow. Buffering substances such as spring onion or ginger juice can be used to avoid skin damage whenever necessary.
2. Pediatric health maintenance tui na should be performed once every day or every other day.

Everyday Exercises

1. How would you distinguish vomiting from normal spitting of milk?
2. How do you differentiate digestive vomiting from vomiting caused by cerebral causes?
3. Master the fundamental principles and methods for pediatric tui na for health maintenance.

INDEX